Board of Certification, Inc.,
Entry-Level
Athletic Trainer
Certification Examination

FOURTH EDITION

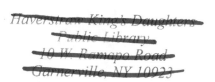

D1412401

Study Guide for the

Board of Certification, Inc.,
Entry-Level Athletic Trainer
Certification Examination

Susan L. Rozzi, Ph.D., ATC, SCAT
Associate Professor
Director, Athletic Training Education Program
Department of Health and Human Performance
College of Charleston
Charleston, South Carolina

Michelle G. Futrell, MA, ATC, SCAT
Senior Instructor
Clinical Coordinator, Athletic Training
Education Program
Department of Health and Human Performance
College of Charleston
Charleston, South Carolina

Douglas M. Kleiner, Ph.D., ATC, CSCS, EMT,
FACSM, FNATA
Wright State University
Boonshoft School of Medicine
Department of Emergency Medicine
Dayton, Ohio

FOURTH EDITION

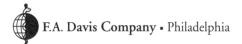

F.A. Davis Company • Philadelphia

F. A. Davis Company
1915 Arch Street
Philadelphia, PA 19103
www.fadavis.com

Printed in the United States of America

Last digit indicates print number: 10 9 8 7 6 5 4 3 2 1

Senior Acquisitions Editor: Quincy McDonald
Developmental Editor: Liz Schaeffer
Manager of Content Development: George Lang
Manager of Art and Design: Carolyn O'Brien

As new scientific information becomes available through basic and clinical research, recommended treatments and drug therapies undergo changes. The author(s) and publisher have done everything possible to make this book accurate, up to date, and in accord with accepted standards at the time of publication. The author(s), editors, and publisher are not responsible for errors or omissions or for consequences from application of the book, and make no warranty, expressed or implied, in regard to the contents of the book. Any practice described in this book should be applied by the reader in accordance with professional standards of care used in regard to the unique circumstances that may apply in each situation. The reader is advised always to check product information (package inserts) for changes and new information regarding dose and contraindications before administering any drug. Caution is especially urged when using new or infrequently ordered drugs.

ISBN 10: 0-8036-0020-8
ISBN 13: 978-0-8036-0020-1

This book is dedicated to all athletic training students who undertake the challenge of our profession's certification examination, aspiring to join the ranks of certified athletic trainers. The future of our profession is in your hands. Make us proud!

Foreword

Taking the Board of Certification (BOC) examination is a culminating event in an athletic training student's professional preparation—an event that often produces a great deal of anxiety and anticipation. I can vividly recall my own experiences as an undergraduate student 14 years ago trying to prepare for a version of the BOC exam very different from what exists today. The exam has evolved in recent years into a computer-based assessment format that challenges students' cognitive understanding of athletic training principles along with their critical thinking and clinical reasoning skills in the five domains of our discipline. In early 2010, the BOC announced revisions to the testing format to include alternative-type questions and "testlets" in addition to the traditional multiple-choice questions. As a result, athletic training educators are faced with the challenge of preparing students for this new testing format.

As a program director I have observed very bright and academically prepared students struggle with the BOC exam due to test anxiety and lack of familiarity with the testing format. That is why I view the *Study Guide for the Board of Certification, Inc., Entry-Level Athletic Trainer Certification Examination,* Fourth Edition, as a much-needed resource for students in preparing for the exam and becoming acquainted with the new format. Susan Rozzi and Michelle Futrell have extended Douglas Kleiner's previous editions of this text into a cutting-edge resource for athletic training students and educators. The *Study Guide* includes a detailed description of the new exam format along with more than 1,000 multiple-choice questions and more than 70 interactive testlets that provide students ample opportunity to practice test taking in a computer-based format. The testlets are a unique component that does not exist in other BOC exam preparation materials and will certainly prove to be a valuable resource for students.

When preparing for the BOC exam, students often feel overwhelmed and wonder how to tackle the seemingly impossible task of reviewing every bit of information they have learned in their academic program. I can personally attest that several of the exam preparation tips provided in the *Study Guide* are quite effective in helping students to overcome this daunting task. For example, using the results of practice tests to guide the development of a study calendar has proved very effective in my own program. Students should use this book to supplement their exam preparation plan. They should still review content-specific textbooks, position statements, and course notes and use the practice questions as a means of formative assessment throughout the review process. Students should not try to "cram" for the exam but rather use a methodical approach to studying based on their personal strengths and weaknesses in each content area.

As an educator, I am very excited about this latest edition of the *Study Guide* and look forward to integrating the extensive collection of practice test items and testlets into my own exam review course. Best of luck to all students who will use this resource in preparing for the BOC exam. You *can* do it!!

Jolene M. Henning, Ed.D., ATC, LAT
Director, Entry-Level Master's Athletic Training
Education Program
Associate Professor
University of North Carolina at Greensboro

Contributor and Reviewers

CONTRIBUTOR

Dennis Trapani
Multimedia Assistant
Department of Athletics
College of Charleston
Charleston, South Carolina

REVIEWERS

Steve Cernohous, Ed.D., ATC, LAT
Assistant Professor/Clinical Education Coordinator
Athletic Training Education Program
College of Health and Human Services
Northern Arizona University
Flagstaff, Arizona

Allison Checchio
Student, Athletic Training
Northeastern University
Boston, Massachusetts

Charles F. Davis, Jr., M.Ed, ATC
Associate Professor/Athletic Trainer
Exercise Science Department
Southern Connecticut State University
New Haven, Connecticut

Richard Frazee, M.Ed., ATC/L
Program Director, Athletic Training Education
Health, Leisure, and Exercise Science
University of West Florida
Pensacola, Florida

Heather LaSasso
Student, Athletic Training
Northeastern University
Boston, Massachusetts

Christopher Metzgier, ATC, CSCS
Certified Personal Trainer
Philadelphia Sports Clubs
Philadelphia, Pennsylvania

Thomas G. Palmer, MS, ATC, CSCS
Clinical Coordinator, Athletic Training
Northern Kentucky University
Highland Heights, Kentucky

Mary Romanello, PT, ATC, SCS, Ph.D.
Department of Sports Medicine
College of Mount St. Joseph
Cincinnati, Ohio

Deborah Swanton, Ed.D., ATC, LAT
Dean, School of Sport Science and Fitness Studies
Chair, Athletic Training
Endicott College
Beverly, Massachusetts

Adam J. Thompson, Ph.D., LAT, ATC
Director of Athletic Training Education
Associate Professor
Indiana Wesleyan University
Marion, Indiana

Robert C. Toth, MS, ATC
Assistant Head Athletic Trainer, Clinical Education
Coordinator, Clinical Instructor
Athletics/Exercise and Sport Science Department
University of Utah
Salt Lake City, Utah

Katie M. Walsh, Ed.D., ATC
Associate Professor
Director, Athletic Training Program
East Carolina University
Greenville, North Carolina

Acknowledgments

We thank all our professional mentors and role models, whose love of learning inspired us to contribute to the education of future professionals. We also thank all our students, who willingly and without question volunteered to assist in the numerous tasks needed to produce this study guide.

Special thanks go to our colleagues at the College of Charleston who provided their creativity, expertise, encouragement, and support from project beginning to end.

Much appreciation to Jolene M. Henning, Ed.D., ATC, LAT, a distinguished educator and proponent of undergraduate education, for writing the foreword to this guide.

Finally, and most importantly, thanks and love go to our families (CJ, Jamie, Tyler, Eric, and Kylie Grace), whose understanding and encouragement made it possible for us to transform an idea into reality.

Susan L. Rozzi, Ph.D., ATC, SCAT
Michelle G. Futrell, MA, ATC, SCAT

Contents

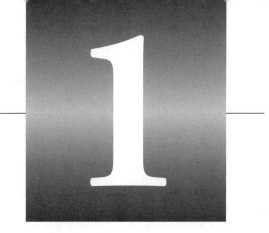

Role of This Study Guide

Most likely you have already completed or are nearing completion of an athletic training education program accredited by the Commission on Accreditation of Athletic Training Education (CAATE), and you are looking toward taking the Board of Certification (BOC) examination. Your goal is probably very similar to that of athletic training students across the country: to use the knowledge, skills, and abilities you have obtained to pass the BOC examination and add the certified athletic trainer (ATC) credential to your résumé.

The purpose of the certification exam is to establish standards for entry into the profession and to ensure that all persons who earn the ATC credential demonstrate similar knowledge and skills required to practice. The ATC credential is also needed to obtain licensure or certification to practice as an athletic trainer in most states. Thus, this credential opens the door to your career in athletic training.

Anticipating the certification examination can be very daunting. However, the more prepared you are going into the exam, the less stressful the process will be. This study guide is designed to walk you through the exam preparation process and build on the knowledge and skills you have already obtained during your educational preparation. It should be used as a supplement to the core reference texts you have used throughout your education.

BENEFITS OF THIS STUDY GUIDE

This study guide will help you identify your strengths and weaknesses in the various exam content areas. You will identify the concepts that you need to review as well as those you have already mastered. This guide also allows you to familiarize yourself with testing procedures and the different types of questions you will see on the test. Knowing what to expect can help reduce anxiety and allows you to focus on completing the exam successfully. benfi

REVIEW TIPS

Expect the questions in this study guide to be challenging. They were written to be as thorough as possible and to cover as many areas of athletic training knowledge as possible. You may be faced with questions for which you do not know the answer immediately. Use these difficult questions to identify areas you need to focus on during study sessions. Similarly, use them to apply the suggestions for approaching the different question types and to practice your critical thinking skills. Helpful hints for analyzing each question type are included. Sample questions then assist you in applying the test-taking strategies you learn.

Treat practice tests as if they are actual tests. Create an environment that is free from distractions. Set aside a block of time during which all you are concentrating on is the test. Turn off your cell phone. Turn off the music. Remove any books or notes that might tempt you to look up an answer. The more closely your practice test environment resembles actual testing conditions, the less anxious you will be on test day.

COMPONENTS OF THIS STUDY GUIDE

This text and its accompanying CD not only offer hundreds of review questions, they also provide you with logistical information about BOC exam eligibility and the administrative policies and procedures associated with signing up for and taking the test. Also included is information on the development of the BOC exam, including the relationship between the *Role Delineation Study* (the job description of a certified athletic trainer) and the exam's content, various components, and scoring. The requirements for maintaining your certification after successful completion of the exam are also discussed.

One important part of preparing for a comprehensive exam, such as this one, is creating a study plan that is well thought out. Pay particular attention to the chapter devoted to this information. An accompanying appendix contains worksheets to assist you in putting your personal study plan into effect.

The appendices include a list of recommended references sorted by practice domain. If you need to find a reference that pertains to a specific content or practice area, this list is a great place to start. As well, there are lists of each of the six practice domains and the main athletic training roles within each domain.

The key advantage of this study guide is the practice questions, which are comparable to those used on the exam. Appendix A contains 800 multiple-choice practice questions by domain. These questions, as well as 255 additional multiple-choice questions, also appear on the enclosed CD-ROM.

The CD allows you to generate a comprehensive practice test to simulate the testing environment or to take practice tests on material from a specific domain. Following a practice test, you will be able to generate a report that outlines your strengths and weaknesses that will assist you in focusing your study efforts. Additionally, the CD provides 73 of the multifaceted focused testlets that are now included in the BOC exam. These testlets allow you to practice critical thinking skills while applying athletic training knowledge to patient-specific scenarios using stand-alone and alternative test item types.

You began preparing for this exam the day you opened your first athletic training text. This study guide will assist you in making your final preparations to enter the doorway to your athletic training career. You control your own outcome. Have a plan. Be prepared. This is your opportunity to prove that you are ready to function as an entry-level certified athletic trainer!

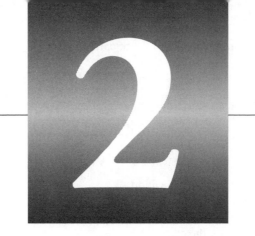

Examination Information From the Board of Certification, Inc.

MISSION OF THE BOARD OF CERTIFICATION

Upon inception in 1969, the Board of Certification (BOC), Inc., was an entity of the professional membership organization of the National Athletic Trainers' Association (NATA) and as such was solely responsible for certification of athletic trainers. However, in 1989 the BOC became an independent not-for-profit corporation to provide a certification program for entry-level athletic trainers and recertification standards for maintaining status as a certified athletic trainer. The BOC is currently the only accredited certification program for athletic trainers in the United States. Every 5 years the BOC undergoes review and reaccreditation by the National Commission for Certifying Agencies (NCCA), the accreditation body of the National Organization for Competency Assurance (NOCA). The BOC is currently governed by an eight-member board of directors, consisting of five athletic trainer directors, one physician director, one public director, and one corporate/educational director.

The mission of the BOC is "to certify Athletic Trainers and to identify, for the public, quality health care professionals through a system of certification, adjudication, standards of practice, and continuing competency programs." The BOC provides a certification program known as the BOC examination for entry-level athletic trainers. The purpose of this exam is to assess candidates' knowledge in the six domains of athletic training as defined by the *Role Delineation Study.*

CERTIFICATION EXAMINATION ELIGIBILITY

According to information provided in the *BOC Exam Candidate Handbook,* which is available free of charge from the BOC, candidates for the BOC certification exam must meet the following requirements:

- The candidate's exam application must be endorsed by the recognized program director of the candidate's Commission on Accreditation of Athletic Training Education (CAATE)–accredited program
- Proof must be provided of current certification in emergency cardiac care (ECC), which includes adult and pediatric cardiopulmonary resuscitation (CPR), airway obstruction, second-rescuer CPR, and use of automatic external defibrillator and barrier device (examples of courses that meet this BOC requirement are in the *BOC Exam Candidate Handbook*)
- The candidate must have graduated from a CAATE-accredited program or be enrolled in the last semester (or quarter) of a CAATE-accredited program, provided all academic and clinical requirements of the CAATE-accredited program have been satisfied or will be satisfied during this last semester (or quarter)

The BOC complies with the Americans With Disabilities Act (ADA, 1990) by providing reasonable and appropriate accommodations to qualified individuals with disabilities who supply appropriate documentation. The BOC follows the guidelines set forth in the *Principles of Fairness* developed by the Council on Licensure, Enforcement and Regulation (CLEAR) and the National Organization for Competency Assurance (NOCA). If the candidate needs to request reasonable accommodations or a change in exam procedures or processes because of a disability, handicap, or other reason, the candidate must complete the Request for Special Exam Accommodations Form, available online at http://www.bocatc.org. Additionally, thoroughly read the Accommodations Requests section of the *BOC Exam Candidate Handbook* and contact the BOC directly should you have questions.

The Three-Step Application Process

You may apply for the BOC certification exam using the BOC Central registration system available at the BOC's Web site. Through this registration system you will complete a three-step application process.

Step 1: Eligibility Approval

The first step is to submit an eligibility application along with any application fees that may apply. (See Appendix C of the *BOC Exam Candidate Handbook* for a list of all fees associated with applying and sitting for the exam.) All submitted applications are reviewed by BOC staff to determine eligibility to register for the exam. If your application is approved, you will be notified by e-mail that you can register for the exam.

Your approved eligibility application is good for 1 year, meaning that once the application is approved you have only 1 year in which to sit for the exam. If you fail to sit for the exam during this year but you still desire to take the exam, you must submit a new application meeting all current fees and eligibility requirements.

If your application is deemed incomplete, you will be notified via e-mail or postal mail of the application's deficiencies. If your application is denied, your entire application packet, with the exam fees, will be returned. You can initiate an appeal of a denied application provided the BOC does not disapprove your application for educational and/or disciplinary reasons. Appeals must be made in writing to the Exam Administration Manager, must demonstrate that the appeal should be granted, and must be received at least 30 days before the exam registration deadline date. Appeals are reviewed by the BOC staff, and you will be notified in writing via postal mail of the decision.

Step 2: Register and Pay Exam Fees

The second step is to register for and pay for the exam. Both components of this step are completed during the registration period (window), which begins at 9:00 a.m. (Central time) the day after the application deadline. The fees for the exam can be paid to the BOC via Visa, MasterCard, American Express, or personal check/money order. (See Appendix C of the *BOC Exam Candidate Handbook* for a list of all fees.)

Step 3: Schedule the Exam

The third step is to schedule your exam site, date, and time. The BOC exam is administered during 2-week testing periods at more than 250 CASTLE Worldwide, Inc., testing centers in the United States and Canada. CASTLE is a professional testing service. Approximately 3 business days after the exam registration deadline date, CASTLE sends each registered and paid exam candidate an e-mail with a link and a unique user name and password to the e-mail address provided on the application. To ensure this and other important e-mails from CASTLE do not end up in your spam or junk-mail folder, add these e-mail addresses to your list of approved senders: exam@bocatc.org and ibt@castleworldwide.com

When you receive the e-mail, log onto the CASTLE Worldwide, Inc., Web site to schedule your exam site, date, and time by selecting from the days provided on the scheduling calendar. The period when the calendar is available to you for selecting exam dates is called the *scheduling window*. This is the only time when you can schedule an exam. The number of days composing the scheduling window varies with each test cycle but, on average, lasts approximately 25 days. The scheduling window is available to you 24 hours a day, 7 days a week until the end of the window.

You should schedule at least 4 hours and 15 minutes for this exam. After scheduling your exam, you will receive a confirmation e-mail from CASTLE detailing your contact information and exam date, time, and address. This confirmation e-mail will also provide important information regarding exam policies (what you can bring, what you can wear, etc.), acceptable forms of required identification, and a user name and password for logging onto the exam. Do not delete this e-mail after you have read it. Instead, print it, and place in a safe location because you must bring this confirmation e-mail to your exam.

In addition to the printed copy of your e-mail confirmation, you will need to bring a valid, government-issued photo identification (ID) (driver's license, passport, state-issued ID) to the exam. The name on the ID must appear *exactly* the same as the name on your e-mail confirmation. Keep in mind that your school ID *is not* considered an accepted form of identification for this exam.

Examination Schedule Changes

If you need to **reschedule your exam,** you can do so provided you do it at least 5 business days before your currently scheduled exam. You may change exam days within the same test window, or you may transfer to a different exam window. However, there is an additional charge for rescheduling your exam. If you fail to schedule an exam location, date, and time within the specified exam scheduling dates for the current exam window, the BOC will charge you an administrative fee, which must be paid prior to re-registering. See the *BOC Exam Candidate Handbook* for specific details and directions regarding rescheduling, rescheduling fees, and failure to schedule an exam.

If you must **cancel your exam** for any reason, you must submit a written request to the BOC, via e-mail, fax, or postal mail. You will be refunded 50% of the exam fee if your letter is received no later than 5:00 p.m. (Central time) on the exam registration deadline date for the exam window in which you have confirmed registration. If your letter requesting cancellation is received by the BOC after the exam registration deadline date for which you have confirmed registration, then you will not be refunded any of your application fees. Therefore, when you confirm your exam date, be certain the date will not need to be changed. If you cancel your exam, the BOC will maintain your application on file for 1 year. If you do not attempt the exam within that 1-year period, the BOC will destroy your application.

Should you decide to **completely withdraw your application** after you have scheduled an exam, you must submit a written withdrawal notice to the BOC prior to your scheduled exam date and time. The notice must be signed and include your scheduled exam date along with your first and last name. As is the policy when canceling your exam, you will be refunded 50% of the exam fee if your withdrawal letter is received no later than 5:00 p.m. (Central time) on the exam registration deadline date for the exam window in which you have confirmed registration. If your letter requesting withdrawal of your application is received by the BOC after the exam registration deadline date for which you have confirmed registration, you will not be refunded any of your application fees.

Once your application has been returned and you have received any refund due to you, the BOC will no longer consider you an eligible exam candidate. Therefore, if in the future you submit a new application to sit for the BOC certification exam, you will be required to satisfy the eligibility and fee requirements in place at that time.

Exam Day

On the day of your scheduled exam, arrive at the exam site far in advance of your scheduled start time. If you arrive late to the exam, you will not be permitted to take the exam on that day.

Make sure you bring to the exam:

* Your confirmation e-mail
* A valid, government-issued photo ID on which the name appears exactly the same as the name on the e-mail confirmation

When you check in at the test site, you will be required to read and sign an examinee agreement and sign-in form.

If at any time during your exam a computer problem or other delay occurs that lasts up to 30 minutes, you must remain at the testing center. Should the delay exceed 30 minutes, you will be given the option of rescheduling your exam. You will not be penalized or charged a fee to reschedule your exam in this situation.

In the case of inclement weather, your testing center will decide whether to remain open. Should the testing center close, the center manager will make every attempt to contact you by phone to alert you of the closing. After being contacted, you should contact CASTLE Worldwide, Inc., or the testing center to reschedule your exam at no cost to you.

If for any reason you fail to appear for your scheduled exam, your exam fee will be automatically forfeited. If your reason for failing to appear is considered an emergency or extenuating circumstance and is one of the BOC's recognized acceptable reasons as listed in the *BOC Exam*

Candidate Handbook, you may appeal the forfeiture of your exam fee. The appeal must be made in writing, supported by appropriate documentation, and must be received by the BOC within 10 business days following the missed exam. If, after review, the appeal is granted, your exam fee will be applied to the next exam window. If you do not submit an appeal for the forfeiture of your exam fee or if your appeal is denied, you may still schedule another exam, but you will be required to pay the exam fee again. Note that this exam must be rescheduled within 1 year of your original application.

Exam Results

Within 2 to 4 weeks from the last day of the exam window for your exam, you will be notified by e-mail that pass/fail results have been posted on the BOC Web site. Log onto your BOC Central account to see whether you have passed the exam. Your exam score will not be posted on BOC Central, but a score report will be mailed to you via postal mail within 2 to 4 weeks from the last day of the exam window. The score report includes:

* The maximum possible score
* The minimum score needed to pass
* The score you obtained

Scores are reported on a scale from 200 to 800, with the passing point being 500. A more detailed explanation of your exam performance can be obtained by requesting a diagnostic report. This report breaks down your total exam score into the areas tested to describe areas of strength and weakness as they relate to the *Role Delineation Study.* To receive this report, download a Diagnostic Report Request form, and mail the completed form along with the required fee to the BOC.

BOC exams are scored by CASTLE. Your exam is scored only on questions that have been aligned to the exam specifications of the *Role Delineation Study* and validated for scoring. Even though each form of the given exam includes field test items (questions included in the exam so their validity and reliability can be assessed), these items are not considered when calculating your exam score. Each question in the exam has its own point value, which is determined as a function of the weight assigned to the question's category as well as the number of questions in that content category. Therefore, it is pointless for you to attempt to figure out prior to or during the exam the number of questions you must get correct in order to pass the exam.

There is currently no mechanism to appeal your exam score. Additionally, your examination is not available for your review, and staff members from the BOC and CASTLE will not discuss a specific exam question with you. However, you do have the option of sending comments regarding specific exam questions to the BOC after completing the exam. The BOC will review your comments, but you will not receive a written response.

If an incident occurred while you were taking your exam, you have the option to appeal the administration of your exam by submitting an administrative complaint or exam challenge. Your appeal must be submitted in writing and specifically indicate the reason(s) for the appeal as well as why the appeal should be granted. The date and location of your exam as well as the name(s) of any persons involved in the incident should be included in the appeal. This written appeal must be sent to the BOC via e-mail, postal mail, or fax and must be postmarked no later than 24 hours after the exam was taken. If you submit an appeal of the exam administration, you will be notified in writing after the BOC investigates the appeal. If you are not satisfied with the decision of the BOC, you may appeal the decision by following the process detailed in the *BOC Exam Candidate Handbook.*

RETAKING THE EXAM

When you receive the score report from your exam, you will find enclosed an Exam Registration Form for retaking the exam in case you failed to receive a passing score. You can also register for a retake exam online via BOC Central. You may register for the next available exam window if desired, and remember that you must take the exam within 1 year of the date of your most recent exam attempt. If you fail to take the exam within this period, you will need to submit a new application and meet the eligibility and fee requirements in place at that point in time. Keep in mind that your ECC certification must be current at the time you register for the retake exam and that you will need to submit the appropriate exam fee.

SUMMARY

Although the BOC examination application process may seem confusing and even a bit overwhelming at first, you should have few problems if you read and follow the step-by-step directions provided by the BOC. The BOC can provide assistance at any point during the process. Now that you have learned about applying for and scheduling an exam, it is time to learn how the test is constructed so you can best prepare to pass the exam and begin your career as a certified athletic trainer.

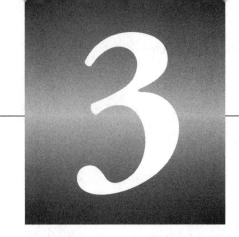

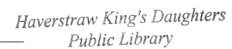

Construction of the Certification Examination

The Board of Certification (BOC) examination is designed to assess a candidate's knowledge in the six domains of athletic training as defined by the current *Role Delineation Study*. Historically, this exam has been a three-section pen-and-paper test consisting of a multiple-choice section, a written simulation section, and a practical examination section. In June 2007, the BOC began administering the test as a completely computerized, integrated examination. Initially, the computer examination was in two parts, lasted 4 hours, and was composed of a multiple-choice section and a hybrid questions section consisting of four problem-based scenarios with numerous multimedia questions. Beginning with the July/August 2009 window, Part I was composed of a minimum of 125 multiple-choice questions, 15 unscored multiple-choice questions, 5 stand-alone "alternative" items, and 2 five-item focused testlets; Part II was composed of four hybrid problems. In February 2010 the BOC announced the construction of the examination was again changing. This new examination format contains a combination of 175 scored and unscored (experimental) items. The items include multiple-choice questions, stand-alone alternative-item types, and focused testlets consisting of alternative item types.

Development and construction of an important credentialing exam, such as the BOC, is complex. Understanding this complex process may assist you in preparing for and successfully completing this exam. Therefore, details of the exam's content and information regarding its construction are discussed in this chapter.

COMPONENTS OF EXAMINATION

When you arrive at the test site and complete the required paperwork, you will input your log-in information to access the exam. You will be presented with an entry screen. The exam contains 175 scored and unscored (experimental)

questions. You will not know which questions are scored and which are experimental. The questions are:

- Multiple-choice items
- Stand-alone "alternative" items
  - Those using newer item types (drag and drop, text-based simulation, multi-select, hot spot)
- Focused testlets
  - A five-item testlet consists of a scenario followed by five key/critical questions relating to that scenario.
  - The questions can include any previously described item type

When you begin your examination, you can select to view a demonstration or you can skip the demonstration and directly enter into the first examination section.

Navigating the Testing Platform

The test questions are on a platform screen that has a series of buttons along the top (Fig. 3-1). The exact layout of these buttons may differ slightly depending on the screen resolution, browser, or operating system of the computer you are using (Box 3-1).

The first five buttons are navigation buttons to assist you in moving through or to subsequent questions. Their labels indicate their function. These buttons may be labeled "First Question" and "Previous Question" and as such will move you backward in the list of questions all the way to the first question (First Question) or just one question back (Previous Question). Likewise, the "Next Question" and "Last Question" buttons move you forward in the list of questions, either to the next question or all the way to the last question. When you have completed a question, click the "Next Question" button to view the next question in the sequence. There may also be a "Go To" button, which permits you to enter a specific question number in the space below the button so you can go directly to that particular question number. After you enter the question number, click

FIGURE 3-1. Test screen navigation buttons.
(Reprinted with permission from the Board of Certification, Inc. All rights reserved.)

Box 3-1	Overview of Button Functions for Testing Screen

- **Navigation arrows:** Allow you to move between the questions.
- **Go-To Button:** Allows you to move to a specific question number if you want to review a question; just type in the question number in the space beneath the button, and click Go To.
- **Flag/Mark Buttons:** Allow you to identify questions you want to review. The total of the number of questions that have been flagged appears in the bottom right corner of the screen. When you have completed a first reading of all the questions, you may navigate between the questions you have flagged by using the right and left flag buttons.
- **Calculator:** Allows you to complete a calculation that you are unable to do easily in your head or on the scrap paper provided.
- **Help Button:** Provides guidance if you have questions about how to use the page logistically.
- **Timer:** Counts down the time remaining for you to complete the entire exam. If watching the timer increases your test anxiety, then you may hide the timer by clicking the **Show/Hide Timer** button to the right of the timer.
- **Status Bar:** Shows a tally of unanswered questions, answered questions, and flagged questions. These tallies will allow you to monitor your progress so you can use your allotted time most effectively.
- **Submit Exam:** Should be clicked only when you are ready to submit your exam. This button looks like all the other buttons on the screen. **DO NOT click this button until you have completed the exam.**

the "Go To" button. Do not hit the "Enter" or "Return" key on your keyboard because this action may take you to the submission confirmation page, the page that prompts you to confirm whether you want to submit your exam for scoring. On your test screen, you may also have three "Flag" or "Mark" buttons. These three buttons are used to flag a question and move to a flagged question. As you progress through the questions, you can use the "Flag" or "Mark" button to mark a question you would like to revisit before you submit your exam for scoring. Flagging a question does not in any way affect your answer to that question and

is a good way to mark a question you have skipped and plan to return to. If you do not flag a skipped question, you will be unable to identify it without reviewing all the questions.

The "Forward" and "Backward" flag buttons move you to the next or previously flagged question.

Among the navigation buttons you may see one labeled "Calculator." Clicking on this button produces a basic function calculator you may use to answer questions. When you are finished with the calculator, close the calculator window by clicking the red circle with a diagonal line or the red X that appears to the right of the "Calculator" label in the attachment screen. The calculator will automatically close when you go to the next question.

Another button you may see on your test screen is the "Help" button. The "Help" button leads you to a demonstration of the test screen features. Unfortunately, the time you spend viewing the help screen information is included in the time you are allotted for completing the BOC exam. You will not get additional time. Therefore, you should be sure to familiarize yourself with the testing platform prior to your test date and use the "Help" button sparingly. Note that, once opened, the help screen may be hidden by the test display screen. Clicking anywhere on the help window should bring it to the forward viewing position.

The last button on top of the examination screen is the "Submit Exam" button. You should click this button *only* when you have completed your examination. After you click this button, you will see a confirmation screen where you will be asked to indicate whether you are finished with the examination or whether you would like to return to the examination. If you accidentally select the "Submit Exam" button, you can still return to your examination by selecting the "Return to Exam" button on the confirmation screen.

In addition to the series of buttons at the top of the exam screen, you may see a digital clock counting down the hours, minutes, and seconds from 4 hours. Keep in mind that the amount of time shown is the time you have left to complete the entire examination. If you do not want to constantly view the examination time remaining and plan to keep track of the time on your own, click the "Show/Hide Timer" button. To reveal a hidden clock, click again on the "Show/Hide Timer" button. When the allotted examination time expires, the test screen will automatically close, and you will be graded on only the questions you have answered.

There may also be an informational toolbar at the bottom of the test window. This section of the window continually updates the number of questions you have not yet answered, the number of answered questions, and the number of answers you have marked or flagged. You can use this information to keep track of your progress and as a double-check before submitting your exam for scoring. (Fig. 3-2).

When you have completed all the questions, you will see a confirmation screen. The purpose of this screen is (1) to inform you of any remaining time, (2) to indicate the number of questions left unanswered, and (3) to remind you that, once you decide to conclude the examination, you then cannot return to answer unanswered questions or edit answered questions. If, after viewing this screen, you decide you would like to return to the exam to review questions, click the "No, Return to Exam" button. This button will bring you back to the first question. If, however, you are ready to end the exam, you will need to type the words "I understand" in a box and then click the "Yes, End the Exam Now" button. This button will submit your questions for scoring.

Question Types

The BOC exam will provide you with 175 questions. These questions will be used to calculate your exam score as well as the validity and reliability of the experimental or field questions. You will not know which questions are experimental and which questions are being scored. Therefore, treat each question as if it is to be scored. In addition to the multiple-choice questions, the BOC exam will include stand-alone "alternative" questions and five-item focused testlets. The stand-alone questions are essentially five unrelated questions.

The focused testlets consist of scenarios followed by five critical thinking questions related to that scenario. Both the alternative questions and focused testlets use question types such as drag-and-drop, text-based simulation, multi-select, and hot-spot questions. These question types are described below.

Multiple-Choice Questions

The first type of question you will be given is the multiple-choice question. Each multiple-choice question will be one of three types of questions: recall, application, or analysis. A recall question is the most basic type: it simply asks you to recall information such as facts, terminology, or definitions. Application questions require you to apply knowledge to a given situation. Analysis questions require you to consider more than one piece of information and recognize the relationships that exist between the pieces of information and the question being asked.

To indicate your answer to a multiple-choice question, place your cursor in the radio button in front of the answer option you are selecting, and click your mouse. Your selected answer will have a black circle in the center of the associated circle, as shown in Figure 3-2. If you wish to change your answer, click your cursor in the new answer option you would like to select. Your new answer will be marked as selected, and your previously selected answer will become deselected.

Your exam may include multiple-choice questions that have additional information, such as a photo or a table, which you will need to view in order to answer the question. If the question refers you to additional information, an attachment link will appear to the right of the question in the test display screen (Fig. 3-3). To view the attachment,

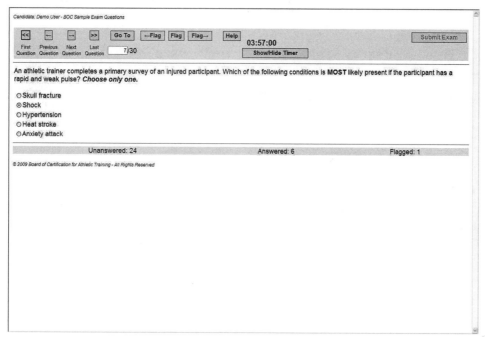

FIGURE 3-2. Full-screen view of questions, including question counts (number of questions).

(Reprinted with permission from the Board of Certification, Inc. All rights reserved.)

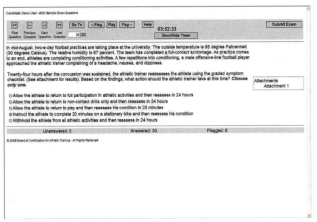

FIGURE 3-3. Attachment link for multiple-choice questions.
(Reprinted with permission from the Board of Certification, Inc. All rights reserved.)

click on this link; a second screen containing the additional information will appear across the top of your current test window. You can move this window around to view the question and the answer options and to answer the question. When you move to the next test question, the attachment window will automatically close. If you need to close the attachment before moving to the next question, click the red circle with a diagonal line or red X that appears to the right of the "Attachment" label in the attachment screen.

When multiple-choice questions are scored, you are penalized the same for answering a question incorrectly as you are for leaving the question unanswered. For tips on answering the multiple-choice questions, see Chapter 5.

Multi-select Questions

Multi-select items are similar to multiple-choice questions, except this type of question allows you to select more than one answer option. That is, you are instructed to choose all the options that apply to the question being asked. To select your answers, use your mouse to click on the checkboxes next to the answer options. Selected answers will show a black checkmark in the center of their associated square. To change an answer, simply click your cursor in the checkmarked square a second time, and the checkmark will disappear (Fig. 3-4).

Drag-and-Drop Questions

Drag-and-drop questions involve clicking on various options presented on a toolbar on one side of the screen and dragging

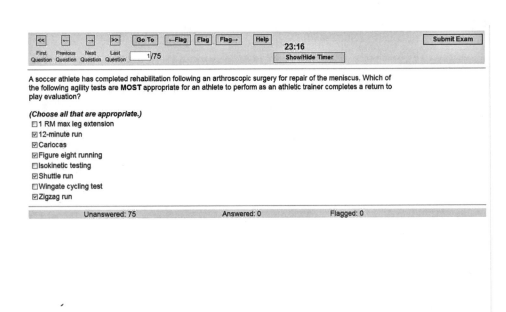

FIGURE 3-4. Multi-select question.
(Reprinted with permission from the Board of Certification, Inc. All rights reserved.)

them to drop boxes on the other side of the screen. This type of question typically asks you to put certain tasks in preferred order or priority order or asks you to rank the toolbar options. For example, the question may ask you to select the exercises an athlete with a 4-day-old second-degree lateral ankle sprain should perform during a visit to the athletic training room and to place these selections in order of difficulty from easiest to most difficult. As with all questions presented in the focused testlets, the lead-in scenario and an item stem or question also appear on the screen (Fig. 3-5).

The drop boxes for drag-and-drop questions are black rectangular fields with labels. The labels provide directions for placement of the drag options as directed by the item stem. For example, if the question asks you to place your selections in the order you would perform them during a rehabilitation program or treatment, then the boxes will be labeled in a sequence such as "Done first," "Done second," and so on.

Additional instructions usually specify the functionality of the toolbar and the drop boxes. For example, the additional instructions may tell you to scroll down the drag options toolbar to view all the available drag options. The instructions may also state that all the toolbar options may not all be used when answering the question.

To answer a drag-and-drop question, use your mouse to click on an answer option in the toolbar. While holding down the mouse button, drag the answer option across the screen until it is over your selected drop box. Releasing the mouse button will drop the dragged answer into the box. Your answer should fill the previously blank box and remain in place after you move your mouse.

If you want to change an answer after you have placed it in a drop box, you can either move it to a different box, or

you can return it to the toolbar. When returning a selected answer to the toolbar, you can drop it anywhere over the toolbar and it will automatically go to its appropriate location. In addition to knowing that you may need to scroll down the toolbar to see all the available answers, it is very important you know that once an answer is removed (dragged away from) the toolbar, it may *not* disappear from the toolbar list. If this situation occurs, it does not automatically indicate that the answer *should* be used again. Therefore, read the question and the additional instructions carefully, and note if answers may be used multiple times.

Prompt-and-Response Questions

A prompt-and-response question consists of an item stem or question followed by a list of answer options labeled "prompts" and a corresponding list of hidden text items labeled "responses." This type of question is commonly used to simulate the process of obtaining an athlete's history or other assessment parameters. For example, it may instruct you to select all the questions that are appropriate to ask the athlete based on the mechanism of the athlete's injury. Upon selecting a prompt, the response to the prompt will appear in the response column. This information may or may not need to be considered when making treatment or management decisions in subsequent focused testlet questions (Fig. 3-6).

To answer a prompt-and-response question, use your mouse to place the cursor over the checkbox in front of the prompt you wish to select. When selected, a black checkmark will appear in the checkbox, and simultaneously a written statement will appear in the associated "Response" column. Unlike multiple-choice, multi-select, and drag-and-drop questions, you *cannot* change a prompt-and-response

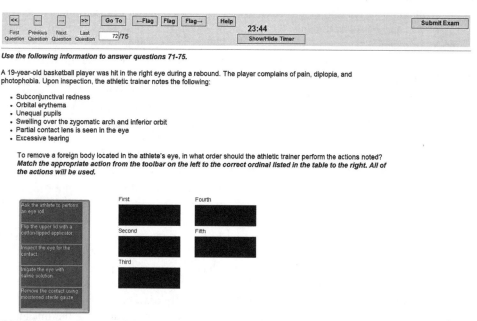

FIGURE 3-5. Drag-and-drop question.
(Reprinted with permission from the Board of Certification, Inc. All rights reserved.)

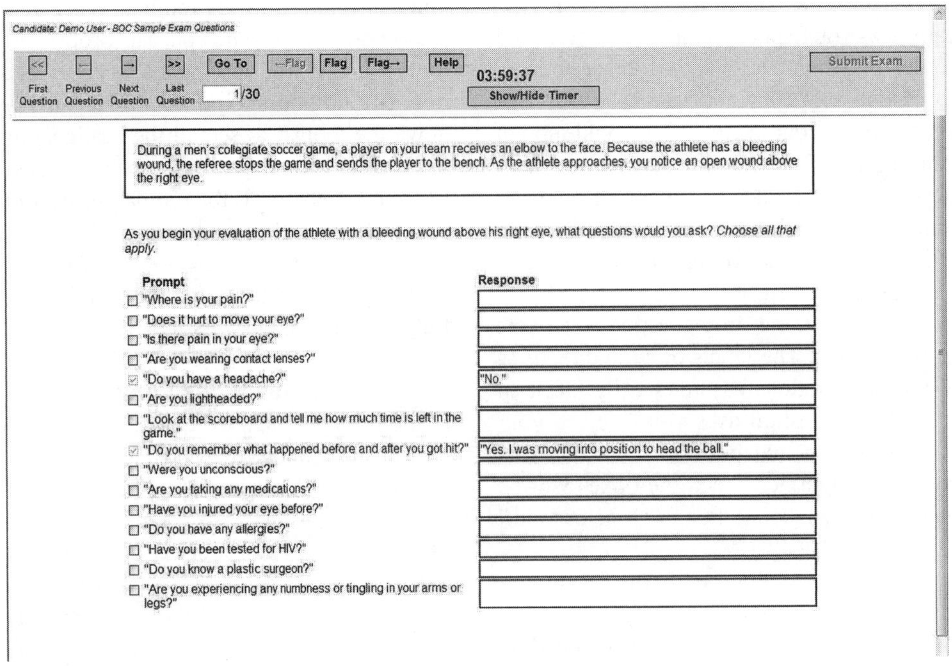

FIGURE 3-6. Prompt-and-response question.
(Reprinted with permission from the Board of Certification, Inc. All rights reserved.)

answer once it has been selected. Therefore, be sure to think through the answer thoroughly before selecting.

Hot-Spot Questions

Hot-spot questions consist of an item stem or question, additional information, and directions for completing the question and submitting your answer. Typically a hot-spot question asks you to identify the location of a structure or landmark on a photograph or figure. For example, you may be asked to locate the dermatome for the C4 nerve root on a photograph of an arm, or you may be asked to locate the tibial tuberosity on a model or diagram.

To answer a hot-spot question, place your cursor over the appropriate location on the image provided and click your mouse button. A circle will appear over the area you have selected. You can reposition the circle until you are satisfied with its placement (Fig. 3-7).

Animated Simulation Questions

An animated simulation (also called a virtual demonstration) consists of an item stem, additional instructions, a toolbar with mini-photos or illustrations as options, and an image. The item stems for these questions instruct you to demonstrate a particular skill or technique. For example, you may be asked to demonstrate the acceptable technique for closing a non-stitchable laceration or for performing joint mobilization of the tibiofemoral joint. The additional instructions that follow the item stem guide you as to how you should answer the question. For example, the instructions may say to select an item from the toolbar to apply to

a wound prior to placing closure strips and instruct you as to the number of action steps that will be scored. The additional instructions may also provide information regarding the functionality of the toolbar and image.

As in drag-and-drop questions, you may need to scroll through the toolbar to see all the possible answer options. If you are unsure of an item depicted in the toolbar's photo or illustration, you can hover your mouse cursor over the photo, and a text label will appear.

To answer an animated simulation, follow the directions provided. You will most likely need to select an item from the toolbar and use that tool to demonstrate a skill or technique. Select a tool from the toolbar by clicking the desired item with your mouse. A pop-up box will appear to confirm your selection. If you inadvertently select the wrong tool or you decide to change your selection, click the "Cancel" button, and you will return to the test item where you can select a different item from the toolbar. Click the "OK" button if you believe you have selected the correct item from the toolbar (Fig. 3-8).

After you have confirmed your toolbar selection, your mouse cursor will return as an arrow or a hand. It may not appear as the item you have selected from the toolbar. Once you have confirmed your toolbar option selection, complete the task directed by the item stem and instructions. For example, you may be instructed to indicate the direction in which you would apply a closure to a wound using three action steps, as if you were applying three adhesive skin closures. To draw on the illustration or photo in the question, place your mouse cursor on the image where you want to start your drawing, and click. Then drag the cursor over the

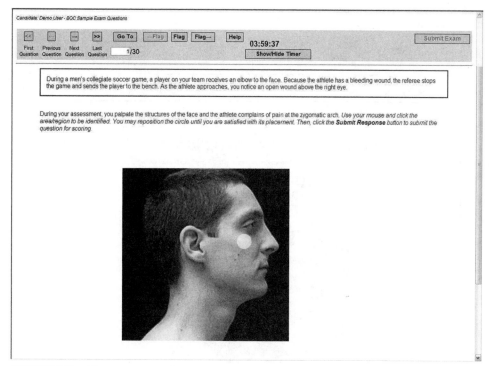

FIGURE 3-7. Hot-spot question.
(Reprinted with permission from the Board of Certification, Inc. All rights reserved.)

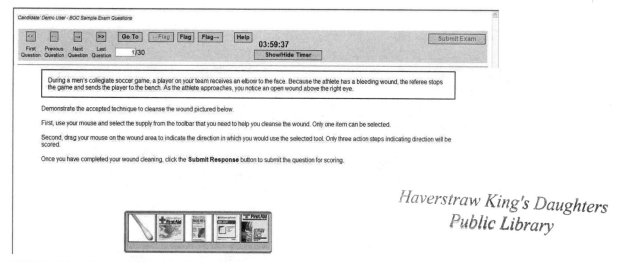

FIGURE 3-8. Animated simulation toolbar.
(Reprinted with permission from the Board of Certification, Inc. All rights reserved.)

image, drawing a line until you reach your end point, and then release the mouse button. The item stem may state that you will be scored on the start and stop locations of your drawing. Once you release the mouse button, a pop-up confirmation box will appear. As you did when you selected the toolbar item, you can either confirm your drawing by clicking "OK," or you can click "Cancel" and return to a screen absent of your earlier drawing and ready for you to start your next attempt (Fig. 3-9).

If the item stem or additional information indicates that more than one drawing will be scored, you will need to return to the image with the first drawing and complete all subsequent drawings, confirming each drawing along the way. For example, in Figure 3-10, three action steps were required to demonstrate the requested technique. When you have answered the question completely, click the "Submit Response" button to submit the test item for scoring and to move on to the next question.

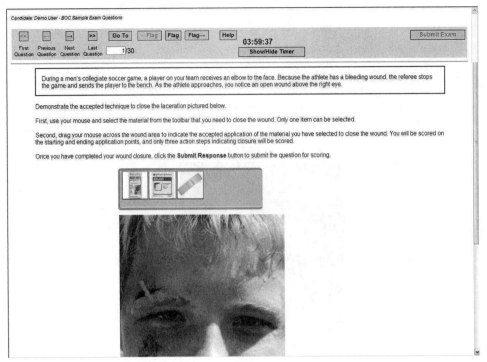

FIGURE 3-9. Action step in an animated simulation.
(Reprinted with permission from the Board of Certification, Inc. All rights reserved.)

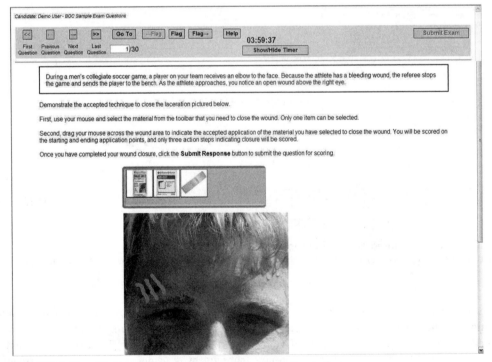

FIGURE 3-10. Three action steps in an animated simulation.
(Reprinted with permission from the Board of Certification, Inc. All rights reserved.)

EXAMINATION ITEM DEVELOPMENT

The *Role Delineation Study*

To be judged *valid,* an exam must relate to some measurable objectives. In college, you are given exams to determine if you are proficient in the objectives of a course. Likewise, the BOC exam is administered to determine whether you show proficiency in the knowledge and skills required to be an athletic trainer. In this model, the *Role Delineation Study* serves as the course objectives.

The *Role Delineation Study* is an integral part of ensuring that the certification exam is valid. In addition, the *Role Delineation Study* serves as a job description of a certified athletic trainer by defining the current entry-level knowledge, skills, and abilities required for practicing athletic trainers. The study achieves these purposes by ensuring that the questions are valid as to their content and that they evaluate the knowledge and abilities needed for someone to function as a competent (entry-level) practitioner. Thus, the BOC certification exam protects the public by ensuring that only competent practitioners who have met specific criteria relevant to the practice of athletic training become certified.

Each question in the BOC certification exam is based on the most current *Role Delineation Study* (Appendix B). Questions are developed to assess the candidate's knowledge on subject matter from each of the six athletic training domains within the study; the domains are distributed according to the following percentages:

- Prevention (15.72%)
- Clinical Evaluation and Diagnosis (22.91%)
- Immediate Care (17.50%)
- Treatment, Rehabilitation, and Reconditioning (23.31%)
- Organization and Administration (11.29%),
- Professional Responsibility (9.27%)

It is important that you read the current *Role Delineation Study,* and use it when preparing for the exam. Do not, however, base your exam preparation on these distribution percentages. Instead, as will be discussed in later chapters of this text, focus your study time on your identified areas of weakness.

Statistical Reliability—Psychometrics: Creating and Validating Examination Questions

Reliability is an index of how accurately the exam measures the candidate's skills, whereas *validity* is the ability of the test to measure what it is supposed to measure. The validity of a certification exam involves the demonstration of at least two major qualities: first, the content of the exam must be shown to be job-related; second, the exam should cover areas in which lack of knowledge would cause harm to the public. These qualities make up some of the defining characteristics of what is called the "content validity" of the exam.

The ability of a certification exam to assess entry-level performance accurately is based in large part on its content validity. The process of validating the content of the BOC certification exam involves the following five rigorous steps: (1) conduct a role delineation study and associated validation study; (2) develop a test blueprint; (3) develop and test items (questions) that pertain to the areas of performance outlined in the test blueprint; (4) create primary and final exams from the validated test items; and (5) review and revise those exams.

After role delineation and associated validity studies have been conducted, the BOC develops a test blueprint, or plan, for the certification exam. Information regarding the importance, harmfulness, and percentage of time devoted to each task in the domains of the *Role Delineation Study* are translated directly into the percentage of items that should be included in the exam for each content area. Once this step is completed, members of a committee of BOC Certified Athletic Trainers who are considered content experts develop the questions. Questions must be referenced to at least two texts on the BOC Examination References list and must be written to a set psychometric standard. For example, the question should: (1) be meaningful, (2) present a definite problem, (3) include as much information as possible, (4) be stated positively whenever possible, and (5) not contain irrelevant material. The five required responses for each test question should: (1) be grammatically consistent with the question, (2) be plausible, (3) contain only one correct or clearly best answer, (4) not use "all of the above" or "none of the above," and (5) not include "never" and "always." All developed test questions are repeatedly edited for clarity, content, and technical adequacy while also being validated by experts from the BOC's testing agency.

In summary, content experts write the questions and validate their appropriateness for the exam, and experts in testing review the questions to ensure that the questions perform as intended. The BOC exam is revised each year to ensure that the exam continues to be a valid measure of candidates' abilities. All items from previous versions of the exam are reviewed carefully and analyzed statistically. Using these analyses, the inappropriate or questionable items are either revised or omitted from future exams.

Examination Scores

The BOC certification exam passing score, the cutoff score that separates examinees who pass from examinees who fail, is determined in a systematic way. The method used by the BOC in its certification exams is a criterion-referenced approach called the Modified Angoff Technique. A criterion-referenced scoring system means that your performance on the exam is measured in relation to standards, not in relation to the performance of others taking the exam. The Modified Angoff Technique relies on the pooled judgments of content experts who determine, for each question, the probability that a "minimally acceptable candidate" will answer the question correctly. They then consider what proportion of a group of minimally acceptable candidates will answer each item correctly. The average of the proportions, also known as the probabilities, is then multiplied by the total number of exam questions. The result represents the "minimally acceptable" score. The final passing point for the exam is based on this pooled judgment, and it includes a statistical adjustment for testing error. This adjustment is provided to give the benefit of the doubt to examinees scoring just below the level judged by the reviewers to be the minimal passing point. Each new exam version is equated to the initial or anchor version to ensure that candidates are not rewarded or penalized for taking different versions of the exam.

The exact point value for each question is determined as a function of the weight assigned to its content category as well as the number of questions in that content category. The range of scores is between 200 and 800, with 500 set as passing the passing point.

Final Preparation for the Examination

You began preparing for this examination the first time you set foot in an athletic training class or covered a practice or game. The certification examination reflects the culmination of your knowledge and clinical skills. Although you should have been exposed to a significant amount of the information that will appear on the examination during the course of your classroom education and practical experience, you should still take time to prepare for it. Your success on test day depends on that preparation.

It is best to begin preparing well in advance of the test date. This process may be considered as "refreshing" the knowledge you have already gained. "Cramming" information just before the examination is discouraged because it could result in more confusion than learning. Do not take the test before you are prepared. Students are often anxious to take the examination as soon as they are eligible, but being eligible is not the same as being prepared. Taking the examination before you are prepared could result in failure, which does nothing to help your confidence, your motivation to study more, or your bank balance. Wait until you have had sufficient time to prepare for the examination, even if that means delaying the examination date. Preparing well will also help you avoid the increased strain on your budget of paying the fees to retake the exam if you are unsuccessful on your first attempt. That being said, it is best to take the examination as close to graduation as your preparation allows while the material is still fresh. Being away from the material for too long may have a negative effect on outcome.

Do not view the examination as an obstacle. Rather, view it as an opportunity to demonstrate your knowledge of athletic training. The right frame of mind is essential for success. You have already started your preparation by familiarizing yourself with the general composition and structure of the test, as discussed in Chapter 3. In this chapter we discuss how to make final preparations for the examination and create a study plan to help you achieve your goals.

CREATE A BUDGET

One of the first steps in preparing is to create a budget. In addition to the approximate $300 cost of registering for the exam, you should also budget for fees to travel to the testing center. (For a complete list of testing center locations, see the CASTLE Worldwide Web site at www.castleworldwide.com.) If the testing site is several hours from your school or home, you may choose to spend the night in a hotel near the testing site the night before. Such planning allows you to arrive at the testing site well rested, and you will not have to worry about missing your test due to unforeseen circumstances, such as oversleeping or travel delays due to weather or accidents.

Your budget should also include the cost of study materials you will need in order to prepare. To help keep these costs to a minimum, hold on to all of your major textbooks. They will be invaluable resources when you are reviewing information you may have forgotten. If you are considering selling a book, check to see whether it is on the Board of Certification's (BOC's) reference list. If the book is on the list, then the BOC deems it to be reliable reference that you should retain as a resource.

Purchase the *Role Delineation Study* from the BOC and at least one study guide. If your budget is tight, Web sites such as Amazon, eBay, or Craigslist may provide low-cost alternatives. Also investigate your school's library or books that your faculty members may be willing to lend you for studying.

Another cost is that of the sample tests available for purchase on the BOC Web site (www.bocatc.org). Currently, there are integrated self-assessments available for purchase, which can be taken in either study mode or test mode. Each integrated self-assessment examination includes 65 multiple-choice questions, 1 focused testlet with 5 alternative item–type questions, and 5 stand-alone alternative item–type questions, all of which are representative of the questions on the test. As of the printing of this text, the cost of each integrated test is $30.

GATHER STUDY MATERIALS

While establishing a budget, begin to gather your study materials. Obtain the *Role Delineation Study,* the document from which the examination is derived. The performance domains portion is included as Appendix B in this book. Choose a review study guide that is most like the actual test (includes interactive computerized options and test review information). If you can purchase additional study guides, the benefit is taking different types of practice tests from different authors, which will prepare you for different question styles and wording. Even if the guides cover the same material, they may ask about it in a completely different way than you are used to.

Make sure you have one broad-based text, such as *Arnheim's Principles of Athletic Training*, and one text in each content area (modalities, rehabilitation, evaluation, general medical, nutrition, organization and administration, and exercise physiology). Refer to the BOC reference list when compiling your study materials. The BOC reference list, organized by practice domains, is in Appendix C. Use the list to search for references specific to the domains for which you need additional information. It is not necessary to collect all the books on the list. Studying information in too many sources may only confuse you.

You many also find it helpful to collect old class notes or lecture outlines and any old tests that you may want to use as practice tests. Ask your professors for assistance; your professors also want you to succeed and might be willing to generate some practice tests from question banks they have. Another way to create a bank of practice test questions is to use review questions found at the end of chapters in textbooks or online as ancillary materials for texts.

In addition, collect exercises that will assist you in honing your critical thinking skills. These types of materials will best prepare you for the focused testlets and stand-alone alternative questions. Written simulation questions from review books, proficiency tests, and practical examinations will assist you the most.

In addition to print materials, you will want to review and perhaps print several electronic resources. The BOC Web site contains valuable information to assist you in preparing for the exam. Review the *Candidate's Handbook* and all the Web pages in the candidate section on the BOC's Web site. The BOC Web site also provides, free of charge, 20 multiple-choice questions, 1 focused testlet (consisting of 5 stand-alone items tied to a common scenario), and 5 alternative items, including multiple choice, multi-select, and drag-and-drop.

When you have gathered your study materials, put them all together in a centralized location so that if you need to verify a piece of information or review a concept, you do not need to waste time searching for your references. An empty milk crate should provide an easy way for you to store your resources. You may want to consider organizing information by practice domain or content area; just remember that some material overlaps in content areas.

IDENTIFY YOUR WEAKNESSES

The next step before creating your study plan is to identify your weaknesses. These weaknesses will guide your study plan. Try the following two exercises to help you identify your weaknesses.

Take a Practice Test

Using the software provided with this book, take a full practice test. It is recommended that you take this and any practice examinations under conditions that closely resemble actual test conditions. That is, you should time yourself, not use any extra material, and resist the temptation to look up an answer to a question until you have completed the practice test. When taking this and any practice test, take notes on vocabulary and content areas with which you are unfamiliar or need to review. Read each question and all the possible answer options thoroughly with this goal in mind. You may find a concept or vocabulary word in an incorrect multiple-choice answer that might be in a question on another practice test or the examination itself. See the Rozzi Web page at http://davisplus.fadavis.com for printable Personal Study Plan Worksheets. After completing the practice test, print the report and your score. This report will tell you the domains in which you missed content. Focus your studies on these areas.

Evaluate Your Knowledge

Using the Athletic Training Practice Domains Worksheet included in Appendix B, rate yourself on each of the content areas using these three criteria:

- **No Clue.** *I've never heard of this word or concept. The material is very unfamiliar to me. I would not be able to answer simple questions related to this content.*
- **Sort of Comfortable.** *I know I have been exposed to this information, but I would have a difficult time answering many questions related to this concept.*
- **I Got That!** *I'm very comfortable with this information and feel well prepared to answers questions related to this content area.*

Be honest with yourself, and try to recall how much education you received on each topic. Consider the quality of the instruction. Everyone has had teachers who skipped a chapter or a section of a course. You may also have been absent on the day when a certain topic was covered.

After you have rated your knowledge on each competency and skill, go back and review your rankings. You know better than anyone else what information you have mastered and what you have not. These results become an index of what you need to study. If you are honest with yourself, you will be able to identify your weaknesses and correct them before facing the certification examination. Being overly confident or overly critical can have negative implications as well. In the first situation, you may miss the opportunity to review key pieces of information; in the latter, you may bog yourself down with excessive information.

Focus on Problem Areas

After you have completed these two exercises, you will have a list of your weak content areas. These areas should be your focus during study sessions. Make sure to study the entire content area of weakness, not just the specific questions that you missed. Studying question content allows you only to review the information specific to the missed question when you most likely have some weakness in the entire content area. As you progress through your study plan, your areas of weakness will become more refined and may change slightly. Your studying should adjust to those changes. Use the weaknesses you have identified as motivators. It should be your goal to become comfortable with these content areas.

CREATE A STUDY PLAN

You are now ready to create a personalized study plan. To be as effective as possible, the plan should be written and organized. The earlier you begin your final study preparations, the more effective your studying will be. A 9- to 12-month study period is recommended. For most students, that means studying throughout their entire senior year with an anticipated mid-April test date.

Begin by determining an anticipated test date. Use this date as the target, and create your study plan by backtracking from this date. The study plan should incorporate information gathered from your self-assessments.

Complete the full practice test in the months leading up to your test date. The practice test should be taken under conditions that most closely resemble testing conditions so that you become more comfortable in a testing situation and obtain better feedback on your potential weaknesses. After completing the practice test, identify the domains and the content areas in which you demonstrated the most weakness, and include them in the worksheets located on the F.A. Davis Web site. These content areas will become the focus of your study sessions.

You should also schedule three to four practical exams, one approximately every other month, with your program director, clinical coordinator, or an approved clinical instructor in your program. Remember, they want to see you succeed. Ask them if they would be willing to administer such practical exams or quiz you on skills or weak content areas. Although the certification examination no longer contains a practical portion, the critical thinking, decision making, and increased stress incurred from these types of exams give you the opportunity to study in a test-like atmosphere.

After you complete each practical examination, ask the person who administered it for feedback, and discuss any questions you had about specific skills as well as the decision-making process. Such practice will assist you with completing the focused testlets and the alternative questions on the BOC test.

The final component of your personalized study plan is engaging in personal and group study sessions. Personal study sessions should occur weekly. These study sessions should be scheduled just as you would schedule any other appointment on your calendar. Find a regular time in your weekly schedule to focus on the weaknesses you have identified during your regular self-assessments. A regular time each week will minimize the chances that studying will be deferred when school, work, or social activities demand your time.

In addition to having a set time, you should also have objectives for each study session. Know going into the session what content areas to review so you can collect the appropriate study materials. A good place to start is the specific content area you identified as being a weakness on the previous practice test. A personal study plan sample and worksheet are included on the F.A. Davis Web site.

Group meetings or study groups with classmates who are also preparing for the exam can enhance the preparation process. Reviewing, teaching, and learning from others are excellent preparation techniques. You are not alone in your preparations, so take advantage of the people around you. Although you may be headed in different directions after graduation, you have all spent many hours together working toward a similar goal—passing the certification examination.

Monthly group study sessions are probably sufficient. Organize into groups no larger than four or five. Select study group members who have similar study habits, but more importantly, select study group members who will do their part by coming to study sessions prepared, focused, and ready to capitalize on the time you have together. You may find that there is one natural leader within the group who will be responsible for scheduling times, locations, and coordinating topics for discussion. If no leader emerges quickly, then the group may decide to schedule the sessions and make different members responsible for facilitating each session.

Create a combined list of content area weaknesses within the group, and focus on those areas during your study sessions. You were all taught from similar teaching philosophies, so you may have similar areas of weakness, but you also have the benefit of having worked with different clinical instructors, which may assist in filling in some of the gaps. Extra time in study sessions can be filled in by quizzing each other on content area, practicing skills, or working through scenarios. Let your goal be "Together, Everyone Achieves Mastery."

EXAM DAY

When the actual examination day arrives, it is important that you enter the test in a confident frame of mind. Do not spend the night before cramming every last bit of information into your head. Cramming is usually not effective and may result in making you more stressed than you need to be. Instead, do something enjoyable. Go out to dinner and to a movie with friends, go bowling, work out, or go to a ballgame, but most of all make sure you get plenty of sleep.

If you are traveling out of town to take the exam, you may want to take a friend with you. Sitting alone in a hotel room or watching television may not make for a restful night. Allow plenty of travel time if you are traveling on the day of the test. Print directions to the testing center before leaving home. Global positioning systems are very accurate, but even sophisticated satellites sometimes make mistakes, and you may require an alternative route. Plan ahead for unforeseen road construction, accidents, or car trouble. If you arrive early, find somewhere to sit, and unwind.

Eat something before going into the test. Glucose is the only energy source your brain can use for fuel, so you want to make sure you are not entering the test in a fasting state. Try to eat a typical breakfast. Even if you do not normally eat breakfast, try to consume something. Consider this your pre-game meal. The same principles that you apply to your athletes apply here as well. You may bring snacks, drinks, and extra clothes into the testing center, but you will be asked to leave them and any other personal items in a locker.

Dress comfortably. Wear layers so you can add or remove clothing as necessary to make yourself comfortable while taking the test. If you take off any clothing, the test administrator may ask you to put it in your locker.

Most of all, try not to be overly anxious about the test. Approach it with confidence. This is your opportunity to demonstrate how well you have prepared and to be rewarded for the studying you have done. In fact, you may find that the test, although very comprehensive, is easier overall than many tests you have taken in college. Strive for relaxed concentration. Be friendly to other candidates in the testing center, but keep your conversations related to events other than the test. Do not discuss preparation techniques or previous test attempts. These topics introduce negative thoughts. Expect some anxiety, but consider it a reminder that you want to do your best and that it is giving you the energy to do so. Relax. Don't be your worst enemy.

When you are taking the test, practice good test-taking strategies. Relax. You are in control. Stay focused on the test and the next task at hand. Make sure to read the directions carefully, especially when facing multimedia questions. This may seem obvious, but it may help you avoid careless errors and allow you to focus on the specific task required.

The exam includes sample questions to familiarize you with the equipment and the actual test. Sample questions will look very similar to practice tests that were available from the BOC during your preparation. You are not required to complete the sample questions, but you might choose to do so to make sure you are comfortable before you start. Decide whether you want to work on the sample questions before you go into the testing center. Many students are prepared and ready to take the test and just get frustrated working through a question that will not be scored.

Budget your test-taking time. A timer is visibly placed on the top of each screen. Some students who are less familiar with computerized testing may find that they constantly focus on the timer. If watching the timer increases your anxiety or pulls your focus away from the test, hide the timer. When taking practice tests, make a mental note of how the timer affects you. This will help you decide whether to use it on the actual test. If you choose to hide the timer, you can make a note of your start time on your scrap paper and refer to your watch during the test so it feels more like a typical classroom test. You can also check with the computerized timer periodically throughout the test. If you choose to hide the timer and use your watch to budget your time, check back for the official time remaining on a regular basis.

Do not be concerned about other candidates who might also be taking tests at the same time. People may be moving around and completing tests at different times. If you need to use the entire 4 hours allotted to you, use it.

Some students find that it helps them to relax by changing positions or even standing up for a minute so they can refocus and return to the test. There are no breaks during the test, but the time allotted is more than adequate for most students, so if you need to take a break and get a snack, a drink, or a sweater, you may do so provided this is allowed by the test site administrator. Strategies for approaching each of the specific question types are included in Chapters 5 and 6 of this text.

Resist the urge to submit your examination as soon as you have completed all of the test items. If you have adequate time remaining, review your test thoroughly to make sure you have answered all of the questions, did not mark any answers incorrectly, and did not make simple mistakes. You may find that you misread a question or that information found elsewhere in the test indicates that the first answer you chose was incorrect. Change answers to questions if you think you made a mistake, but if you are unsure, it is usually wise to go with your first response.

If some unforeseen problem arises while you are taking the test, consult with the staff at the testing center immediately. Their goal is to keep the testing conditions standard and fair for all candidates, and they can assist with most operational issues that might arise. Any issues that the testing center staff cannot handle must be addressed to the BOC.

Finally, approach the examination like the credentialed professional you are soon to become. Think like a certified athletic trainer. Approach the test as you would approach caring for your athletes every day—with a sound knowledge base and good clinical skills. You control your own outcome. Have a plan. Be prepared. This is your opportunity to prove that you are ready to function as an entry-level certified athletic trainer!

Multiple-Choice Questions of the Examination

This chapter focuses on the multiple-choice items of the Board of Certification (BOC) entry-level athletic trainer examination. These questions are taken from the six performance domains of athletic training identified by the *Role Delineation Study* (Table 5-1). Strategies for approaching the focused testlet stand-alone alternative items are discussed in Chapter 6.

STRUCTURE AND TYPES OF MULTIPLE-CHOICE QUESTIONS

Each multiple-choice question consists of a stem and five answer options. The stem presents the basic idea, or premise, of the question. Of the five possible answer options, *only one is the correct answer;* the other four are incorrect and are called distractors.

You will be faced with three types of multiple-choice questions designed to measure your ability to recall, apply, or analyze information. These three types of questions can be placed on a continuum whereby *recall* questions are the most basic; *application* questions require an additional level of thought; and *analysis* questions require the highest levels of processing.

Recall Questions

Recall questions require only that you remember facts, definitions, rules, and so on. Following are some examples.

Which of the following muscles is responsible for elbow flexion and forearm supination?

○ **A. Triceps**

○ **B. Supinator**

○ **C. Biceps brachii**

○ **D. Anconeus**

○ **E. Brachioradialis**

Option C is correct, because the biceps brachii is the only muscle that performs elbow flexion and forearm supination. This question tests your ability to recall basic anatomy.

Of the following joints, which one is proximal to the knee?

○ **A. Subtalar**

○ **B. Calcaneocuboid**

○ **C. Tarsometatarsal**

○ **D. Hip**

○ **E. Tibiofibular**

Option D is correct, because the hip is the only articulation above the knee. Note that some questions will test more than one type of knowledge. In this question, two skills are being tested: vocabulary, because the definition of proximal is needed, and anatomy, because knowledge of each of these joints is required.

Application Questions

Application questions require that you apply knowledge to a given situation. For instance, by rewording the preceding question, it becomes an application question.

An athlete displays pain and weakness during flexion and supination of the forearm. Which of the following muscles would you suspect was injured?

○ **A. Triceps**

○ **B. Supinator**

○ **C. Coracobrachialis**

○ **D. Anconeus**

○ **E. Biceps brachii**

Option E is correct, as you apply your knowledge of muscle actions to a given set of facts.

Analysis Questions

Analysis questions require that you consider more than one piece of information and recognize the relationship between the variables. By expanding the previous application question, it can be developed into an analysis question.

An athlete reports to the athletic training room following a shoulder injury with a marked decrease in right elbow flexion and forearm supination strength as well as paresthesia along the lateral and medial upper arm, elbow, and forearm. Which of the following nerves would you suspect is involved?

- ○ **A.** Musculocutaneous
- ○ **B.** Axillary
- ○ **C.** Long thoracic
- ○ **D.** Median
- ○ **E.** Radial

This question requires that you recognize the muscle involved in the injury, the nerve that innervates it, and the nerve that supplies the dermatome. Therefore, the correct answer is option A, the musculocutaneous nerve.

There will be questions whose answers you will know immediately, whereas others will require more thought. You may come across a question to which the correct response is immediately apparent, but it is still important that you take your time and select the correct response carefully. When you encounter a more challenging question, context clues can help you arrive at the correct answer.

STRATEGIES FOR APPROACHING MULTIPLE-CHOICE QUESTIONS

When approaching multiple-choice questions, there are some strategies you can use that will assist you in making an educated selection, especially if you are unsure of the correct answer immediately (Box 5-1). Remember, there is *only one correct answer* per question. This may be slightly different from other multiple-choice tests you have taken and is different from the multi-select questions in the focused testlets and stand-alone alternative questions.

In some cases, one key phrase or word may separate the correct response from a nearly correct one. Reread the question, and hunt for key terms that may assist you in finding the correct answer. One strategy is to *eliminate the obviously incorrect responses to narrow down your choices* to two or three.

When you read the question for the first time, *read it carefully*. Test-takers often make the mistake of rushing

---

TABLE 5-1 | **Distribution of Multiple-Choice Questions by Domains Identified by the 1999 Role Delineation**

Performance Domain	Percentage of Questions	Number of Questions*
Prevention	15%	~26
Recognition, Evaluation, and Assessment	23%	~40
Immediate Care	21%	~37
Treatment, Rehabilitation, and Reconditioning	22%	~39
Organization and Administration	10%	~18
Professional Development and Responsibility	9%	~16

*Based on 175 scored and unscored test items

Box 5-1 | **Multiple-Choice Question Strategies**

- There is only one correct response.
- Eliminate the obviously incorrect responses to narrow down your choices.
- Read the entire question before answering.
- Rephrase a question in your own words.
- Cover up the answer options before you read the question.
- Eliminate responses that you immediately know are incorrect.
- Question answer options that are totally unfamiliar to you.
- Question answer options that do not grammatically fit with the stem.
- Question answer options that contain absolute words, such as "always" and "every."
- Toss out high and low number options.
- Carefully consider "look-alike" options.
- Carefully consider opposite-answer options.
- Favor answer options that contain qualifiers.
- Give each option the true-false test.
- If two options seem correct, compare them for differences.
- If two answer options seem correct, identify which option is worse.
- Identify distractors.

through the question to get to the possible responses. In doing so, they tend to read only part of the question and anticipate what it is asking. Read the question thoroughly, and then determine what the question is asking. You may find it helpful to *rephrase it into your own words*. For example, try changing a question to a statement. Be careful, however, not to lose sight of the original meaning.

Thinking critically may improve your odds of answering correctly. One way to implement this strategy is to *cover the responses before you read the question*. Read the question carefully, and process what it is asking, and try to predict an answer. Then, uncover and read all the responses, and mark the answer that most closely matches your predicted answer.

If you are still having difficulty answering the question, apply some of the following strategies.

Eliminate responses that you know are incorrect. Doing so will allow you to narrow the possible responses you have left to be considered. For example, consider the following question.

What is the name of cranial nerve IV?

○ **A.** Abducens

○ **B.** Optic

○ **C.** Trochlear

○ **D.** Olfactory

○ **E.** Oculomotor

If you know that abducens is cranial nerve VI and that olfactory is cranial nerve I, then you can narrow the possible correct responses to B, C, or E. Then, evaluate the other three responses to arrive at the correct response, C.

Question the responses that are totally unfamiliar to you. All students graduating from accredited athletic training education programs have been exposed to similar competencies during their educational process. These competencies are extremely detailed, so the likelihood of your seeing a term that is completely new to you is low. The certification examination tests knowledge and skills that have been identified as key to the practice of entry-level athletic trainers. If a response is completely unfamiliar to you, then it is probably beyond the scope of an entry-level athletic trainer and may be eliminated from consideration. If you are taking a practice test and come upon a concept or term that is completely unfamiliar to you, make note of that concept, and then go back and look it up. Consider a question such as the following.

When the three energy-yielding nutrients are completely oxidized, what product(s) is/are common to all three?

○ **A.** Pyrovic acid

○ **B.** Urea

○ **C.** Carbon dioxide, water, and adenosine triphosphate

○ **D.** Adenosine triphosphate

○ **E.** Carbon dioxide, water, adenosine triphosphate, and urea

---

Suppose that you have never heard of pyrovic acid. You should question the validity of this response. In doing so, you would be correct. Pyrovic acid does not exist and is placed there to distract you from the correct answer, C.

Question the responses that do not grammatically fit with the question. Read the question with each response. If there is a grammatical inconsistency, most likely the answer is incorrect. Consider the following question.

When implementing a conditioning program for individuals ages 45 years and older, what should be your first step?

○ **A.** Cooper's 12-minute walk-run test

○ **B.** Assess the athlete's flexibility

○ **C.** Ensure that the athlete has been cleared by a physician through a preparticipation medical screen

○ **D.** Determine the athlete's maximal oxygen consumption

○ **E.** Harvard step-test

If you read the question with each possible response, you will find that options A and E are merely names of tests and not an action step that could be taken, so these options can be eliminated. You are then left with three responses to evaluate in coming to the correct answer, C.

Question responses that contain absolute words. These types of words often indicate that the statement is incorrect. Try substituting nonabsolute words, such as frequently for always or typical for every, to see if you can eliminate a response. Evaluate the following question.

Which of the following statements regarding taping joints is correct?

○ **A.** Taping has been proved to be the only effective way to protect joints against injury.

○ **B.** Taping has been used with little knowledge of its effectiveness.

○ **C.** Taping has been shown to be a must in all postsurgical situations.

○ **D.** Taping has demonstrated little effectiveness in athletics.

○ **E.** Taping has been proved to give athletes a false sense of security.

Evaluate each of the responses that contain absolute words. Option A can be reevaluated by substituting "one of" for "only" so the response reads: Taping has been proved to be one of the effective ways to protect joints against injury. Written this way, the option is more correct, so option A is incorrect as written. In option C, substitute "some" or "most" for "all." The option now reads: Taping has been shown to be a must in some postsurgical situations. With this change, option C is now a correct statement, meaning that the option as currently written is incorrect. Eliminating A and C, you can now evaluate the remaining responses and determine that option B is the correct statement.

Eliminate high- and low-number responses. If the responses to a question are numbers, give more consideration to those with middle-range numbers. Here is an example.

A person who wants to lose at least 1 pound a week should reduce daily caloric intake by how many calories?

○ **A.** 100

○ **B.** 200

○ **C.** 500

○ **D.** 1000

○ **E.** 2000

When evaluating responses with numbers, it is highly unlikely that the high and low ends of the range are correct. It is more likely one of the responses in the middle of the range is correct. In this example, the correct answer is C, right in the middle of the range.

Carefully rule out "look-alike" responses, those that are phrased differently but mean the same thing, therefore canceling each other out. You might see a question such as the following.

A physician holds a weekly clinic in your athletic training room two mornings a week. He has requested permission to store and dispense a few select prescription medications from the athletic training room. How would you best respond to his request?

○ **A.** You agree, with the stipulation that a Drug Enforcement Agency (DEA) facility certificate be obtained and that in the signed physician agreement you are listed as an agent assigned by the DEA.

○ **B.** You agree, with the stipulation that a locked cabinet be installed for which the physician has the only key and the physician is the only one to dispense medications.

○ **C.** You decline, stating that athletic training rooms are not permitted to house prescription drugs; doing so would put the facility in violation of DEA laws.

○ **D.** You decline, stating you believe this would put the staff in violation of state pharmacology laws.

○ **E.** You decline, stating that dispensing medication is outside the scope of practice of an athletic trainer.

In this question, you are provided a set of thorough, difficult distractors. All five possible responses are structured in basically the same grammatical format, with three carrying a negative response and two carrying a positive response and associated rationale. In addition, options D and E are worded differently, but they are "look-alikes," saying almost exactly the same thing. Each multiple-choice question has only one correct answer, so these responses are incorrect, allowing you to narrow your choices to options A, B, or C. After careful review, you determine that option A is correct.

Carefully consider opposite answer responses. If two responses are opposite to each other, chances are one of them is correct. Consider this example.

Negative feedback control is illustrated by decreased production of which of the following hormones?

○ **A.** Testosterone as a result of low luteinizing hormone (LH) blood levels

○ **B.** LH as a result of low testosterone levels in the blood

○ **C.** LH as a result of high testosterone levels in the blood

○ **D.** LH because of inherent rhythmicity of specialized neurosecretory cells

○ **E.** Estrogen as a result of low testosterone and high LH blood levels

---

Of the possible responses to this question, LH is listed as a result in three of them, so most likely one of the three is correct. One can further narrow the responses because options B and C are opposite responses, so one of the two is probably correct. In fact, the correct option is C.

Favor responses that contain qualifiers. Responses that contain qualifiers tend to be longer and therefore more inclusive. These responses are more likely to be correct, and they answer the question better than the others. Look at the following question.

Which of the following statements regarding selection of tape size and type is correct?

○ **A.** Narrow tape is used for large body parts.

○ **B.** Nonelastic tapes are chosen to encircle a muscle belly for better conformity.

○ **C.** Waterproof tape is used for athletes who have a high sweat rate.

○ **D.** Elastic tapes are chosen for joints to ensure better conformity to the bony processes.

○ **E.** Correction tape is more adhesive, is more rigid, has greater tensile strength, and is more expensive than cloth tape.

Several of the possible responses to this question contain qualifiers, but option E contains the most qualifiers, making it the most thorough and therefore the best response.

Give each response the true-false test. Search for one true statement among the possible responses. If nothing else, this approach will allow you to reduce your choices to the best possible answer. Consider the following question.

When evaluating a knee joint injury, what is an important anatomical consideration that might contribute to a possible meniscal injury?

○ **A.** Medial and lateral menisci are attached to their respective collateral ligaments and become distorted during tibial rotation.

○ **B.** Medial and lateral menisci are firmly attached to the joint capsule and tibial plateau and therefore are unable to move during tibial rotation.

○ **C.** The medial meniscus is attached to the medial collateral ligament and becomes distorted during tibial rotation.

○ **D.** The lateral meniscus is attached to the lateral collateral ligament and becomes distorted during tibial rotation.

○ **E.** Medial and lateral menisci are not attached to ligaments and are free to move during tibial rotation.

Reread each option independently, and decide whether the statement is true or false.

Option A. False; the lateral meniscus is not attached to the lateral collateral ligament.

Option B. False; although the medial meniscus has some attachment to the joint capsule through the medial collateral ligament, the lateral meniscus does not.

Option C. True.

Option D. False; the lateral meniscus is not attached to the lateral collateral ligament.

Option E. False; the medial meniscus is attached to the medial collateral ligament.

From your analysis, you can correctly conclude that the only true answer is option C, making it the correct answer.

If two responses seem correct, compare them for differences. There is only one correct answer to each question. Therefore, if two responses seem correct, read carefully for the differences between them, and refer back to the question to find the best response. If you are unable to determine any difference between the two responses, both are most likely incorrect. Consider the following question.

A tooth sits in a bony cavity. The periodontal membrane surrounds it. This membrane is likened to "tiny springs" for each tooth. What is its function?

○ **A.** It serves as a cushion and allows for better chewing ability.

○ **B.** It serves as a cushion and protects the nerve and blood supply from impingement.

○ **C.** It serves as a cushion and protects the bony cavity from fracture.

○ **D.** It serves to hold the tooth firmly in the socket.

○ **E.** It is an anatomical structure but serves no real function.

After evaluating each of the responses, you have narrowed your choices to options A, B, or C. Each of these options seems correct. Look at each one, and compare them closely, looking for differences. When you have determined the differences, evaluate portions of each response in reference to the question to determine the correct response. When you look closely at option B, you can determine that both functions listed are correct as opposed to options A and C. Therefore, the correct option is B.

If two responses seem correct, identify which one is worse. As students, you are conditioned to look for the best answer. Approaching a question from a different perspective can help you clarify the underlying purpose of the question. For example:

The anterior cruciate ligament stabilizes the knee joint to prevent which motion?

○ **A.** The femur gliding anteriorly on the tibia

○ **B.** The tibia gliding anteriorly on the femur

○ **C.** The tibia gliding posteriorly on the femur

○ **D.** The femur gliding posteriorly on the tibia

○ **E.** The patella gliding anteriorly over the tibia

On your first reading, you determine that not only are there two sets of opposite responses but also that options A and C and options B and D seem very similar. You quickly eliminate options E, A, and C because you know that the anterior cruciate ligament (ACL) restricts anterior tibial translation. That means that either option B or D is correct, but you could argue that no matter whether the tibia is gliding anteriorly or the femur is gliding posteriorly, they are the same basic motion. In this situation, it might be helpful to look at the question in a different way and attempt to clarify what the question is really asking by concluding which of the two remaining options is incorrect.

The question is asking specifically about the ACL and the motion it restricts based on its anatomic position and attachments. Although it attaches on the femur and tibia, its position and line of pull restrict tibial, not femoral, motion. Therefore, option D is incorrect, and option B is correct.

Identify distractors. Distractors are extraneous pieces of information that are intended to distract you from the real purpose of the question. In fact, when multiple-choice questions are created for the BOC exam, the incorrect answer options are called distractors because they attempt to distract you from the correct answer. To avoid being distracted by the incorrect options, focus on the question, and break it down so you clearly understand what the question is asking. Then evaluate each response for its accuracy. Consider the following example.

Which of the following factors are contraindications to the use of diathermy?

○ **A. Metal implants, sensory loss, and hemorrhage**

○ **B. Metal implants, chronic inflammation, and hemorrhage**

○ **C. Chronic inflammation, sensory loss, and hemorrhage**

○ **D. Metal implants, sensory loss, and chronic inflammation**

○ **E. Chronic inflammation, metal implants, and pain**

Each option has three components that must be evaluated for accuracy. Evaluate each component, and make a determination. If the component is correct in one response, it is correct in another. It only takes one incorrect component to make the entire response a distractor. Evaluating each of these components individually will allow you to determine that A is the correct option.

No matter what strategies you employ as you dissect each multiple-choice question and arrive at an educated answer, remember that *you are looking for the best response,* not only a correct one. You are also not looking for a response that must be true all the time, in all cases and without exception. Each response must be evaluated in the context of the individual question.

Strategies for Approaching the Multiple-Choice Questions as a Section

Just as there are strategies for approaching individual multiple-choice questions, there are strategies for approaching the multiple-choice questions as a whole. These strategies should be employed during practice tests so that when you take the actual test you are comfortable with the techniques.

- **Answer easy questions first.** Doing so will allow you to build confidence, score points, orient yourself to test structure and vocabulary, and allow you to make associa-

tions that will help you formulate answers to more difficult questions.

- **Do not dwell on a question if the answer does not occur to you immediately.** Use scrap paper to note in a column the question numbers for which you are unable to make even an educated guess. If you think you can make an educated guess, but you are still unsure, note these question numbers in a separate column. This approach allows you to make more efficient use of your allotted testing time.

- **Rethink difficult questions.** After you have worked through all the questions one time, return to the questions you were unsure of on first reading. You may find that you have picked up clues from your first complete reading or that you have become more comfortable in the testing situation, thus allowing the answers to become more apparent. First address the questions for which you made an educated guess but were unsure which response was correct. Employ the strategies for approaching difficult questions listed in the previous section of this chapter to narrow your responses to the one best response (see Box 5-1). You can then approach the questions that were completely unfamiliar to you on first reading. Work through each question, and attempt to reach an educated guess.

- **Guess. There is no penalty.** If, after carefully reading and working through a question, you are still unable to come up with one clear answer, then guess. If you have employed the strategies discussed, you will most certainly be able to eliminate some responses, narrowing your odds and increasing your ability to make an educated guess. You will not be penalized for guessing. *Do not leave any questions blank.* Your score is based on the number of correct responses, so an educated guess is better than leaving a question unanswered.

- **Resist the urge to submit your test as soon as you finish the last question.** If you have time remaining, go back and review the test to make sure that you have answered all the questions and did not mismark any answers. This is not the time to reevaluate specific responses for each question. You have already done that. Instead, you are looking for simple mistakes. *Change answers only if you made a mistake.*

HOW TO USE SAMPLE MULTIPLE-CHOICE QUESTIONS TO PREPARE FOR THE EXAM

The sample multiple-choice questions contained in this study guide will help you prepare for the multiple-choice questions on the exam, but they will also help you prepare for the other questions on the exam. The material is all athletic training! Everyone says some question types are more difficult than the others, but not everyone agrees which type is harder. This is a product of candidate individuality. Everyone learns in different ways. Some people are more visual, others are more analytical, and still others are kinesthetic learners. The same holds true for testing preferences. Some people prefer multiple-choice questions, and others enjoy the critical thinking or simulation skills tested in the multimedia question types. However, it is all athletic training knowledge, so it is just a matter of how you prefer to receive the questions. If you know that multiple-choice questions are not your preference, commit to spending extra time with these sample questions so that your comfort level increases before you take the actual examination.

If you follow the sample study plan provided in Chapter 4, you will take numerous practice questions during your examination preparation. Treat each of these practice questions as if it were an actual examination. Take the practice question in one sitting, and do not use study aids. The more comfortable you become with the computerized testing system and working under a time limit while taking practice questions, the less stressful the actual examination will be. Taking the practice questions in this manner will also give you a more accurate picture of your strengths and weaknesses and areas on which you should focus your studies.

Sample multiple-choice questions are in Appendix A. These questions are divided into the six performance domains, with correct answers included at the end of each domain. Use the questions in this format to study the domains that you have identified as weaknesses. Although you should not disregard your areas of strength totally, most of your studying should focus on your weaker areas. There is little point in rereading information that you have already mastered.

In addition to using the questions as a group, you can use information from individual questions to direct your preparations. Your study habits should not focus only on the exact questions you missed. Rather, you should focus your attention on the content area of the question. Simply finding the correct answer to a single question will do little to strengthen your knowledge in the entire subject area. For example, read the following question.

A recreational tennis player has been diagnosed with vitamin D deficiency. Which of the following conditions is this athlete most likely to exhibit?

○ **A. Xerophthalmia**

○ **B. Rickets**

○ **C. Osteomalacia**

○ **D. Beriberi**

○ **E. Osteoporosis**

The correct option is C. If you did not easily identify this answer, then you need to review information related to vitamin deficiencies. Keep in mind that this is only a sample examination and that you will not see the same questions on the actual examination. You might instead see a question related to a vitamin A or vitamin K deficiency. If you studied just the vitamin D information, you would not be prepared for those questions.

While taking practice questions or working through the written multiple-choice questions, you should also make notes of vocabulary or concepts that are foreign to you. This strategy should include foreign information found in incorrect responses to questions. Look at the following question.

Injury to the spleen often results in referred pain in the upper left quadrant. How is this occurrence documented correctly?

○ **A. Tinel's sign**

○ **B. Kehr's sign**

○ **C. Battle's sign**

○ **D. Murphy's sign**

○ **E. Romberg's sign**

Suppose that you knew quickly that the correct option is B but you are only somewhat familiar with Tinel's sign and completely unfamiliar with Murphy's sign. You should make note of these terms so you can look them up later.

This text is purposely constructed as a study guide. Therefore, the questions are written to be challenging and to prompt you to investigate areas that you might need to review.

Focused Testlets and Stand-Alone "Alternative" Questions

This chapter discusses the question types used in the focused testlets and as the stand-alone "alternative" items on the Board of Certification (BOC) entry-level athletic trainer certification examination. These questions may be presented in any of these formats:

• Multiple choice
• Multi-select
• Drag and drop
• Prompt and response
• Hot spot
• Animated simulation

Regardless of question type, all questions will be presented on the testing platform as described in Chapter 3. Each question has a stem and associated answer options. The item stem is the specific question to be answered and includes any instructions you may need to answer the item, such as "select all that apply." Some question types may provide additional information, such as directions for using toolbars, drop boxes, and your keyboard mouse. Questions in the focused testlets include a lead-in problem scenario. Note that the scenario text may change slightly through the five questions, based on events or situations that appeared in earlier questions. A detailed description of each question type is provided in Table 6-1.

STRATEGIES FOR APPROACHING FOCUSED TESTLET AND STAND-ALONE ALTERNATIVE QUESTION TYPES

An important consideration when responding to the focused testlets and stand-alone alternative questions is how the questions will be scored. Multiple-choice questions are scored as right or wrong. This means you can accumulate points for correct answers, but you are not penalized for incorrect answers. Therefore, when answering multiple-choice questions, you are instructed to answer all the questions and encouraged to guess if you are unsure of the correct answer. This approach contrasts with how the questions in focused testlets and the stand-alone "alternative" items are scored. These latter questions are scored by awarding points for correct answers and for correct order of answers. Points are lost when contraindications are selected or dangerous procedures are performed. Therefore, if you are unsure of an answer to one of these questions, you should not guess.

Multiple-Choice and Multi-Select Questions

Of the various question types in the focused testlets and the stand-alone alternative items, two are multiple choice and multi-select. A multiple-choice question includes the problem scenario, a question, and a statement directing you to choose *only one* response from the options. If you have not already done so, read Chapter 5 to learn more about the structure of and strategies for approaching multiple-choice questions. Like multiple-choice questions, multi-select questions include the problem scenario, a question, and a selection statement. However, multi-select questions differ in that they instruct you to *choose all* response options that apply to the item.

When you are presented with a multi-select question, carefully read the problem scenario, the question, and any additional instructions to be sure you know what the question is actually asking. Instead of immediately reading through the response options, decide how you would answer the question if you were instructed to make a list of your actions instead of selecting from a provided list. For example, if a multi-select question asks about the actions you should take to determine the correct size of a running shoe, use your scrap paper to make your list of actions, such as "measure both feet" and "ensure the toe box is wide enough to allow for toe movement." When you have completed your

TABLE 6-1 | **Question Types**

Question Type	Description
Multiple Choice	Consists of a question and five possible responses; question asks you to select only one response to answer the question; selected answers *may be changed* until question submitted for scoring
Multi-Select	Consists of a question and multiple possible responses; question asks you to select all responses that apply; selected answers *may be changed* until question submitted for scoring
Drag and Drop	Consists of a question, additional instructions, a toolbar with drag options, and drop boxes with labels; question asks you to select drag options and place them in drop boxes according to specific instructions; selected answers *may be changed* until question submitted for scoring
Prompt and Response	Consists of an item stem, a column of answer options labeled "prompts," and a corresponding column labeled "responses"; select the appropriate prompts that apply to the item stem; after a prompt item is selected, its associated response column will reveal previously hidden text; revealed text provides information for answering subsequent testlet questions; selected answers *may not be changed* once selected
Hot Spot	Consists of an item stem, additional information, and directions for completing the question and submitting your response; question asks you to identify a particular location on a photograph or figure; selected answers *may be changed* until question submitted for scoring
Animated Simulation (Virtual Demonstration)	Consists of an item stem, additional instructions, a toolbar with mini-photos or illustration as options, and an image or figure; question asks you to demonstrate a particular skill or technique; selected answers *may be changed* until question submitted for scoring

list, you can compare it with the question's answer options and select options accordingly. If you read a response option you did not initially think of when writing your list, then you need to decide if the response is a distractor or a correct answer you did not initially consider. If you are completely unfamiliar with the response, it is most likely a distractor. Keep in mind that distractors are intended to draw your attention away from the correct answers.

Another strategy for completing multi-select questions is to disregard the number of answer options you have selected. Do not feel you need to select a certain percentage of the available answer options. For example, if a question provides 10 answer options, and you initially determine only two of the options apply to the question, do not select additional items just because there are eight unselected answer options. Instead, re-read the scenario and the item question and decide if additional options are warranted. Be sure you can justify each selected response item.

Drag-and-Drop Questions

Drag-and-drop questions consist of a problem scenario, an item question, additional instructions needed to answer the item question, a toolbar with drag options, and drop boxes with labels. The additional instructions usually indicate functionality of the toolbar and the drop boxes. For example, the additional instructions may let you know that you will need to scroll down the drag options toolbar to view all the available drag options. The drop boxes are black rectangle shapes with labels. The labels provide directions for placement of the drag options.

When you are presented with a drag-and-drop question, carefully read the problem scenario, the question, and any additional instructions to be sure you know what the question is actually asking. Initially, look at the labels of the drop boxes. Are they labeled as a sequence (i.e., done first, done second, etc.) or labeled as titles (such as injuries, conditions, medication names, etc.)? Also note the number of drop boxes provided and whether the directions indicate that all of the boxes should be used when answering the question. For example, you may be provided with nine boxes for placing steps in order for treating an injury. If the instructions state that all steps will be used, you know that you must select all nine options from the toolbar.

Scroll through the answer options in the toolbar. Count the options, and then try to differentiate the viable answers from the distractors. If the number of options in the toolbar equals the number of drop boxes and the directions indicate all steps will be used without indicating that options may be used more than once, you know each option will be used in your answer. Therefore, it is just a matter of placing those options into the correct sequence. However, if there are more possible options than drop boxes, you will need to determine the best answers. In this case, re-reading the question and additional information may assist you in ruling out possible distractors.

After you have familiarized yourself with the question's components, use your scrap paper to write down your answer to the question. This approach is recommended because once you drag an answer from the toolbar, it may *not* disappear from the toolbar list, forcing you to see the answer you have already selected every time you scroll through the answer options. Additionally, the answer options toolbar may contain an extensive list of options so that you will be unable to see all of your options at one time. Therefore, organizing your answer on paper initially may minimize the potential for confusion.

Prompt-and-Response Questions

Prompt-and-response questions consist of the problem scenario, a question, a column of answer options labeled "prompts" and a corresponding column labeled "responses." In addition to posing the question, the item question will provide you specific instructions for answering the question as it relates to the scenario.

This type of question is similar to a multi-select question because you will be instructed to select all answers that are appropriate or that apply. However, on selecting a prompt, the corresponding response will appear, providing you with more information about the problem scenario.

When you are presented with a prompt-and-response question, carefully read the problem scenario, the question, and any additional instructions, and make sure you know what the question is asking you to do. Then carefully read through all of the prompt answer options *before* you make your first selection. Try to determine which answers are potential correct answers and which are distractors. Before you make a selection, use your scrap paper to organize the prompt answers into two columns. In the first column, write down all the potentially correct prompts. In the second column, write down the prompt options you consider to be distractors. Then, number the answers in the first column in the order that you would complete them.

For example, if a prompt-and-response question is asking you to gather a medical history on an athlete who has sustained an acute lateral ankle sprain, you might write the following prompt options in column one and number them 1, 2, and 3:

1. "What happened?"
2. "Did you hear anything when you injured your ankle?"
3. "Can you point to the area of pain?"

Next, you might write the following prompt options in the second column:

- "Have you ever been diagnosed with patellofemoral pain syndrome?"
- "Do you take a multipurpose vitamin and mineral supplement?"

After you have completed your lists, click on the first prompt option that you listed as appropriate, and read the response. Information in the response will provide you additional information regarding the problem scenario and may assist you in answering the other questions in the focused testlet. Keep in mind that you *cannot change* a prompt-and-response answer after you have selected it.

Continue working through the question by clicking on the remaining prompts in the order listed on your scrap paper and reading the revealed responses. If the revealed response to one of your selections indicates your selection was inappropriate, do not panic or think you have immediately failed. Re-read the question and any additional information, and then return to your written list and make adjustments as necessary. Try to avoid letting this small incident negatively affect the remainder of your test. Focus your efforts on accumulating points toward your total score by answering upcoming questions correctly.

Hot-Spot Questions

Hot-spot questions consist of a problem scenario, a question, and additional information and directions for completing the question and submitting your answer. Typically, a hot-spot question asks you to use your mouse to identify a particular location on a photograph or figure.

Carefully read the problem scenario, the question, and any additional instructions, and make sure you know what the question is asking you to do. Before you move your mouse over the figure to answer the question, locate the question answer on your own body. You are used to identifying anatomical landmarks and performing skills on your own body, so this step may help you make an easier transition between seeing the words in the test question and finding its location on the figure. When you return to the test screen to place the hot-spot circle, keep in mind that you can reposition the circle until you are satisfied with its placement. When you are satisfied with the circle's placement, reclick your mouse to set the circle and then proceed to the next question item.

Animated Simulation Questions

Animated simulations (also called virtual demonstrations) consist of the problem scenario, a question, additional instructions, a toolbar with mini-photos or illustrations as options, and an image. This type of question will have you demonstrate a particular skill or technique. The additional instructions will explain how to answer the question along with information regarding the functionality of the toolbar and image.

When you are presented with an animated simulation question, carefully read the problem scenario, the question, and any additional instructions and make sure you know what the question is asking you to do. Scroll through the options in the toolbar to ensure you see all the possible answer options. Keep in mind that hovering your mouse over the toolbar produces a text label on each image.

Resist the urge to select a tool immediately. Instead, write down the names of the tools on your scrap paper. You can even make notes as to the most appropriate uses for these items. Re-read the question and any additional instructions. Look at your written list, and circle the tool that can best assist you in answering the question. Next, determine exactly how you will use the tool. You can use your finger on the computer screen to simulate the action(s) you plan to perform on the image. Be sure to note the number of actions that will be scored (as described in the question's additional instructions). After you have visualized your answer and decided on a tool, use your mouse to select the tool from the toolbar, confirm your selection, and then perform the requested task to answer the question.

Before you submit your answer for scoring, re-read the question and the additional instructions. If a question states that more than one drawing will be scored, you will need to return to the image with the first drawing and complete all subsequent drawings, confirming each drawing along the way.

HOW TO PREPARE FOR THE EXAMINATION USING THE SAMPLE FOCUSED TESTLETS

Utilize all the information available to you in this text, on the accompanying CD, and at the BOC's Web site. The CD contains more than 1000 multiple-choice questions and over 70 focused testlets. These focused testlet questions use more than 130 photos, images, and videos to present the questions on a testing platform that simulates the one used to deliver the BOC exam. Additionally, the focused testlets incorporate all of the question types. Let's take a close look at how you can use these sample focused testlets to your advantage when preparing for the examination.

Gain Confidence in Navigating the Test

The sample focused testlets will familiarize you with the various question types as well as the testing platform, navigation features, and answering methods. The more familiar you are with the test delivery system, the more likely the test will assess your abilities and skills instead of your degree of comfort with the test technology.

Identify Weak Content Areas

While working through the focused testlet questions, you will be able to identify unfamiliar content areas and topics in which you lack confidence. Look beyond the question presentation and the media delivering the question, and focus on the question's content. For example, when a hot-spot question asks you to identify the distal insertion of the sartorius muscle, it is helpful if you know this muscle is one of three muscles that have a common insertion at the pes anserinus, but can you locate the pes anserinus on an anatomical model?

If you are confident in your answer to the above question, use the question to further test your knowledge of this area. For example, ask yourself to name the other two muscles that also form the pes anserinus. Also, ask yourself the function and innervation for each of these muscles. You can use the study plan on the F.A. Davis Web site to record the unfamiliar concepts and vocabulary words you have identified while working through the focused testlets. You can also use this form to note the practice domains in which you have identified weak areas.

Sharpen Your Critical Thinking Skills

The third way the sample focused testlets can assist you is by providing a means for sharpening your critical thinking and decision-making skills. These practice testlets have been set up so you can logically progress through a scenario, answering questions whereby you must prioritize your actions and critically select from possible choices. As you work through each testlet, think about the factors you consider when making your selections. Try to determine if there are factors you failed to consider that you need to incorporate into future choices. For example, if the problem scenario states that during the first tournament of the season, a 10-year-old soccer player reports trouble catching her breath, should you immediately call emergency medical services, or should you assess the athlete's condition? Perhaps more important than knowing the correct answer is knowing the factors that determine the correct answer, because these are the factors that you can apply to decisions in other testlet questions.

Also visit the BOC's Web site to learn more about the question types comprising the focused testlets and stand-alone alternative questions. You can view a free sample of the examination. To reach these free samples, go to the Candidates section, and click on the link "Sample Exam Questions."

SUMMARY

You have now familiarized yourself with the BOC testing platform, the various question types, and strategies for reviewing content and answering the exam questions. Now it is time to apply all that you have learned to the practice questions in Appendix A and on the CD and move closer toward your goal of becoming a certified entry-level athletic trainer.

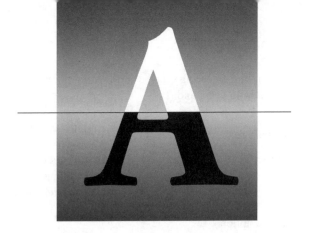

Sample Multiple-Choice Questions

Domain I: Prevention

1. In athletes, which factor is most likely to result in anemia?

○ **A.** An elevated hemoglobin level

○ **B.** Insufficient dietary iron intake

○ **C.** Loss of iron due to chronic heel strike

○ **D.** Red blood cell loss secondary to irritation of the lining of the urinary bladder

○ **E.** A vegetarian diet

2. An athlete has recently undergone a splenectomy. Which of the following functions are most impacted by this surgical procedure?

○ **A.** Ability to filter poisons out of the blood and produce mediators for blood clotting

○ **B.** Ability to filter toxins from the blood and regulate the body's electrolyte level

○ **C.** Ability to produce and destroy blood cells during systemic infection

○ **D.** Ability to produce estrogen and progesterone

○ **E.** Capacity to store vitamins A, E, and K and produce vitamin D

3. One of the most comprehensive approaches to sports injury research involves applying the principles of epidemiology. Which of the following best describes the science of epidemiology?

○ **A.** Study of the distribution of diseases, injuries, or other health states in human populations for the purpose of identifying and implementing measures to prevent their development and spread

○ **B.** Study of the efficacy of specific injury evaluation and treatment measures

○ **C.** Study of the distribution and injury exposure rates of humans participating in sports in diverse environmental settings

○ **D.** Study of individual sport risk factors and the impact of those factors on participation rates

○ **E.** Study of the prevention of the spread of disease in the physically active population

4. Identify the intrinsic factor that most likely influences the onset of athletic injuries.

○ **A.** Being a female high-school athlete

○ **B.** Practicing when the temperature is 85°F and the humidity is 85%

○ **C.** Running on a cross-country wooded trail

○ **D.** Using an inflatable bladder football helmet

○ **E.** Exercising during the early morning and evening hours

5. Osteoporosis is a condition that predominantly afflicts older women. Which of the following factors decreases the chance of developing this condition?

○ **A.** Moderate swimming and increased vitamin C intake

○ **B.** Weight-bearing activities and increased calcium intake

○ **C.** Maintaining 10% body fat and using a minimal-resistance stationary bike

○ **D.** Increased electrolytes and use of nonsteroidal anti-inflammatory medication

○ **E.** Avoidance of physical activity and dairy products

6. What should be your first step when implementing conditioning programs for individuals 45 years and older?

○ **A.** Complete Cooper's 12-minute walk-run test.

○ **B.** Determine the athlete's flexibility.

○ **C.** Ensure a pre-participation medical screen has been completed.

○ **D.** Determine maximal oxygen consumption.

○ **E.** Complete a Harvard step test.

7. How is the word *trauma* defined?

○ **A.** Any injury involving progressive increase in tissue death

○ **B.** Any injury with a rapid onset

○ **C.** Any injury involving internal bleeding

○ **D.** Any injury or wound

○ **E.** Any injury with rapid onset of swelling

8. Which of the following statements best describes the knee joint in comparison to the hip joint?

○ **A.** The knee joint is more dependent on ligamentous structures for stability.

○ **B.** The knee joint is more dependent on bony alignment for support.

○ **C.** The knee joint is more stable in a lower extremity open chain position.

○ **D.** The knee joint is less likely to disarticulate.

○ **E.** The knee joint is inherently less susceptible to degenerative forces.

9. Which of the following athletes is most at risk for developing Sever's disease?

○ **A.** 11-year-old competitive male soccer player

○ **B.** 12-year-old female breast stroker

○ **C.** 8-year-old elite female gymnast

○ **D.** 13-year-old male interior lineman

○ **E.** 12-year-old female track athlete

10. Sports can be classified based on their comparative risk of injury. According to the American Academy of Pediatrics, in which of the following categories would soccer be classified?

○ **A.** Contact/collision

○ **B.** Non-contact

○ **C.** Intermittent contact

○ **D.** Non-collision

○ **E.** Limited contact

11. An athlete demonstrates limited dorsiflexion at the pre-participation screening. Which of the following factors is *most* likely restricting this motion?

○ **A.** Excessive fat

○ **B.** Neural tissue tightening

○ **C.** Bony structures of the joint

○ **D.** Flexibility of the Achilles tendon

○ **E.** Flexibility of the anterior tibialis muscle

12. Which hormone or hormones are secreted by the corpus luteum?

○ **A.** Only estrogen

○ **B.** Only progesterone

○ **C.** Estrogen and progesterone

○ **D.** Neither estrogen nor progesterone

○ **E.** Follicle-stimulating hormone

13. Which of the following conditions is the most common leading to the onset of cardiac problems in middle-aged and older athletes?

○ **A.** Cystic fibrosis

○ **B.** Marfan's syndrome

○ **C.** Cardiac arrhythmia

○ **D.** Atherosclerosis

○ **E.** Hypertrophic cardiomyopathy

14. Which of the following paths constitutes the normal route for conduction of electrical activity through the heart?

○ **A.** Sinoatrial node to atrioventricular node to atrioventricular bundle to Purkinje's fibers to ventricular musculature

○ **B.** Sinoatrial node to atrial musculature to atrioventricular node to atrioventricular bundle to bundle branches to ventricular musculature

○ **C.** Sinoatrial node to atrial musculature to atrioventricular node to atrioventricular bundle to bundle branches to Purkinje's fibers to ventricular musculature

○ **D.** Sinoatrial node to atrioventricular node to atrioventricular bundle to bundle branches to Purkinje's fibers

○ **E.** Sinoatrial node to atrioventricular bundle to atrial musculature to atrioventricular node to bundle branches to ventricular musculature to Purkinje's fibers

15. Which of the following records should aid an athletic trainer in identifying disqualifying abnormalities and correctable or treatable physical conditions in an athlete?

○ **A.** Medical referral records

○ **B.** Athletic injury records

○ **C.** Preseason medical evaluation

○ **D.** Daily medical reports

○ **E.** Athletic injury reports

16. You are the athletic trainer at a high school that sponsors 22 sports. There are approximately 500 athletes. Which type of pre-participation exam would be the most effective and efficient?

○ **A.** Provide a station-based exam with the assistance of multiple medical and health-care professionals prior to the start of each sport season (i.e., fall, winter, spring).

○ **B.** Provide individual exams with the assistance of five family practice physicians stationed in individual exam rooms.

○ **C.** Provide a station-based exam with the assistance of multiple medical and health-care professionals in the summer prior to the start of the school year.

○ **D.** During the summer months, schedule individual appointments for each athlete with the team physician.

○ **E.** Require each athlete to obtain a physical exam through a licensed health-care provider.

17. According to NCAA guidelines, which of the following athletes must complete a comprehensive pre-participation medical evaluation?

○ **A.** A baseball player transferring from a similar-division NCAA institution who reports no injuries or health concerns on his medical history form

○ **B.** A junior basketball player who has not completed a comprehensive exam since his freshman year

○ **C.** A junior football player who has not completed a cardiovascular screening as part of the pre-participation exam since his freshman year

○ **D.** A senior sprinter who had only history and blood pressure measurements taken as part of the cardiovascular screening during the pre-participation physical exam

○ **E.** A senior field hockey player who tore her anterior cruciate ligament in her sophomore season and participated during her junior year

18. According to the American Academy of Pediatrics Guidelines for Sport Participation, which of the following athletes should be recommended for clearance to participate?

○ **A.** An athlete recently diagnosed with carditis wishing to participate in lacrosse

○ **B.** An athlete with atlantoaxial instability wishing to participate in cross country

○ **C.** An offensive lineman with one kidney

○ **D.** An athlete with an enlarged spleen wishing to participate in swimming

○ **E.** An athlete with an enlarged liver wishing to participate in basketball

19. A swimmer notes Wolff-Parkinson-White syndrome. Which statement best characterizes this condition?

○ **A.** Currently the leading cause of sudden death in athletes

○ **B.** Characterized by a prolonged PR interval and a shortened QRS complex

○ **C.** Results in atrial pre-excitation and bradycardia due to accessory pathway electrical activity

○ **D.** Rarely occurs in athletes but is often provoked by exercise bouts

○ **E.** Characterized by ventricular pre-excitation and tachycardia due to electrical conduction over accessory pathways

20. A properly fitted mouth guard has not been shown to be effective in reducing the risk of which of the following injuries?

○ **A.** Tooth fractures

○ **B.** Temporomandibular joint sprains

○ **C.** Fractured zygomatic bone

○ **D.** Intruded teeth

○ **E.** Cerebral concussions

21. One of your soccer players who wears a custom derotation brace while playing is complaining of gastrocnemius cramping. You choose to remove the most superior calf strap in an attempt to relieve her cramping. In a subsequent practice, she sustains a noncontact ligamentous knee injury because the brace failed to provide appropriate stability. Who might be deemed negligent in this situation?

○ **A.** Brace manufacturer

○ **B.** Sales representative who initially measured and fit the brace

○ **C.** Athletic trainer

○ **D.** Coach

○ **E.** Institution that employs the coach and the athletic trainer

22. How often must helmets be recertified and reconditioned using a vendor approved by the National Operating Committee on Standards for Athletic Equipment if no warranty exists or after the warranty expires?

○ **A.** Every year

○ **B.** Every 2 years

○ **C.** At the end of the playing season

○ **D.** Every 4 years

○ **E.** Recertification/reconditioning not recommended after warranty expires

23. A football helmet bears the National Operating Committee on Standards for Athletic Equipment (NOCSAE) mark. What does this mark imply about the helmet?

○ **A.** It is a warranty that the helmet will protect the athlete from potential head injuries.

○ **B.** This helmet has met the requirements of NOCSAE performance testing when it was manufactured or reconditioned.

○ **C.** The helmet will minimize the severity of a head injury such as a concussion.

○ **D.** It states that there is risk inherent in playing football and that a serious injury can occur as a result of participation in the sport.

○ **E.** The helmet can be safely removed during an on-field emergency care situation.

24. You have determined that a player's football helmet does not fit correctly. Which of the following descriptions indicates an incorrectly fitted helmet?

○ **A.** The back of the helmet covers the base of the skull.

○ **B.** The ear holes line up with the ears.

○ **C.** The jaw pads are ¾″ from the skin of the jaw.

○ **D.** The helmet does not recoil on impact.

○ **E.** The front edge of the helmet stays above the eyebrows when downward pressure is applied.

25. Which of the following persons is/are required to wear a helmet during a baseball game?

○ **A.** The batter only

○ **B.** The on-deck batter and the batter only

○ **C.** The batter, the on-deck batter, and the base coaches only

○ **D.** The batter, the on-deck batter, the base coaches, and the base runners only

○ **E.** The batter, the on-deck batter, the base coaches, the base runners, and all the umpires

26. Which international organization has a number of committees concerned with sports products that focus on testing materials and products used throughout industry, recreation, and leisure among other areas?

○ **A.** ASTM

○ **B.** NOCSAE

○ **C.** HEEC

○ **D.** ISO

○ **E.** ANSI

27. You observe a lacrosse player cutting down his mouthpiece so that it covers only his front six teeth. What should you communicate to this athlete regarding the primary risk associated with his actions?

○ **A.** His actions have invalidated the manufacturer's warranty.

○ **B.** He has predisposed himself to dental injury.

○ **C.** He has increased his risk of an airway obstruction.

○ **D.** He has increased his risk of sustaining a concussion.

○ **E.** He is at increased risk of incurring a team penalty.

28. Your athlete is unable to wear contact lenses. What type of corrective eyewear would you recommend for participation?

○ **A.** Polycarbonate lenses

○ **B.** Plastic lenses

○ **C.** Polyethylene lenses

○ **D.** Fiberglass lenses

○ **E.** Ethyl vinyl acetate lenses

29. Which football player would be most likely to wear a cantilevered shoulder pad?

- **A.** Quarterback
- **B.** Punter/Kicker
- **C.** Youth football player
- **D.** Linebacker
- **E.** Wide receiver

30. Which of the following indicates a correctly fitted shoulder pad for a football running back?

- **A.** The epaulets and cups cover distally to 2″ above the olecranon process.
- **B.** The inferior border of the shoulder pad is aligned with the spine of the scapula when the arms are raised above the head.
- **C.** The neck opening allows the athlete to achieve no more than 90° of abduction.
- **D.** The inside shoulder pad covers the tip of the shoulder in direct line with the lateral aspect of the shoulder.
- **E.** The shoulder pads contact the base of the helmet.

31. According to NCAA guidelines, for which sport can a player opt to wear soft headgear pending game approval even though headgear is not required by sport regulations?

- **A.** Field hockey
- **B.** Women's lacrosse
- **C.** Fencing
- **D.** Basketball
- **E.** Soccer

32. An evaluation of a cross-country runner reveals that she has excessive supination bilaterally. Her coach would like to purchase shoes that most effectively address her biomechanical alignment. Which type of shoe would you recommend for this athlete?

- **A.** Shoe with a flared heel, curved last, and moderate-to-high degree of shock absorption
- **B.** Shoe with little to no flare, straight last, and moderate-to-high degree of shock absorption
- **C.** Shoe with a flared heel, straight last, and low-to-moderate degree of shock absorption
- **D.** Shoe with no heel flare, curved last, and moderate-to-high degree of shock absorption
- **E.** Shoe with a flared heel, board last, and low-to-moderate degree of shock absorption

33. An athlete reports to the athletic training room wearing a neoprene knee brace with medial and lateral supports. What is the intended purpose of this brace?

- **A.** To provide support for a patellofemoral condition and enhance proprioception
- **B.** To allow for controlled progressive immobilization
- **C.** To provide enhanced proprioception to minimize risk of initial injury
- **D.** To provide restriction against rotational forces
- **E.** To provide additional support subsequent to a collateral ligament injury

34. An athlete complains of chronic corn and callus formation bilaterally on her feet. After evaluation, you determine that the athlete has ill-fitting footwear. Which of the following actions should you recommend this athlete take to minimize future corn and callus formation?

- **A.** Select shoes with a lateral heel wedge, a straight last, and soft heel counter.
- **B.** Wear properly fitted socks, and select shoes that have ½″ to ¾″ distance between the longest toe and the front of the shoe and are fitted to the appropriate width.
- **C.** Wear properly fitted socks; powder feet daily; and select shoes with a flared heel.
- **D.** Select shoes with a lightweight breathable upper, extra padding at the Achilles tendon area and a minimum of ¾″ distance between the longest toes and the front of the shoe.
- **E.** Try on shoes late in the day when feet are the largest; select shoes that feel snug in the store because they will stretch with wear and that have a deep grooved tread.

35. Which of the following pieces of equipment are mandated by the NCAA?

- **A.** Protective eyewear for female lacrosse players
- **B.** Rib protection for baseball catchers
- **C.** Protective cups for wrestlers
- **D.** Intra-oral mouthpiece for male basketball players
- **E.** Helmet with face mask for softball batters

36. What type of material is capable of absorbing force through deforming its shape and then quickly returning to its original form?

- **A.** Low-density foam
- **B.** Moleskin
- **C.** High-density foam
- **D.** Felt
- **E.** Thermo-moldable plastic

37. An athlete has sustained a humeral exostosis. Which of the following is the best material for constructing a functional protective device?

○ **A.** Plaster cast material and orthopedic felt

○ **B.** Thermo-moldable plastic and adhesive moleskin

○ **C.** Fiberglass roll and orthopedic felt

○ **D.** Thermo-moldable plastic and high-density foam

○ **E.** Adhesive Sorbothane and adhesive felt

38. One objective in blister care is to reduce friction. Which of the following supplies is least effective in reducing friction?

○ **A.** Moleskin

○ **B.** Skin lube

○ **C.** 1½ ˝ white tape

○ **D.** Gel circle

○ **E.** Heel and lace pad

39. Which of the following statements most accurately describes the effectiveness of tape in supporting a joint?

○ **A.** Effectiveness is currently unknown, pending further outcome data.

○ **B.** Support is most effective after 15 minutes of warm-up.

○ **C.** Support is more effective in adolescent athletes compared with senior athletes.

○ **D.** Taping is a key component in an injury prevention program.

○ **E.** Effectiveness is attributed solely to its ability to limit range of motion.

40. Which of the following statements is true regarding selection of tape size and type?

○ **A.** Elastic adhesive tape is used for bodily areas requiring high tensile strength.

○ **B.** Tape is qualified based on the grade of backing, the quality of adhesive mass, and the winding tension.

○ **C.** Large-width tape is used for bodily areas requiring high tensile strengths.

○ **D.** The more acute the angles required, the wider the tape must be to fit the contours.

○ **E.** Elastic tape is used for joints that do not expand with motion.

41. Which of the following athletes would most benefit from using custom foot orthotics during sport participation?

○ **A.** A field hockey player with turf toe

○ **B.** A softball player with pes planus and posterior medial tibial stress syndrome

○ **C.** A runner with Sever's disease

○ **D.** A soccer player with weak evertors

○ **E.** A gymnast with pes cavus and a plantar-flexed first ray

42. Which of the following athletes is effectively treated with an off-the-shelf, ready-made orthotic?

○ **A.** A field hockey player with turf toe

○ **B.** A softball player with excessive pronation and history of stress fractures

○ **C.** A distance runner with pes cavus, rigid mid-foot, and a plantar-flexed first ray

○ **D.** A soccer player with a history of Jones' fractures

○ **E.** An aerobics instructor with pes planus and exercise-induced compartment syndrome

43. Which type of soft orthotic material has a high energy-absorbing quality with a high density, making it effective for preventing blisters and absorbing ground reaction forces in multiple directions?

○ **A.** Sorbothane

○ **B.** Orthopedic felt

○ **C.** Sponge rubber

○ **D.** Gauze padding

○ **E.** Closed-cell foam

44. An interior lineman is placed in a hard cast after sustaining a severe wrist sprain. According to NCAA rules pertaining to protective equipment, how can this athlete legally participate in a football game?

○ **A.** The cast must be covered with no less than ½˝-thick closed-cell, slow-recovery foam.

○ **B.** The cast must be removed before the athlete can legally participate.

○ **C.** The cast must be covered completely with a 6˝ elastic bandage and secured with tape.

○ **D.** The cast must be covered with no less than ¾˝-thick foam.

○ **E.** The cast must be covered with at least 1˝ of open-cell, quick-recovery foam.

45. Which of the following wraps should you select to most effectively apply a shoulder spica to a female collegiate volleyball player?

○ **A.** 6″ × 10-yd elastic bandage

○ **B.** 6″ × 6-yd elastic bandage

○ **C.** 4″ adhesive elastic tape

○ **D.** 6″ adhesive elastic tape

○ **E.** 4″ × 10-yd elastic bandage

46. Which of the following is the *least* important use for adhesive tape in the sporting venue?

○ **A.** Retention of wound dressings

○ **B.** Stabilization of compression bandages

○ **C.** Support of recent injuries

○ **D.** Stabilization of an injury during rehabilitation and return to play

○ **E.** Prevention of musculoskeletal injuries

47. When taping a wrist to limit hyperextension, you must place three strips in an X pattern. Where should the X pattern be placed to limit hyperextension most effectively?

○ **A.** Over the dorsal aspect of the wrist, with the center of the X over the radiocarpal joint

○ **B.** Over the radial aspect of the wrist, with the center of the X over the first carpometacarpal joint

○ **C.** Over the palmar aspect of the wrist, with the center of the X over the radiocarpal joint

○ **D.** Over the ulnar aspect of the wrist, with the center of the X over the fifth carpometacarpal joint

○ **E.** Over the dorsal aspect of the wrist, with the center of the X over the carpometacarpal joint

48. Body tissues that sustain a shearing force are most likely to result in which of the following injuries?

○ **A.** Ligament tears, spiral fractures, and lacerations

○ **B.** Ligament tears, blisters, and abrasions

○ **C.** Blisters, comminuted fractures, and contusions

○ **D.** Spiral fractures, ligament tears, and blisters

○ **E.** Comminuted fractures, tendon injuries and contusions

49. Taping for which of the following conditions would be enhanced through the use of a commercially produced teardrop pad or similarly shaped pad constructed from commercial padding?

○ **A.** Transverse arch strain/sprain

○ **B.** Longitudinal arch strain/sprain

○ **C.** Plantar fasciitis

○ **D.** Achilles tendonitis

○ **E.** Hallux valgus

50. During a prophylactic ankle taping application using a closed basket-weave procedure, heel locks are applied to the medial and lateral aspects of the ankle in a continuous manner incorporating a figure-eight pattern. What is the primary goal of this procedure?

○ **A.** Limit subtalar dorsiflexion and plantar flexion

○ **B.** Limit talar joint dorsiflexion and plantar flexion

○ **C.** Limit ankle joint pronation and supination

○ **D.** Limit subtalar inversion and eversion

○ **E.** Limit forefoot adduction and abduction

51. A soccer team will be playing on artificial turf during an upcoming match. What injuries should you be most prepared to treat during the match?

○ **A.** Abrasions and turf toe

○ **B.** Concussions and arch sprains

○ **C.** Contusions and ankle sprains

○ **D.** Tibial fractures and concussions

○ **E.** Blisters and hamstring strains

52. Which of the following actions would be most helpful in minimizing injuries common to participation on artificial turf?

○ **A.** Encourage athletes to wear longer cleats.

○ **B.** Apply extra padding and taping to exposed skin of each athlete.

○ **C.** Encourage athletes to wear heel cups inside their cleats.

○ **D.** Tape longitudinal arches of each athlete.

○ **E.** Encourage athletes to wear two pair of socks with the outside pair inside out.

53. Which of the following concerns is of lowest priority when ensuring a risk-free playing environment?

○ **A.** Goal supports are not padded.

○ **B.** Bleachers are within 1′ of the playing area.

○ **C.** A sprinkler head on the playing surface is flush to or below the playing surface.

○ **D.** A pothole is located along the goal line.

○ **E.** A wall just beyond the end of the basketball court is not padded.

54. When meeting with the host team's athletic trainer at the start of a softball tournament, which of the following pieces of information will assist you the most in minimizing injuries to your players?

○ **A.** Name of team physician, accessibility to athletic training room, and type of lightning detector being used

○ **B.** Facility-specific emergency action plan protocols, location of spine board, and host athletic trainer's cell phone number

○ **C.** Directions to nearest hospital, host athletic trainer's cell phone number, and type of surface the tournament will be played on

○ **D.** Location of automated external defibrillator, location of biohazard supplies, and directions to nearest hospital

○ **E.** Safe shelter in the event of a lightning delay, facility-specific emergency action plan protocols, and the host athletic trainer's cell phone number

55. Which of the following rules governing play is correct?

○ **A.** The athletic trainer treating an injured tennis player during a match is limited to 3 minutes for evaluation and treatment.

○ **B.** The athletic trainer may enter the field to care for an injured soccer player as long as play is on the other end of the field.

○ **C.** An athletic trainer called out on the field for a football injury must decide in the first 15 seconds whether the player is going to come off the field.

○ **D.** A player removed from a basketball game for injury must sit out at least 3 minutes before returning.

○ **E.** An athletic trainer called onto the mat to treat a bleeding wrestler has an unlimited amount of time for evaluation and treatment.

56. Which of the following athletes would most likely suffer a injury because of faulty ergonomics?

○ **A.** An offensive lineman with excessive lordosis suffering from chronic low back pain

○ **B.** A male lacrosse player with shoulder pain

○ **C.** A volleyball player with genu recurvatum who sustains a contact-related anterior cruciate ligament tear

○ **D.** A field hockey player returning from lunch who inverts her ankle on the curb

○ **E.** A baseball player who suffers a zygomatic arch fracture after being hit by a line drive

57. Which of the following groups should be included in an ergonomic risk assessment?

○ **A.** The worker's direct supervisor, stockholders in the company, and the risk management coordinator

○ **B.** The worker, company management, and the director of human resources

○ **C.** The facility nurse, the director of human resources, and the worker

○ **D.** The worker, the worker's direct supervisor, and the facility's nurse

○ **E.** The safety engineer, the risk management coordinator, and the director of facility security

58. What information should you include in your emergency action plan to instruct athletic trainers in communicating information to the 911 dispatcher?

○ **A.** Caller's title and position, condition of injured persons, and medical history of injured persons

○ **B.** Telephone number calling from, date of caller's most recent cardiopulmonary resuscitation training, and location of the victim

○ **C.** Caller's name, number of individuals injured, and first-aid treatment being provided

○ **D.** Number of individuals injured, name of the person meeting the ambulance, and directions to location

○ **E.** Number of persons on site who are certified in cardiopulmonary resuscitation, first-aid treatment being provided, and caller's name

59. Which of the following statements best characterizes prevention of catastrophic cervical spine injuries?

○ **A.** A football helmet is designed to reduce the risk of axial loading.

○ **B.** Catastrophic cervical spine injury resulting from axial loading is neither caused nor prevented by players' standard equipment.

○ **C.** Proper training in tackling and blocking techniques is not as effective as protective equipment in minimizing the risk of a catastrophic cervical spine injury.

○ **D.** Players who initiate contact with their head down are less at risk for sustaining a catastrophic cervical spine injury if a cowboy collar is added to the shoulder pads.

○ **E.** Players who are on the receiving end of head-down, helmet-to-helmet contact are not at risk for a catastrophic cervical spine injury.

60. Your school has a gymnastics program, and you are assisting the athletics director in formulating a policy for the use, storage, and maintenance of the school's trampoline and mini-tramps. Which of the following components is *least* likely to be in your policy?

○ **A.** Athletes may freely use the trampoline without supervision once they are able to demonstrate skill proficiency.

○ **B.** Trampolines should be supervised by persons familiar with the routine and skills being practiced.

○ **C.** Coaches, student athletes, and managers should be trained in the principles of spotting with the overhead harness.

○ **D.** A mat being used with the mini-tramp should be sufficiently wide and long to prevent athletes from landing on the mat's edge.

○ **E.** All users of the trampoline should be taught proper procedures for unfolding, folding, transporting, storing, and locking the trampoline.

61. Which NCAA committee is responsible for establishing policies and recommendation on safe sport participation?

○ **A.** Committee on the Medical Aspects of Sports

○ **B.** Committee on Sport Safety

○ **C.** Committee on Risk Management in Intercollegiate Athletics

○ **D.** Committee on Injury Surveillance and Prevention

○ **E.** Committee on Competitive Safeguards of Sports

62. Why are regulations governing younger players more strict than those governing professional athletes?

○ **A.** To reduce liability

○ **B.** To encourage young athletes to comply with sport rules

○ **C.** To encourage coaches of young athletes to teach proper technique

○ **D.** To provide extra protection for young, skeletally immature athletes

○ **E.** To address higher injury rates seen in youth sports as compared with professional sports

63. According to NCAA policies, how frequently are sports rules reviewed and potentially revised?

○ **A.** Annually

○ **B.** Biannually

○ **C.** Every other year

○ **D.** Every 5 years

○ **E.** When requested by an NCAA member institution

64. An athletic trainer for a collegiate ice hockey team has requested in writing that protective barriers be constructed around the rink to protect spectators and to comply with local regulations. The request was denied by the administration of the institution due to lack of available funding. During a game, an inattentive fan is struck in the head by a puck and suffers a skull fracture. What liability factor might the school be found guilty should the spectator choose to sue for damages?

○ **A.** Failure to act

○ **B.** Failure to warn

○ **C.** Ignoring the law

○ **D.** Ignorance of the law

○ **E.** Intentional harm

65. The women's soccer team is unable to use the practice field and has been relocated to a new practice site. A fire hydrant is found to be located 1´ from the sideline of the temporary practice field. What would be the best action to address this safety hazard?

○ **A.** Apply warning cones around the area.

○ **B.** Apply mats/padding to the hydrant, and place warning cones around the area.

○ **C.** Inform the athletes about the hydrant and ask them to use caution when playing nearby.

○ **D.** Stand beside the hydrant during the entire practice.

○ **E.** Place your kit in front of the hydrant, and ask the coach to limit practice time on that end of the field.

66. When an individual chooses to participate in a sport, the knowledge of potential risks is in most cases clearly understood. Should an injury situation arise, when would the injured athlete assume none of the risk?

○ **A.** When the athlete does not fully comprehend the school's assumption of risk policy

○ **B.** When the athlete has never played the sport before the season in which the injury occurs

○ **C.** When the athlete makes no effort to determine hazards associated with the sport

○ **D.** When the athlete chooses not to sign the assumption of risk statement

○ **E.** When the athlete is not warned of the dangers associated with participation

67. According to the Bloodborne Pathogen Standards, which statement best describes the persons required to receive training through their employer in regard to occupational exposure to bloodborne pathogens?

○ **A.** Any employee who has the potential for occupational exposure to blood or other potentially infectious materials

○ **B.** Only employees involved in direct patient care who might be exposed to blood or other potentially infectious materials

○ **C.** All federal and state employees

○ **D.** Only health-care providers dealing with high-risk patient populations

○ **E.** Persons completing a first-aid and cardiopulmonary resuscitation course

68. An exposure control plan for eliminating or minimizing exposure to bloodborne pathogens and other potentially infectious materials is required to meet Bloodborne Pathogen Standards. The exposure control plan must include plans for exposure prevention; education regarding bloodborne pathogens, including signs and symptoms; and action steps to take if exposure occurs. What additional component must also be included in the plan?

○ **A.** Location of sharps containers and other personal protective equipment

○ **B.** An accurate record of employees' bloodborne pathogen and cardiopulmonary resuscitation/first-aid certifications

○ **C.** An accurate record of every occupational exposure

○ **D.** An accurate record of employees' hepatitis B vaccinations

○ **E.** An accurate record of HIV status of employees

69. Which of the following bloodborne pathogens is most commonly contracted by health-care workers?

○ **A.** Hepatitis C

○ **B.** Syphilis

○ **C.** HIV

○ **D.** Hepatitis D

○ **E.** Hepatitis B

70. An athletic trainer has been exposed to a potentially infectious material. What is the *first* step the athletic trainer should take to minimize side effects?

○ **A.** Cleanse the exposed body area with soap and water.

○ **B.** Inform a supervisor about the exposure incident.

○ **C.** Seek medical care within 2 hours as designated in the exposure control plan.

○ **D.** Request medical information or testing from the involved source person.

○ **E.** Complete an exposure report.

71. As the sole athletic trainer providing patient care in the athletic training room, you are unexpectedly called to another area of the building to care for an injured person. Which of the following athletes receiving treatment can you most safely leave unsupervised?

○ **A.** An athlete with Achilles tendonitis completing a cold whirlpool treatment

○ **B.** An athlete with patellar tendonitis receiving electrical stimulation treatment

○ **C.** An athlete with iliotibial band syndrome completing a conditioning session on the treadmill in the therapy pool

○ **D.** An athlete with an acute ankle sprain receiving cryotherapy and elevation

○ **E.** An athlete with a facet joint lock in the middle of a continuous mechanical traction session

72. When designing a hydrotherapy area, which design elements are recommended to reduce the risk of patient injury?

○ **A.** Electrical outlets must be at least 3′ off the floor and equipped with GFIs, and hydrotherapy tanks should be connected directly to a floor drain.

○ **B.** Electrical outlets must be at least 2′ off the floor; hydrotherapy tanks should be connected directly to a floor drain; and floors should be carpeted to reduce slippage.

○ **C.** Electrical outlets must be equipped with GFIs; floors should be sloped toward the drains to minimize puddling; and lighting should be a minimum of 140 watts.

○ **D.** The area should be a minimum of 60 square feet per athlete being serviced; walls should be constructed from cinderblock; and floors should be carpeted to reduce slippage.

○ **E.** The area should use only natural lighting and should be a minimum of 10 square feet per athlete being serviced, and plumbing fixtures should include mixing valves and foot pedal activators.

73. Which of the following components of a therapeutic modality treatment protocol enhances patient safety?

○ **A.** Thoroughly clean and prepare the skin before applying electrodes for electrical stimulation.

○ **B.** Turn off the machine before removing electrodes following cessation of an electrical stimulation treatment.

○ **C.** Screen the patient for established contraindications to modality use.

○ **D.** Apply conductive gel before beginning an ultrasound treatment.

○ **E.** Apply lotion following an iontophoresis treatment.

74. Which government agency has developed national guidelines for the safety and efficacy of low-level lasers?

○ **A.** Occupational Health and Safety Administration

○ **B.** Department of Health and Environmental Control

○ **C.** American Medical Association Committee on Medical Safeguards

○ **D.** United States Department of Health and Human Services

○ **E.** United States Food and Drug Administration

75. Which of the following acts may an athletic trainer be accused of committing if he or she proceeds with a therapeutic treatment before gaining patient consent?

○ **A.** Failure to inform

○ **B.** Negligence

○ **C.** Failure to comply

○ **D.** Criminal battery

○ **E.** Criminal assault

76. Which is the only therapeutic modality for which federal performance standards currently exist?

○ **A.** Ultrasound

○ **B.** Electrical stimulation

○ **C.** Phoresor

○ **D.** Paraffin bath

○ **E.** Mechanical cervical traction

77. At what governmental level are the laws and policies regarding the use of therapeutic modalities by athletic trainers established and regulated?

○ **A.** State

○ **B.** National

○ **C.** District

○ **D.** Local

○ **E.** International

78. On what does reabsorption of electrolytes and water by the kidney most depend?

○ **A.** Facilitated diffusion

○ **B.** Pinocytosis

○ **C.** Active transport

○ **D.** Osmosis

○ **E.** Passive transport

79. A middle-distance runner suffers from exercise-induced asthma. Which of the following environments is most likely to reduce the intensity and number of episodes of wheezing during activity?

○ **A.** Cold and dry

○ **B.** Warm and dry

○ **C.** Cold and moist

○ **D.** Warm and moist

○ **E.** Hot and dry

80. Which of the following athletes would be *most* at risk for developing a heat-related illness?

○ **A.** An athlete recovering from a recent bout of the stomach flu

○ **B.** An athlete recently diagnosed with asthma

○ **C.** An athlete who is a vegetarian

○ **D.** An athlete with blonde hair and fair skin

○ **E.** An athlete with a body fat percentage below the recommended range

81. During preseason, your football players regularly submerge themselves in cold water tubs in the locker room to cool off after practice. Which method of heat exchange is being employed?

○ **A.** Convection

○ **B.** Conduction

○ **C.** Radiation

○ **D.** Evaporation

○ **E.** Conversion

82. As a high-school athletic trainer, you have multiple practice sessions occurring simultaneously. Which group of athletes is *most* at risk for developing a heat-related illness?

○ **A.** Cross-country team completing speed drills

○ **B.** Field hockey team preparing for tomorrow's game

○ **C.** Soccer team working on corner kicks

○ **D.** Football team running through offensive plays

○ **E.** Volleyball team completing conditioning drills

83. A linebacker weighs 200 lb at the pre-practice weigh-in and weighs 192 lb after practice. What conclusion and recommendation will you make for this athlete?

○ **A.** The athlete is at increased risk for heat illness and must gain all 8 lb back prior to the next practice session.

○ **B.** The athlete should be encouraged to drink as much fluid as possible in the next 24 hours.

○ **C.** The athlete is at extreme risk for heat illness and should be referred for IV fluid replacement.

○ **D.** The athlete's weight loss falls below the point of increased risk of heat illness, and the athlete is cleared for participation at the next practice session.

○ **E.** The athlete is at increased risk for heat illness and must gain a minimum of 2 lb prior to the next practice session.

84. According to the NATA position statement on environmental cold injuries, three layers of clothing are recommended to minimize risk of hypothermia. Which of the following is correct regarding these layers?

○ **A.** The external layer allows evaporation of sweat with minimal absorption.

○ **B.** The internal layer allows evaporation of sweat with minimal absorption.

○ **C.** The middle layer provides resistance against wind.

○ **D.** The external layer provides insulation.

○ **E.** The internal layer provides insulation.

85. Which of the following athletes is demonstrating that he is acclimatized to a hot and humid environment?

○ **A.** The athlete who produces the least amount of sweat after 1 hour of participation

○ **B.** The athlete who consumes the least amount of water during the practice session

○ **C.** The athlete who is the first team member to begin sweating during an outdoor practice session

○ **D.** The athlete who has the highest heart rate during the exercise session

○ **E.** The athlete who demonstrates the highest percentage of sodium loss on the team

86. While you are working in a baseball tournament, a storm approaches. The flash-to-bang count is 30 seconds. How should you apply this information?

○ **A.** The storm is 6 miles away, and all individuals should immediately seek safe shelter.

○ **B.** The storm is 6 miles away, and individuals should be informed of the possibility of lightning and should begin making plans for eventual evacuation of the field.

○ **C.** The storm is 5 miles away, and officials should be alerted of a possible storm in the area.

○ **D.** The storm is 5 miles away, and players should be removed from the field and kept in the dugouts until the flash-to-bang number increases.

○ **E.** The storm is 30 miles away, and officials, coaches, and spectators should be informed of the possibility of lightning and instructed to keep an eye to the sky and await further instructions.

87. A soccer player weighed 165 lb (75 kg) prior to practice and 160.6 lb (73 kg) after practice. He consumed 1200 mL of fluid in a 2-hour practice session. Assuming the athlete has not urinated during the practice, calculate this athlete's sweat rate.

○ **A.** 3200 mL/hr

○ **B.** 1600 mL/hr

○ **C.** 800 mL/hr

○ **D.** 400 mL/hr

○ **E.** 2400 mL/hr

88. Myosin cross-bridges contain active sites for which of the following?

○ **A.** Calcium and adenosine triphosphate

○ **B.** Troponin-tropomyosin and adenosine triphosphate

○ **C.** Actin and adenosine triphosphate

○ **D.** Only adenosine triphosphate

○ **E.** Calcium and troponin-tropomyosin

89. What is the largest structural feature of a muscle?

○ **A.** Myofilament

○ **B.** Myofibril

○ **C.** Sarcomere

○ **D.** Cross-bridge

○ **E.** Z line

90. Lactic acid is a byproduct of which metabolic process?

○ **A.** Krebs cycle

○ **B.** Electron transport chain

○ **C.** Anaerobic glycolysis

○ **D.** Gluconeogenesis

○ **E.** Aerobic glycolysis

91. The radius in flexion of the wrist is an example of which type of lever?

○ **A.** First-class

○ **B.** Second-class

○ **C.** Third-class

○ **D.** Fourth-class

○ **E.** Fifth-class

92. Which option describes the sequential application of the velocities of the hips, shoulders, and arms while executing the tennis forehand groundstroke?

○ **A.** Trading distances for forces

○ **B.** Angular and linear velocity change with length of lever

○ **C.** Greatest linear velocity perpendicular to axis of rotation

○ **D.** Moment of force

○ **E.** Summation of forces

93. To what is the magnitude of muscular force available in the rectus femoris muscle directly proportional?

○ **A.** Pain threshold

○ **B.** Number and size of fibers

○ **C.** Length of fibers

○ **D.** Elasticity of fibers

○ **E.** Number of antagonists

94. What is the importance of the elasticity of the large circulatory vessels?

○ **A.** Determining amount of peripheral resistance

○ **B.** Determining distribution of blood volume to major areas of the body

○ **C.** Autoregulating blood flow

○ **D.** Maintaining blood pressure and flow during heart relaxation

○ **E.** Maintaining heart rhythm

95. An athlete with a pre-conditioning stroke volume of 70 mL/beat has just completed an 8-week cardiovascular training program. His stroke volume is now 105 mL/beat. How would you characterize this value?

○ **A.** Normal secondary to training effects

○ **B.** High secondary to overtraining

○ **C.** Low secondary to training effects

○ **D.** Unexplainable because stroke volume should not change with training

○ **E.** Normal only for power anaerobic athletes

96. Which is the *most* potent agent regulating respiration?

○ **A.** Oxygen concentration of the blood

○ **B.** Carbon dioxide levels at the respiratory center

○ **C.** Lactic acid levels in the blood

○ **D.** Glucose levels in the blood

○ **E.** Oxygen levels in the hypothalamus

97. Which statement best describes the pressures present during inhalation?

○ **A.** Atmospheric pressure is lower than intrapleural pressure.

○ **B.** Intra-alveolar pressure is lower than intrapleural pressure.

○ **C.** Intra-alveolar pressure is lower than atmospheric pressure.

○ **D.** Intra-alveolar pressure is higher than atmospheric pressure.

○ **E.** Intrapleural pressure is higher than atmospheric pressure.

98. In which of the following respiratory system components is pressure normally negative?

○ **A.** Alveoli

○ **B.** Bronchi

○ **C.** Intrapleural space

○ **D.** Atmosphere

○ **E.** Blood

99. An athlete would like to decrease body fat percentage. What advice would you give?

○ **A.** Include cardiovascular training in aerobic training zone for prolonged periods

○ **B.** Work intensely for short periods with rest in between

○ **C.** Work for prolonged periods with a slight oxygen debt

○ **D.** Discontinue any resistance training programs

○ **E.** Exercise for prolonged periods above lactate threshold

100. What percentage of a given amount of lactic acid must be oxidized to carbon dioxide and water to provide the energy to generate glucose from the remaining lactic acid?

○ **A.** 30%

○ **B.** 45%

○ **C.** 60%

○ **D.** 15%

○ **E.** 25%

101. What does the second messenger hypothesis suggest?

○ **A.** Cyclic adenosine monophosphate stimulates receptor molecules at the surface of target cells.

○ **B.** Adenyl cyclase stimulates interior cell responses for particular hormones.

○ **C.** Hormones combining with receptor molecules stimulate adenyl cyclase, which increases cyclic adenosine monophosphate production.

○ **D.** There are two messengers by which cyclic adenosine monophosphate is transported to target cells.

○ **E.** Multiple enzymes contribute to cellular responses for specific hormones.

102. To what does the renal fraction refer?

○ **A.** Amount of blood flowing through the capillary system of the kidneys

○ **B.** Total volume of blood pumped by the heart each minute that ends up in the renal circulation

○ **C.** Amount of blood filtered at the glomeruli of the kidneys

○ **D.** Amount of blood entering the renal artery divided by that which passes out of the renal vein

○ **E.** Amount of blood leaving the renal vein as it is filtered at the glomeruli of the kidneys

103. What is the *most* important function of basophils?

○ **A.** Combat certain parasitic infections and allergic reactions

○ **B.** Extreme mobility and quick response to invasion of microorganisms

○ **C.** Extreme phagocytic activity

○ **D.** Release heparin into the bloodstream

○ **E.** Retain heparin

104. What physiological action occurs during ventricular systole?

○ **A.** The second heart sound is heard.

○ **B.** The aortic valves open.

○ **C.** The atrioventricular valves open.

○ **D.** The P-wave can be recorded.

○ **E.** A T-wave can be recorded.

105. Which of the following lists contains only disaccharides?

○ **A.** Glucose, maltose, lactose

○ **B.** Lactose, galactose, glucose

○ **C.** Galactose, fructose, glucose

○ **D.** Sucrose, fructose, maltose

○ **E.** Maltose, lactose, sucrose

106. What is considered a cause of mineral deposits in the kidneys, blood vessels, and other soft tissues in the body?

○ **A.** Excessive dietary vitamin A

○ **B.** Inadequate dietary vitamin D

○ **C.** Excessive dietary vitamin D

○ **D.** Excessive dietary vitamin K

○ **E.** Inadequate dietary vitamin K

107. Distribution of oxygen and usable metabolic materials occurs through which vessels?

○ **A.** Arteries

○ **B.** Veins

○ **C.** Glands

○ **D.** Capillaries

○ **E.** Venules

108. You suspect that a swimmer may be experiencing symptoms of overtraining. Which of the following situations is a significant indicator of overtraining?

○ **A.** Athlete demonstrates increased whole-body muscle tone.

○ **B.** Athlete complains of being easily agitated.

○ **C.** Athlete reports increased urinary output.

○ **D.** Athlete's blood pressure is below pre-participation baseline.

○ **E.** Athlete's resting heart rate is elevated above pre-participation baseline.

109. What substance is contained in a higher percentage in white (anaerobic) muscle fibers compared with red (aerobic) muscle fibers?

○ **A.** Glycogen

○ **B.** Fat

○ **C.** Myoglobin

○ **D.** Protein

○ **E.** Hemoglobin

110. How should you instruct an athlete to breathe while performing a bench press?

○ **A.** Inhale as the bar is thrust upward and exhale as the bar is lowered.

○ **B.** Hold the breath as the bar is lowered and inhale as the bar is thrust upward.

○ **C.** Inhale as the bar is lowered and exhale as the bar is thrust upward.

○ **D.** Hold the breath until one repetition is complete.

○ **E.** Inhale as the bar is lowered and hold the breath as the bar is thrust upward.

111. Which of the following foods is the *most* reliable source for iron?

○ **A.** Tuna

○ **B.** Pork chop

○ **C.** Spinach

○ **D.** Steamed broccoli

○ **E.** Raisins

112. What is the primary function of the gallbladder?

○ **A.** Secrete digestive enzymes

○ **B.** Store bile

○ **C.** Release insulin into the bloodstream

○ **D.** Produce hormones for regulating carbohydrate metabolism

○ **E.** Store glucose

113. Which of the following statements is *most* accurate regarding the gastroesophageal sphincter?

○ **A.** Serves to regulate the movement of swallowed materials into the stomach

○ **B.** Serves to prevent stomach contents from being forced back into the esophagus

○ **C.** Represented by the first 4 cm of the esophagus

○ **D.** Also called the pyloric sphincter

○ **E.** Found at the junction between the stomach and the small bowel

114. An athlete has chosen this typical fast food meal. Calculate the total calories contained in this meal for the athlete.

Food	Protein	Fat	Carbohydrates
Hamburger	17 g	22 g	40 g
Large cola			25 g
Order of French fries	4 g	14 g	40 g

○ **A.** 162

○ **B.** 324

○ **C.** 648

○ **D.** 828

○ **E.** 933

115. Which nutrient requires gastric intrinsic factor for absorption?

○ **A.** Calcium

○ **B.** Vitamin B_{12}

○ **C.** Vitamin A

○ **D.** Iron

○ **E.** Vitamin D

116. In general terms, metabolism consists of basically two types of biochemical reactions. What do these reactions include?

○ **A.** Activation and energy-trapping reactions

○ **B.** Isomerase and mutase reactions

○ **C.** Degradative and synthetic reactions

○ **D.** Oxidation and reduction reactions

○ **E.** Productive and reduction reactions

117. Which vitamin deficiency usually occurs only in neonates, persons taking certain drugs, or individuals with faulty fat absorption?

○ **A.** Vitamin D

○ **B.** Vitamin K

○ **C.** Vitamin B_{12}

○ **D.** Folic acid

○ **E.** Vitamin A

118. What product is formed when two carbon units from fatty acids are released during oxidation?

○ **A.** Ketones

○ **B.** Glycogen

○ **C.** Acetylcoenzyme A

○ **D.** Oxaloacetic acid

○ **E.** Pyruvic acid

119. Which two enzymes are capable of completing protein digestion in the small intestine?

○ **A.** Pancreatic amylase and salivary amylase

○ **B.** Pancreatic lipase and bile salts

○ **C.** Pepsin and trypsin

○ **D.** Carboxypeptidase and aminopeptidase

○ **E.** Bile salts and salivary amylase

120. Which substance in the human body can be converted to vitamin A?

○ **A.** Tryptophan

○ **B.** Glucose

○ **C.** Vitamin D

○ **D.** Carotene

○ **E.** Tretinoin

121. An athlete whose daily energy expenditure is 2350 kcal is consuming approximately 2100 kcal daily. If this intake and expenditure continues for 8 weeks, what change in body weight will occur?

○ **A.** Body weight will decrease by 4 lb.

○ **B.** Body weight will increase by 4 lb.

○ **C.** Body weight will decrease by 8 lb.

○ **D.** Body weight will increase by 8 lb.

○ **E.** Body weight will maintain set point.

122. In which form do fats primarily occur in food?

○ **A.** Triglycerides

○ **B.** Sterols

○ **C.** Phospholipids

○ **D.** Glycerols

○ **E.** Fatty acids

123. An athlete consuming a diet low in carbohydrates but with enough protein and fat to meet theoretical energy needs may produce which of the following effects?

○ **A.** Positive nitrogen balance

○ **B.** Buildup of ketones

○ **C.** Less reliance on protein as an energy source

○ **D.** Negative nitrogen balance

○ **E.** Increased conversion of amino acids to proteins

124. The need for which vitamin is influenced by the presence of tryptophan in the diet?

○ **A.** Thiamine

○ **B.** Pantothenic acid

○ **C.** Niacin

○ **D.** Biotin

○ **E.** Riboflavin

125. What is the function of the pancreas after an athlete has ingested a high glycemic index food?

○ **A.** Releases bile to digest the carbohydrate

○ **B.** Secretes insulin to uptake blood glucose

○ **C.** Secretes glucagon to store blood glucose

○ **D.** Releases tryptophan to stimulate serotonin release

○ **E.** Releases salivary amylase to initiate carbohydrate digestion

126. What occurs during protein digestion?

○ **A.** Water molecules are removed from peptide bonds, thereby splitting the amino acids apart.

○ **B.** Pepsin is inhibited by the high acidity of the stomach.

○ **C.** Hydrochloric acid secretion is decreased because of the action of pancreatic amylase.

○ **D.** Hydrochloric acid secretion is increased because of the hormone gastrin.

○ **E.** Sodium bicarbonate secretion is increased because of the acidity in the stomach.

Answers for Domain I: Prevention

Role A: Educate the appropriate patient(s) about the risks associated with participation and specific activities using effective communication techniques to minimize the risk of injury and illness.

1. B
2. C
3. A
4. A
5. B
6. C
7. D
8. A
9. A
10. A

Role B: Interpret pre-participation and other relevant screening information in accordance with accepted guidelines to minimize the risk of injury and illness.

11. D
12. C
13. D
14. C
15. C
16. A
17. A
18. B
19. E

Role C: Instruct the appropriate patient(s) about standard protective equipment using effective communication techniques to minimize the risk of injury and illness.

20. C
21. C
22. B
23. B
24. C
25. D
26. A
27. A
28. A
29. D
30. D
31. A
32. A
33. E
34. B
35. A

Role D: Apply appropriate prophylactic/protective measures using commercial products or custom-made devices to minimize the risk of injury and illness.

36. C
37. D
38. C
39. A
40. B
41. B
42. A
43. A
44. B
45. E
46. E
47. C
48. B
49. A
50. D

Role E: Identify safety hazards associated with activities, activity areas, and equipment by following accepted procedures and guidelines in order to make appropriate recommendations and to minimize the risk of injury and illness.

51. A

52. B

53. C

54. E

55. E

56. A

57. D

58. C

59. B

60. A

61. E

62. D

63. A

64. A

65. B

66. E

Role F: Maintain clinical and treatment areas by complying with safety and sanitation standards to minimize the risk of injury and illness.

67. A

68. C

69. E

70. A

71. D

72. A

73. C

74. E

75. D

76. A

77. A

Role G: Monitor participants and environmental conditions by following accepted guidelines to promote safe participation.

78. C

79. D

80. A

81. A

82. D

83. E

84. B

85. C

86. A

87. B

Role H: Facilitate physical conditioning by designing and implementing appropriate programs to minimize the risk of injury and illness.

88. C

89. A

90. C

91. C

92. E

93. B

94. D

95. A

96. B

97. C

98. C

99. A

100. D

101. C

102. B

103. D

104. B

105. E

106. C

107. D

108. E

109. A

110. C

Role I: Facilitate healthy lifestyle behavior using effective education, communication, and interventions to reduce the risk of injury and illness and promote wellness.

111. B

112. B

113. B

114. D

115. B

116. C

117. B

118. C

119. D

120. D

121. A

122. A

123. B

124. C

125. B

126. D

Domain II: Clinical Evaluation and Diagnosis

1. The bat swing in baseball (movement of the arms) takes place in which of the following planes?

○ **A.** Frontal

○ **B.** Transverse

○ **C.** Sagittal

○ **D.** Reverse

○ **E.** Supine

2. The final motion of a top-spin forehand stroke in tennis involves which forearm motion?

○ **A.** Rotation

○ **B.** Pronation

○ **C.** Supination

○ **D.** Circumduction

○ **E.** Adduction

3. What is the function of the bladder?

○ **A.** Establishing acid-base relationships

○ **B.** Being a reservoir for urine

○ **C.** Being a reservoir for urine and helping to expel urine

○ **D.** Collecting urine and establishing acid-base relationships

○ **E.** Accumulating electrolytes before urination

4. Which of the following statements about bradycardia is the most correct?

○ **A.** Bradycardia is characterized by a resting heart rate faster than 100 beats per minute.

○ **B.** Bradycardia is characterized by a resting heart rate slower than 60 beats per minute.

○ **C.** Bradycardia is characterized by palpitations.

○ **D.** Bradycardia is characterized by a resting heart rate faster than 100 beats per minute and an increased stroke volume.

○ **E.** Bradycardia is characterized by a threefold decrease in cardiac output.

5. A tennis player reports experiencing shoulder pain during the mid-portion of her forehand stroke. Which of the following muscles are responsible for this joint motion and should therefore be screened for potential injury?

○ **A.** Pectoralis major and subscapularis

○ **B.** Anterior deltoid and latissimus dorsi

○ **C.** Infraspinatus and posterior deltoid

○ **D.** Anterior deltoid and pectoralis major

○ **E.** Coracobrachialis and pectoralis minor

6. Which of the following is classified as a saddle joint and is capable of 2° of freedom?

○ **A.** Fourth carpometacarpal joint

○ **B.** First metacarpophalangeal joint

○ **C.** First carpometacarpal joint

○ **D.** Fifth carpometacarpal joint

○ **E.** Fifth metacarpophalangeal joint

7. Which structure returns deoxygenated blood to the heart?

○ **A.** Aortic arch

○ **B.** Pulmonary artery

○ **C.** Pulmonary vein

○ **D.** Superior and inferior vena cava

○ **E.** Left ascending coronary artery

8. Which cavities comprise the dorsal cavity?

○ **A.** Cranial and abdominal cavities

○ **B.** Cranial and thoracic cavities

○ **C.** Spinal and abdominal cavities

○ **D.** Cranial and spinal cavities

○ **E.** Thoracic and abdominal cavities

9. In the initial phase of throwing a ball, as the shoulder girdle and arm move from a posterior retracted position to a forward, internally rotated position, what are the primary muscles responsible for moving the scapula and the arm forward?

○ **A.** Subscapularis, anterior deltoid, coracobrachialis, and serratus anterior

○ **B.** Supraspinatus, teres major, rhomboids, and pectoralis major

○ **C.** Serratus anterior, subscapularis, anterior deltoid, and pectoralis major

○ **D.** Serratus anterior, upper trapezius, latissimus dorsi, and pectoralis major

○ **E.** Subscapularis, upper trapezius, latissimus dorsi, and triceps

10. How many degrees of freedom are allowed by the glenohumeral joint?

○ **A.** 1

○ **B.** 2

○ **C.** 3

○ **D.** 4

○ **E.** 5

11. An athlete has been diagnosed as having myositis ossificans. Which of the following factors most likely contributed to the development of this condition?

○ **A.** Excessive resistance training

○ **B.** Use of continuous ultrasound during the inflammatory phase of the healing process

○ **C.** Excessive plyometric training

○ **D.** Use of high-volt pulsed stimulation during the repair phase of the healing process

○ **E.** Intramuscular bleeding following a severe contusion

12. When evaluating an athlete 3 days after sustaining a mild head injury, which of the following symptoms would lead you to suspect the athlete is experiencing post-concussion syndrome?

○ **A.** Persistent headache, lack of concentration, and fatigue

○ **B.** Steady gait, visual disturbances, and insomnia

○ **C.** Behavior changes, impaired memory, and tinnitus

○ **D.** Fatigue, nystagmus, and anoxia

○ **E.** Tinnitus, dyspnea, and depression

13. Which of the following findings is the greatest health risk associated with bulimia?

○ **A.** Gastrointestinal disturbances

○ **B.** Increased incidence of caries

○ **C.** Electrolyte imbalance

○ **D.** Inflammation of the esophagus and parotid glands

○ **E.** Menstrual irregularities

14. Following trauma, what is the initial response at the vascular level?

○ **A.** Margination followed by vasoconstriction

○ **B.** Transient vasodilation followed by vasoconstriction

○ **C.** Continual vasoconstriction

○ **D.** Transient vasoconstriction followed by vasodilation

○ **E.** Margination followed by vasodilation

15. An axial compression fracture in football players most commonly results from which of the following mechanisms of injury?

○ **A.** Contact with the top of the helmet while the cervical spine in a partially flexed position

○ **B.** Contact with the face mask, forcing the cervical spine into hyperextension

○ **C.** Contact with the helmet, pushing the cervical spine into lateral flexion and depressing the shoulder

○ **D.** Contact with the chin strap, forcing the cervical spine into partial extension

○ **E.** Contact with the side of the helmet, resulting in lateral rotation of the cervical spine

16. A softball player with epilepsy reports experiencing heightened senses of smell and hearing during a game. Which stage of an epileptic seizure is this athlete currently experiencing?

○ **A.** Aura

○ **B.** Clonic

○ **C.** Postictal

○ **D.** Status epilepticus

○ **E.** Tonic-clonic

17. At which level of the spine is rotation in the transverse plane the greatest?

○ **A.** Thoracic vertebrae

○ **B.** Cervical vertebrae

○ **C.** Thoracolumbar junction

○ **D.** Lumbar vertebrae

○ **E.** Lumbosacral junction

18. Which of the following injurious factors is the most significant determiner as to whether an athlete will sustain a first- or second-degree lateral ankle sprain?

○ **A.** The amount of eversion at the subtalar joint

○ **B.** The amount of inversion at the subtalar joint

○ **C.** The amount of eversion combined with torsion at the subtalar joint

○ **D.** The amount of inversion at the subtalar joint combined with plantar flexion at the talocrural joint

○ **E.** The amount of plantar flexion at the talocrural joint

19. An athlete reports to the athletic training room complaining of burning, numbness, and shooting pain between the third and fourth metatarsal heads. He reports that the pain increases when he wears cleats and lessens when he is sitting or wearing sandals. Which of the following conditions is most closely associated with these symptoms?

○ **A.** Peroneal nerve palsy

○ **B.** Morton's neuroma

○ **C.** Tarsal tunnel syndrome

○ **D.** Medial plantar nerve compression syndrome

○ **E.** March fracture

20. While reviewing an athlete's injury report, you note his diagnosis is an anterior dislocation of the glenohumeral joint. How should the mechanism for this injury be documented in the injury report?

○ **A.** In the objective section, document that the athlete stated that his arm was cocked to throw the football when he was hit.

○ **B.** In the subjective section, document that the athlete reports a mechanism of shoulder abduction and external rotation.

○ **C.** In the subjective section, document that the athlete states he fell on an outstretched arm.

○ **D.** In the objective section, document that you determined that he has pain when the arm is forced into horizontal adduction and external rotation.

○ **E.** In the subjective section, document that you determine he has limited internal rotation and abduction.

21. An athlete has sustained a hamstring strain. Which of the following characteristics indicates the fibroplastic repair phase of the healing process for this injury?

○ **A.** Immediate vasoconstriction followed by reflex vasodilation, stagnation, and stasis

○ **B.** Formation of an insoluble fibrin clot and phagocytosis

○ **C.** Synthesis of intracellular matrix and formation of granulation tissue

○ **D.** Formation of fibroblasts, decrease in type III collagen fiber, and increase in type I collagen fibers

○ **E.** Conversion of prothrombin to thrombin and production of collagen fibers

22. An athlete with a tibial fracture reports to the athletic training room following a follow-up appointment with the orthopedic surgeon. The physician has told her that a fibrocartilage soft callus has formed about the area of the fracture. Physiologically, what is the next step in the healing process?

○ **A.** Fibrocartilage becomes ossified and forms a bony callus made of spongy bone.

○ **B.** A fracture hematoma forms.

○ **C.** Osteoclasts remove excess tissue from the bony callus.

○ **D.** Chondroblasts begin to proliferate and enter the callus, forming cancellous bone.

○ **E.** Osteoblasts reabsorb bone fragments and clean up debris.

23. Diagnosis of acute concussion usually involves the assessment of a range of domains. Which of the following clinical domains should be considered in this diagnosis?

○ **A.** Cognitive symptoms, physical signs, and age of the athlete

○ **B.** Angle of head impact, amnesia, and sleep disturbances

○ **C.** Somatic symptoms, behavioral changes, and cognitive impairment

○ **D.** Behavioral changes, type of protective equipment, and emotional symptoms

○ **E.** Anthropometric measures, cognitive symptoms, and physical signs

24. During a concussion evaluation, the athlete becomes annoyed with assessment questions. In which of the following clinical domains would you classify this exhibited symptom?

○ **A.** Behavioral changes

○ **B.** Physical signs

○ **C.** Cognitive symptoms

○ **D.** Cognitive impairment

○ **E.** Emotional symptoms

25. When conducting a knee evaluation, you suspect an athlete has injured his lateral meniscus. Due to its attachment to the lateral meniscus, what other structure should you suspect may be involved?

○ **A.** Head of the fibula

○ **B.** Biceps tendon

○ **C.** Plantar muscle

○ **D.** Popliteal muscle

○ **E.** Patella

26. The classic mechanism of injury for a medial collateral ligament sprain of the knee is valgus stress with external tibial rotation. When this force occurs, what other soft-tissue damage may occur simultaneously?

○ **A.** Medial meniscus sustains compressive forces

○ **B.** Iliotibial band sustains tensile forces

○ **C.** Lateral meniscus sustains compressive forces

○ **D.** Popliteus muscle sustains tensile forces

○ **E.** Posterior cruciate ligament sustains compressive forces

27. Which of the following terms is matched correctly?

○ **A.** Neurapraxia: axon undergoes wallerian degeneration

○ **B.** Axonotmesis: mildest form of peripheral nerve injury

○ **C.** Paresthesia: abnormal sensation

○ **D.** Neurotmesis: complete disruption of the nerve

○ **E.** Neurodynia: degeneration of nerve cells

28. The brachial plexus consists of nerves that are derived from which of the following nerve roots?

○ **A.** C2–C6

○ **B.** C3–C7

○ **C.** C4–C8

○ **D.** C5–T1

○ **E.** C5–T3

29. Which of the following symptoms is most closely associated with carpal tunnel syndrome?

○ **A.** Tingling of the dorsum of the hand

○ **B.** Tingling of the fourth and fifth fingers

○ **C.** Tingling of the tip of the thumb and index and middle fingers

○ **D.** Weakness of the muscles of the hypothenar eminence

○ **E.** Weakness of the wrist extensors

30. Absence of which of the following signs and symptoms following a hard blow to the right side of the rib cage would raise suspicion of a liver laceration?

○ **A.** Decreased blood pressure

○ **B.** Referred pain located in the anterior left side of the chest

○ **C.** Referred pain just below the right scapula and substernal area

○ **D.** Elevated heart rate

○ **E.** Severe abdominal pain

31. Which of the following joints and its associated ligaments are involved in a shoulder separation?

○ **A.** Sternoclavicular joint, anterior and posterior sternoclavicular ligaments, costoclavicular ligament, interclavicular ligament

○ **B.** Acromioclavicular joint, acromioclavicular ligament, conoid and trapezoid ligaments

○ **C.** Glenohumeral joint; superior, middle, and inferior glenohumeral ligaments; coracohumeral ligaments

○ **D.** Acromioclavicular joint; costoclavicular, acromioclavicular, and coracoclavicular ligaments

○ **E.** Glenohumeral joint; coracohumeral, superior, and posterior glenohumeral ligaments

32. Chondromalacia patella is most often the result of biomechanical changes affecting the lower extremity. Which of the following factors may result in abnormal patellar tracking?

○ **A.** Genu valgum, patella alta, and Q angle greater than 15° to 20°

○ **B.** Deep femoral groove, external tibial torsion, and foot pronation

○ **C.** Femoral anteversion, shallow femoral groove, and Q-angle less than 15°

○ **D.** Genu varum, foot pronation, and external tibial torsion

○ **E.** Femoral retroversion, external tibial torsion, and foot supination

33. A 12-year-old basketball camper reports anterior knee pain focused at the inferior insertion of the patellar tendon. What apophyseal injury should you suspect?

○ **A.** Sever's disease

○ **B.** Osgood-Schlatter disease

○ **C.** Salter Harris II fracture

○ **D.** Larsen-Johansson disease

○ **E.** Legg-Calvé-Perthes disease

34. You are reviewing medical records and note that an athlete has sustained an osteochondral fracture. In which joint does this injury most commonly occur?

○ **A.** Ankle

○ **B.** Knee

○ **C.** Hip

○ **D.** Shoulder

○ **E.** Pelvis

35. An 18-year-old diver reports low back pain exacerbated with lumbar extension and relieved with lumbar flexion. Pain is described as localized and primarily dull and achy. She denies radiating or radicular pain. Based on this athlete's sport and history, what injury would you suspect?

○ **A.** Disc herniation

○ **B.** Spondylolysis

○ **C.** Scoliosis

○ **D.** Sacroiliac joint dysfunction

○ **E.** Lumbar facet joint lock

36. An athlete is suspected of having a corneal abrasion. Which of the following questions would give you the most information to confirm your evaluative conclusion?

○ **A.** Are you experiencing double vision?

○ **B.** Do you feel as though a curtain fell over your field of vision?

○ **C.** When you close your eyelid, do you feel like you have something rubbing in your eye?

○ **D.** Were you hit with an object such as a tennis ball or racquetball?

○ **E.** Have you experienced any discharge coming from your eye?

37. A basketball player is undercut while dunking and uses his outstretched hand to break his fall. He reports immediate pain in his wrist and fracture is suspected. Which carpal bone is most commonly fractured?

○ **A.** Lunate

○ **B.** Capitate

○ **C.** Trapezium

○ **D.** Pisiform

○ **E.** Navicular

38. An athlete suspects she may have been exposed to viral hepatitis. In the prodromal stage, which of the following signs and symptoms could the athlete exhibit?

○ **A.** Fatigue, myalgia, and jaundice

○ **B.** Headache, rash, and increase in appetite

○ **C.** Malaise, mild abdominal pain, and arthralgias

○ **D.** Jaundice, anorexia, and vomiting

○ **E.** Headache, fatigue, and increased urinary output

39. The vertebral border of the spine of the scapula normally aligns with the spinous process of which vertebra?

○ **A.** C8

○ **B.** T1

○ **C.** T2

○ **D.** T3

○ **E.** T4

40. An athlete is being evaluated for metatarsalgia. Which of the following signs are you most likely to observe?

○ **A.** Supination and lateral foot callus formation

○ **B.** Hallux valgus with associated bunion formation

○ **C.** Shortening of the mid-stance phase of the gait cycle

○ **D.** Polydactyly

○ **E.** A stiff mid-foot and a plantar-flexed first ray

41. Which of the following best defines kyphosis?

○ **A.** A convex curve of the upper thorax

○ **B.** A concave curve of the lumbar area

○ **C.** A lateral curve often combined with rotation

○ **D.** A concave curve of the cervical area

○ **E.** A lateral curve of the cervical area

42. A pole vaulter misses the pit and makes contact with his head against the base of the support pole. Upon initial observation, you note bleeding from a small head laceration and blood and cerebrospinal drainage from the nose and ears. What condition do you suspect?

○ **A.** Subdural hematoma

○ **B.** Epidural hematoma

○ **C.** Concussion

○ **D.** Skull fracture

○ **E.** Ruptured tympanic membrane

43. A women's basketball player is elbowed in the jaw during a practice session. Observation reveals a portion of the tooth is broken, some bleeding, and the pulp chamber is exposed producing a great deal of pain. With which type of tooth fracture are the signs most closely associated?

○ **A.** Uncomplicated crown fracture

○ **B.** Root fracture

○ **C.** Complicated crown fracture

○ **D.** Complicated pulp fracture

○ **E.** Uncomplicated periodontal fracture

44. While inspecting an athlete's pupils, you note that one pupil is larger than the other. Prior to concluding that this is a symptom of this athlete's acute injury, you need to rule out which previously existing or congenital condition?

○ **A.** Anisocoria

○ **B.** Astigmatism

○ **C.** Myopia

○ **D.** Nystagmus

○ **E.** Glaucoma

45. An athlete reports anterior knee pain. On inspection you note the athlete has squinting patellae. Which of the following is most likely the potential cause of this patellar malalignment?

○ **A.** Hip anteversion

○ **B.** External femoral rotation

○ **C.** External tibial rotation

○ **D.** Abnormally short patellar tendon

○ **E.** Abnormally long patellar tendon

46. An offensive lineman exhibits lumbar hyperlordosis. Which of the following is the typical anatomical profile for an athlete with excessive hyperlordosis?

○ **A.** Weakened back extensor muscles with tightened or shortened hip extensors and abdominals

○ **B.** Tightened or shortened hip flexor muscles or back extensors with weakened or elongated hip extensors or abdominals

○ **C.** Tightened or shortened hip extensor muscles with weakened hip flexor muscles

○ **D.** Weakened hip flexors with weakened back extensors and shortened hip extensors

○ **E.** Tightened or shortened abdominals with tightened or shortened hip extensors and weak back extensors

47. During the observation-inspection phase of injury assessment, it is important for the athletic trainer to gather which of the following pieces of information?

○ **A.** The severity of pain

○ **B.** The presence of crepitation

○ **C.** The amount of swelling or ecchymosis

○ **D.** The presence of paresthesia

○ **E.** The type of activity that caused the pain

48. Pale skin color indicates which of the following conditions?

○ **A.** High blood pressure

○ **B.** Poisoning

○ **C.** Asphyxia

○ **D.** Heatstroke

○ **E.** Shock

49. An athlete who underwent surgical repair of the anterior cruciate ligament is unable to achieve the final degrees of extension, as she "locks out" her knee in the open kinetic chain position. What should you advise for this athlete to complete the "screw home motion" and achieve full extension?

○ **A.** The vastus medialis oblique must contract to internally rotate the tibia.

○ **B.** The quadriceps must contract to externally rotate the tibia.

○ **C.** The popliteus must contract to externally rotate the tibia.

○ **D.** The iliotibial band must contract to internally rotate the tibia.

○ **E.** The medial hamstrings must contract to internally rotate the tibia.

50. Which of the following calcaneal alignments is most commonly observed in patients with pes planus?

○ **A.** Calcaneal varus

○ **B.** Calcaneal inversion

○ **C.** Calcaneal valgus

○ **D.** Calcaneal pronation

○ **E.** Calcaneal supination

51. Which observation would lead you to believe an athlete has functional as opposed to structural scoliosis?

○ **A.** Scoliosis is observed during erect posture and during forward trunk flexion.

○ **B.** Scoliosis is observed during forward trunk flexion and disappears during erect posture.

○ **C.** Scoliosis is observed during erect posture and disappears during forward trunk flexion.

○ **D.** Scoliosis is observed during erect posture and disappears during trunk extension.

○ **E.** Scoliosis is observed during trunk extension and disappears during erect posture.

52. Which of the following deformities would lead you to suspect Colles' fracture?

○ **A.** Madelung's deformity

○ **B.** Dinner fork deformity

○ **C.** Smith's deformity

○ **D.** Volkmann's ischemic contracture

○ **E.** Sugar-tong deformity

53. Which term describes a constant, involuntary movement of the eyeballs that often accompanies a concussion?

○ **A.** Anisocoria

○ **B.** Pupil accommodation

○ **C.** Nystagmus

○ **D.** Tinnitus

○ **E.** Diplopia

54. While evaluating an athlete's facial injury, you observe that the athlete is unable to look upward toward the ceiling. Which of the following conditions would you suspect?

○ **A.** Orbital blow-out fracture with entrapment of the inferior rectus muscle

○ **B.** Orbital blow-out fracture with entrapment of the superior rectus muscle

○ **C.** Ruptured globe with spontaneous rupture of the inferior rectus muscle

○ **D.** Ruptured globe with spontaneous rupture of the buccinator muscle

○ **E.** Orbital blow-out fracture with entrapment of the infraorbital nerve

55. Which of the following areas should be noted during the observation portion of the injury evaluation?

○ **A.** Demeanor, posture, and deformity

○ **B.** Movement, swelling, and mechanism of injury

○ **C.** Abnormal end feels, crepitus, and asymmetry

○ **D.** Posture, sensation, and swelling

○ **E.** Movement, asymmetry, and reflexes

56. A volleyball player has inverted and plantar-flexed her ankle. She complains of lateral ankle pain. On inspection, you note the presence of two tendons posterior to the lateral malleolus. What anatomical structures maintain these tendons in this position?

○ **A.** Superior and inferior peroneal retinacula

○ **B.** Superior and inferior tibial retinacula

○ **C.** Lateral and posterior fibular retinacula

○ **D.** Superior and inferior extensor retinacula

○ **E.** Lateral and inferior calcaneal retinacula

57. Which of the following normal lower extremity alignment patterns is present in females as compared with males?

○ **A.** Normal females present with wider pelvis and genu varum.

○ **B.** Normal females present with hyperflexibility and a narrower intercondylar notch of the femur.

○ **C.** Normal females present with genu valgum and lateral tibial torsion.

○ **D.** Normal females present with genu recurvatum and neutral tibial torsion.

○ **E.** Normal females present with a wider intercondylar notch of the femur and femoral anteversion.

58. An athlete reports falling directly on his knee and presents with a golf-ball–size lump just below the skin over the patella. Which bursa is most associated with this presentation?

○ **A.** Deep infrapatellar

○ **B.** Suprapatellar

○ **C.** Superficial infrapatellar

○ **D.** Pes anserine

○ **E.** Prepatellar

59. An athlete is seated with his lower legs hanging freely. Observation reveals the tibial tuberosity is more than 10° lateral to the inferior patellar pole. Based on this tubercle sulcus angle, to what condition may this athlete be predisposed?

○ **A.** Lateral patellar tracking

○ **B.** Medial compartment osteoarthritis

○ **C.** Anterior cruciate ligament tear

○ **D.** Iliotibial band syndrome

○ **E.** Medial meniscus tear

60. During observation of an athlete's hip and pelvis, you note that while the athlete is standing erect her left anterior superior iliac spine (ASIS) is slightly inferior to her right ASIS. What condition might be associated with this observation?

○ **A.** Normal pelvic alignment

○ **B.** Anteriorly rotated left ilium

○ **C.** Anteriorly rotated right ilium

○ **D.** Posteriorly rotated left sacrum

○ **E.** Posteriorly rotated right sacrum

61. You are observing the gait cycle in an athlete who is postoperative for anterior cruciate ligament repair. The athlete lacks the last 10° of extension. In which phase of the gait cycle would this deficit be most apparent?

○ **A.** Mid-stance

○ **B.** Pre-swing

○ **C.** Initial contact

○ **D.** Mid-swing

○ **E.** Terminal stance

62. Which of the following statements best describes how normal running gait differs from normal walking gait?

○ **A.** Running gait has a greater stride length and less stride width.

○ **B.** Running gait requires less range of motion and strength.

○ **C.** The running gait cycle contains the dual phases of double limb support.

○ **D.** Pre-swing is absent from the running gait cycle.

○ **E.** The running cycle has less total upward and downward motion of the body.

63. Weakness or reflex inhibition of the psoas major muscle causes this compensatory gait whereby, during the swing phase, lateral rotation and flexion of the trunk occur with hip adduction. The trunk and pelvic movements are exaggerated. What is this compensatory gait?

○ **A.** Leg-length discrepancy

○ **B.** Severe weakness or paralysis of the gluteus maximus

○ **C.** L4–L5 nerve root compression

○ **D.** Weakness of the gluteus medius muscle

○ **E.** Legg-Calvé-Perthes disease

64. In which anatomical position are the rotator cuff muscles in their optimal length-tension relationship?

○ **A.** With the humeral head in 90° of abduction and maximal external rotation

○ **B.** With the glenoid fossa angled 30° from the frontal plane

○ **C.** With the humeral head in 90° of abduction

○ **D.** With the glenoid fossa perpendicular to the sagittal plane

○ **E.** With the glenoid fossa angled 10° from the frontal plane and the humeral head abducted 10°

65. You are observing a swimmer complete forward shoulder flexion. How should the scapula be moving after the first 60° of forward flexion of the glenohumeral joint?

○ **A.** The scapula should be upwardly rotating, moving 2° for every 1° of glenohumeral motion.

○ **B.** The scapula should be elevating, moving 1° for every 2° of glenohumeral motion.

○ **C.** The scapula should be elevating, moving 2° for every 1° of glenohumeral motion.

D. The scapula should be upwardly rotating, moving 1° for every 2° of glenohumeral motion.

E. The scapula should be abducting, moving 1° for every 2° of glenohumeral motion.

66. A football player walks off the field toward you, and you observe his right arm being held against his torso and his head looking away from the injured shoulder. What pathology is most associated with this observation?

A. Acromioclavicular joint sprain

B. Anterior glenohumeral joint dislocation

C. Posterior glenohumeral joint dislocation

D. Brachial plexus injury

E. Humeral fracture

67. During an elbow evaluation, the athlete points to the lateral aspect of his elbow and reports feeling pain about this area. Which of the following conditions should be considered in your differential diagnosis?

A. Radial nerve trauma, biceps brachii tendonitis, and ulnar collateral ligament sprain

B. Avulsion of the common flexor tendon, radial collateral ligament sprain, and median nerve trauma

C. Radiocapitellar chondromalacia, avulsion of the common extensor tendon, and annular ligament sprain

D. Olecranon bursitis, radial head fracture, and osteochondral fracture

E. Osteophyte formation, rupture of the biceps brachii tendon, and radial head dislocation

68. Which structure is located medial to the biceps tendon at the elbow?

A. Ulnar nerve

B. Extensor carpi radialis

C. Radial head

D. Annular ligament

E. Brachioradialis

69. Which of the following groups of muscles insert into the medial aspect of the tibia just distal to the medial condyle?

A. Vastus medialis, gracilis, and semimembranosus

B. Semitendinosus, sartorius, and vastus medialis

C. Biceps femoris, semitendinosus, and semimembranosus

D. Sartorius, gracilis, and semitendinosus

E. Sartorius, gracilis, and semimembranosus

70. Which of the following groups of bones comprise the distal row of carpal bones from the radius to the ulna?

A. Scaphoid, lunate, triquetral, pisiform

B. Trapezoid, trapezium, lunate, scaphoid

C. Scaphoid, capitate, trapezoid, hamate

D. Trapezium, trapezoid, triquetral, pisiform

E. Trapezium, trapezoid, capitate, hamate

71. Which four palpable bony prominences define the carpal tunnel?

A. Radial styloid, navicular, ulnar styloid, and hook of the hamate

B. Radial styloid, base of the first metacarpal, base of the fifth metacarpal, and ulnar styloid

C. Pisiform, tubercle of the navicular, hook of the hamate, and tubercle of the trapezium

D. Tubercle of the navicular, lunate, pisiform, and ulnar styloid

E. Lister's tubercle, tubercle of the trapezium, capitate, and base of the fifth metacarpal

72. Which ligaments comprise the lateral ligaments of the elbow?

A. Radial collateral ligament, lateral ulnar collateral ligament, anterior oblique band, posterior oblique band

B. Transverse oblique band, annular ligament, accessory collateral ligament, radial collateral ligament

C. Radial collateral ligament, lateral ulnar collateral ligament, accessory collateral ligament, anterior oblique band

D. Anterior oblique band, posterior oblique band, transverse oblique band, annular ligament

E. Annular ligament, accessory collateral ligament, radial collateral ligament, lateral ulnar collateral ligament

73. The mobile wad of three consists of which three muscles?

A. Extensor carpi ulnaris, extensor carpi radialis brevis, and extensor carpi radialis longus

B. Flexor carpi ulnaris, flexor carpi radialis, and palmaris longus

C. Extensor carpi radialis brevis, extensor carpi radialis longus, and brachioradialis

D. Flexor carpi radialis, pronator teres, and palmaris longus

E. Brachioradialis, brachialis, and biceps brachii

74. What structure makes up the medial border of the femoral triangle?

◯ **A.** Adductor longus muscle

◯ **B.** Inguinal ligament

◯ **C.** Sartorius muscle

◯ **D.** Gracilis muscle

◯ **E.** Pectineus muscle

75. Which bone lies directly proximal to the first metacarpal?

◯ **A.** Trapezoid

◯ **B.** Pisiform

◯ **C.** Trapezium

◯ **D.** Navicular

◯ **E.** Lunate

76. In a contusion of the medial epicondyle of the humerus, which nerve is most likely to sustain a compressive force?

◯ **A.** Median

◯ **B.** Radial

◯ **C.** Brachial

◯ **D.** Ulnar

◯ **E.** Musculocutaneous

77. When completing a shoulder evaluation, which muscle of the rotator cuff is unable to be palpated?

◯ **A.** Supraspinous

◯ **B.** Infraspinous

◯ **C.** Teres minor

◯ **D.** Subscapularis

◯ **E.** Biceps

78. What is the term used to describe the intense pain experienced by an athlete when an examiner presses into the abdomen and then quickly releases?

◯ **A.** Reflex tenderness

◯ **B.** Bounding tenderness

◯ **C.** Reflex pain

◯ **D.** Rebound phenomenon

◯ **E.** Rebound tenderness

79. Which of the following best describes the location of the sinus tarsi?

◯ **A.** Just posterior to the lateral malleolus

◯ **B.** Just posterior to the medial malleolus

◯ **C.** Just anterior to the lateral malleolus

◯ **D.** Just anterior to the medial malleolus

◯ **E.** Just inferior to the lateral malleolus

80. A softball player sustains a line drive to the face. Which facial bone should be palpated to rule out a fracture because it is the most commonly fractured bone in the face?

◯ **A.** Mandible

◯ **B.** Orbital rim of the eye

◯ **C.** Zygomatic bone

◯ **D.** Nasal bone

◯ **E.** Temporal bone

81. The proximity of the fibular attachments of which of the following ligaments causes some difficulty in differentiation during palpation?

◯ **A.** Calcaneofibular and anterior talofibular

◯ **B.** Tibiofibular and anterior talofibular

◯ **C.** Deltoid and posterior talofibular

◯ **D.** Posterior talofibular and calcaneofibular

◯ **E.** Deltoid and calcaneofibular

82. You suspect that an athlete has sustained a spontaneous pneumothorax. While palpating tactile fremitus, which of the following findings would confirm your suspicions?

◯ **A.** Decreased fremitus is palpable unilaterally.

◯ **B.** Decreased fremitus is palpable bilaterally.

◯ **C.** Increased fremitus is palpable unilaterally.

◯ **D.** Increased fremitus is palpable bilaterally.

◯ **E.** Fremitus is absent bilaterally.

83. An athlete has sustained an ankle dislocation. Which pulse should be palpated to determine involvement of vascular structures?

◯ **A.** Dorsal pedal pulse

◯ **B.** Posterior tibial pulse

◯ **C.** Saphenous pulse

○ **D.** Plantar pedal pulse

○ **E.** Fibular pulse

84. An athlete presents with acute palpable cervical adenopathy. What does this finding indicate?

○ **A.** Lymphedema

○ **B.** A cervical injury

○ **C.** Mononucleosis

○ **D.** An active infection

○ **E.** A cervical nerve root injury

85. When evaluating a visibly upset child with an acute ankle injury, which of the following palpation schemes would be most appropriate?

○ **A.** Palpate the contralateral side first, and then palpate the injured ankle with light pressure beginning away from the injury.

○ **B.** Palpate the contralateral side first, and then palpate the injured ankle beginning at the injury site and working away using light pressure.

○ **C.** Palpate the injured side first, beginning away from the injury with light pressure, working toward the injured site; then palpate the contralateral side only as needed for comparison.

○ **D.** Palpate the injured side first, beginning at the injury site with light pressure, working away from the injury; then palpate the contralateral side only as needed for comparison.

○ **E.** Palpate only the structures on the involved limb necessary to gather information.

86. Which of the following best describes the feeling of palpating a ballotable patella?

○ **A.** The patella bounces back to its original position following downward pressure.

○ **B.** The patella remains at its downward compressed location.

○ **C.** The patella feels thick and boggy with compression.

○ **D.** The patella produces crepitus with downward pressure.

○ **E.** The patella feels solid and immovable with downward pressure.

87. Which of the following components can be palpated during the evaluation of an acute joint injury?

○ **A.** Heat, redness, and swelling

○ **B.** Muscle guarding, swelling, and deformity

○ **C.** Redness, muscle spasm, and ligament laxity

○ **D.** Point tenderness, crepitus, and redness

○ **E.** Heat, swelling, and deformity

88. Which of the following demonstrates the order of bony palpation from proximal to distal?

○ **A.** Peroneal tubercle, cuboid, third cuneiform, styloid process at base of the fifth metatarsal

○ **B.** Calcaneus, sustentaculum tali, talar head, navicular tuberosity, first cuneiform

○ **C.** Sinus tarsi, dome of the talus, second cuneiform, navicular, third metatarsal

○ **D.** Medial calcaneal tubercle, first cuneiform, navicular tubercle, first metatarsal, medial sesamoid of the great toe

○ **E.** Calcaneus, talar head, navicular, sustentaculum tali, sinus tarsi, first cuneiform

89. When palpating soft tissue on the medial aspect of the ankle, in which order are the flexor tendons palpated moving from anterior to posterior?

○ **A.** Tibialis posterior, flexor digitorum longus, and flexor hallucis longus

○ **B.** Tibialis anterior, flexor hallucis longus, and flexor hallucis brevis

○ **C.** Peroneus brevis, flexor digitorum longus, and flexor hallucis brevis

○ **D.** Plantaris, lumbricals, and tibialis posterior

○ **E.** Flexor digiti minimi, flexor digitorum longus, and flexor hallucis longus

90. Which position is most advantageous for palpating the dome of the talus?

○ **A.** Dorsiflexion and inversion

○ **B.** Plantar flexion and eversion

○ **C.** Plantar flexion and inversion

○ **D.** Dorsiflexion and eversion

○ **E.** Dorsiflexion without inversion or eversion

91. Where is the common peroneal nerve palpable?

○ **A.** At the peroneal tubercle

○ **B.** At the neck of the fibula

○ **C.** In the popliteal fossa

○ **D.** At the base of the fifth metatarsal

○ **E.** At the lateral malleolus

92. In which position is the medial meniscus most easily palpated?

○ **A.** Knee in full extension and the tibia locked in external rotation

○ **B.** Knee flexed to at least 45° and the tibia internally rotated

○ **C.** Knee flexed to at least 90° and the tibia externally rotated

○ **D.** Knee in at least 120° of flexion and the tibial internally rotated

○ **E.** Knee in no more than 15° of flexion and tibia externally rotated

93. Which bony landmark should be palpated in order to palpate the proximal insertion of the rectus femoris muscle?

○ **A.** Anterior inferior iliac spine

○ **B.** Anterior superior iliac spine

○ **C.** Greater trochanter of femur

○ **D.** Linea aspera of the femur

○ **E.** Iliac tubercle

94. When fitting an athlete for a cane, which structure should be palpated and aligned with the top of the cane?

○ **A.** Anterior superior iliac spine

○ **B.** Superior arc of the iliac crest

○ **C.** Ischial tuberosity

○ **D.** Lesser trochanter of the femur

○ **E.** Greater trochanter of the femur

95. Where should the proximal attachment for the muscle group responsible for decelerating knee extension and hip flexion during running be palpated?

○ **A.** Anterior inferior iliac spine

○ **B.** Iliac crest

○ **C.** Pubic symphysis

○ **D.** Greater trochanter

○ **E.** Ischial tuberosity

96. When palpating the clavicle for a suspected fracture, at which location should attention be focused because most fractures occur at this area?

○ **A.** Approximately ⅓ the distance from the medial attachment

○ **B.** Approximately ⅔ the distance from the medial attachment

○ **C.** Within a few millimeters from the center of the bone

○ **D.** Within a few millimeters of the medial attachment

○ **E.** Within a few millimeters of the lateral attachment

97. To palpate the rotator cuff muscle responsible for initiating shoulder abduction, how should the patient be positioned?

○ **A.** With the glenohumeral joint in maximal internal rotation

○ **B.** With the glenohumeral joint in maximal external rotation

○ **C.** With the glenohumeral joint in 90° of abduction

○ **D.** With the glenohumeral joint in 30° of forward flexion

○ **E.** With the glenohumeral joint in 30° of extension

98. How would the athletic trainer best assess possible cervical nerve root involvement subsequent to trauma?

○ **A.** Passive neck range of motion

○ **B.** Unilateral sensory and motor function in the upper extremities

○ **C.** Bilateral sensory and motor function in the upper extremities

○ **D.** Resisted neck range of motion

○ **E.** Active neck range of motion

99. During a cranial nerve assessment, the athlete is unable to look laterally. Which cranial nerve is demonstrating a deficit?

○ **A.** Trigeminal

○ **B.** Vagus

○ **C.** Abducens

○ **D.** Olfactory

○ **E.** Facial

100. During a manual muscle test, the athlete demonstrates weakness of the primary hip flexors. Which muscles are weak?

○ **A.** Iliacus, psoas major, psoas minor, rectus femoris, and sartorius

○ **B.** Iliopsoas, pectineus, gluteus minimus, and piriformis

○ **C.** Gluteus minimus, psoas major, psoas minor, gracilis, and sartorius

○ **D.** Iliacus, gluteus maximus, rectus femoris, and pectineus

○ **E.** Psoas major, rectus femoris, gracilis, iliacus, and sartorius

101. Which of the following muscles contribute to scapular elevation?

○ **A.** Levator scapulae and pectoralis major

○ **B.** Rhomboid major and upper portion of the serratus anterior

○ **C.** Lower portion of the trapezius and rhomboid minor

○ **D.** Middle trapezius and lower portion of the serratus anterior

○ **E.** Pectoralis minor and teres minor

102. What occurs before the T-wave of a normal electrocardiogram?

○ **A.** Closing of the atrioventricular valves

○ **B.** Closing of the aortic valves

○ **C.** Opening of the aortic valves

○ **D.** First heart sound

○ **E.** Opening of the atrioventricular valves

103. When completing a manual muscle test for the middle deltoid muscle, in what position should the athlete be placed if unable to hold the test position against gravity?

○ **A.** Semi-recumbent, with examiner standing anterior to the athlete

○ **B.** Seated, with the examiner standing at the side of the athlete

○ **C.** Supine, with the examiner standing caudally

○ **D.** Seated, with the examiner standing behind the athlete

○ **E.** Semi-recumbent, with the examiner standing behind the athlete

104. During a hand evaluation, the athletic trainer instructs the athlete to move from a clenched fist to an open hand with fingers spread. Which muscle group is responsible for this action?

○ **A.** Lumbricals

○ **B.** Volar interossei

○ **C.** Extensor digitorum longus

○ **D.** Extensor digitorum brevis

○ **E.** Dorsal interossei

105. The radial extensor muscles of the wrist and the radial flexor muscles of the wrist working together cause which motion of the wrist and forearm?

○ **A.** Flexion

○ **B.** Extension

○ **C.** Abduction

○ **D.** Adduction

○ **E.** Supination

106. When completing a manual muscle break test for the gluteus maximus muscle, where should the examiner's hands be placed?

○ **A.** The stabilizing hand on the contralateral posterior superior iliac spine and the hand providing resistance on the lower part of the posterior thigh in the direction of hip flexion

○ **B.** The stabilizing hand on the ipsilateral posterior superior iliac spine and the hand providing resistance on the lower part of the posterior thigh in the direction of hip flexion

○ **C.** The stabilizing hand on the upper thigh and the hand providing resistance on the posterior ankle in the direction of knee extension

○ **D.** The stabilizing hand on the ipsilateral posterior superior iliac spine and the hand providing resistance on the posterior mid-lower leg in the direction of hip flexion

○ **E.** The stabilizing hand on the contralateral posterior superior iliac spine and the hand providing resistance on the anterior thigh in the direction of hip extension

107. While evaluating a football player for a brachial plexus injury on the sideline, the athletic trainer determines that the athlete is unable to extend his elbow against resistance. A deficit in which nerve root is most associated with this impairment?

○ **A.** C3

○ **B.** C4

○ **C.** C5

○ **D.** C6

○ **E.** C7

108. Which of the following descriptions is the best example of the coordination between dynamic and isometric contractions of opposing muscle groups to perform movement at a joint?

○ **A.** Tibialis posterior pulling the talus toward the calcaneus while the tibialis anterior pulls the talus anteriorly during dorsiflexion of the talocrural joint

○ **B.** Pectineus pulling the femur into internal rotation while the sartorius pulls the femur into external rotation during flexion of the hip joint

○ **C.** Supraspinatus pulling the head of the humerus toward the glenoid fossa while the deltoid pulls the head of the humerus superiorly during glenohumeral abduction

○ **D.** Popliteus pulling the tibia posteriorly toward the femur while the quadriceps muscle group rotates the tibia externally during extension of the knee joint

○ **E.** Biceps brachii supinating the forearm while the triceps muscle group pulls the ulna toward the humerus during elbow extension

109. What muscles comprise the hypothenar eminence?

○ **A.** Flexor digitorum superficialis, flexor digitorum profundus, and lumbricals

○ **B.** Abductor pollicis brevis, flexor pollicis brevis, and opponens pollicis

○ **C.** Abductor pollicis longus, abductor pollicis brevis, and tendon of the flexor pollicis longus

○ **D.** Abductor digiti minimi, opponens digiti minimi, and flexor digiti minimi brevis

○ **E.** Extensor digiti minimi, adductor digiti minimi, and dorsal interossei

110. A quick and easy method to determine the shoulder's active range of motion is to have the athlete touch the opposite scapula from behind the head and/or up the center of the back. What is this test commonly called?

○ **A.** Apley's scratch test

○ **B.** Allen's test

○ **C.** Drop arm test

○ **D.** Apprehension test

○ **E.** Crossover test

111. An athletic trainer who is evaluating a knee asks the athlete to lie supine with the quadriceps relaxed. He then gently pushes the patella laterally. What condition is the athletic trainer attempting to rule out with this special test?

○ **A.** Chondromalacia

○ **B.** Jumper's knee

○ **C.** Patellofemoral stress syndrome

○ **D.** Patellar instability

○ **E.** Patellar osteochondritis

112. During your examination of an adolescent pitcher, you have the athlete make a fist and extend the wrist against resistance while stabilizing the forearm. If you elicit pain at the lateral epicondyle of the athlete's elbow, which of the following conditions would you suspect?

○ **A.** Little League elbow

○ **B.** Lateral epicondylitis

○ **C.** Occlusion of the brachial artery

○ **D.** Osteophyte formation

○ **E.** Triceps tendinitis

113. Which orthopedic special test is performed with the examiner resisting glenohumeral external rotation and forearm supination, and what finding constitutes a positive test?

○ **A.** Empty can test; athlete is unable to hold test position against resistance

○ **B.** Yergason's test; pain or snapping in the bicipital groove

○ **C.** Speed's test; tenderness or pain in the bicipital groove

○ **D.** Hawkins-Kennedy test; shoulder pain and apprehension

○ **E.** O'Brien's test; pain or clicking within the glenohumeral joint

114. Which orthopedic special test is performed by internally rotating the tibia with one hand while applying a valgus force to the knee with the other hand as the knee is slowly flexed, and what finding constitutes a positive test?

○ **A.** Jerk test; femur moves anteriorly and rotates internally on the tibia

○ **B.** Jerk test; shift or clunk is felt at 30° of knee flexion

○ **C.** Pivot shift test; anterior translation of the tibia

○ **D.** Pivot shift test; palpable clunk or shift at 20° to 30° of knee flexion

○ **E.** Flexion-reduction drawer test; femur moves anteriorly and rotates internally on the tibia

115. During an ankle evaluation, the athletic trainer notes the athlete is able to invert and dorsiflex the ankle through a partial range of motion against gravity. How will the athletic trainer grade this test on a scale of 0–10?

○ **A.** The athletic trainer grades this test as a 4.

○ **B.** The athletic trainer must position the athlete in an antigravity position and retest to confirm grade.

○ **C.** The athletic trainer must position the athlete in the horizontal plane and retest to confirm grade.

○ **D.** The athletic trainer grades this test as a 2.

○ **E.** The athletic trainer grades this test as a 5.

116. An athlete with medial tibial stress syndrome reports pain along the medial tibia traversing behind the medial malleolus and medial longitudinal arch. To assess the muscle most likely associated with this pain, which motions should you assess?

○ **A.** Resisted plantar flexion and inversion

○ **B.** Passive plantar flexion and inversion

○ **C.** Resisted dorsiflexion and inversion

○ **D.** Active dorsiflexion and inversion

○ **E.** Resisted plantar flexion and eversion

117. After completing a patient history and range-of-motion assessment, the athletic trainer is concerned that the athlete's pain may be related to vertebral disc damage. Which of the following groups of special tests would best assist the athletic trainer in ruling out this pathology?

○ **A.** Well straight leg raise test, Kernig-Brudzinski test, and Valsalva's maneuver

○ **B.** Hoover test, bowstring test, and Milgram's test

○ **C.** Lasegue's test, quadrant test, and spring test

○ **D.** Tension sign, stork standing test, and long sit test

○ **E.** Gaenslen's test, bilateral straight leg raise test, and slump test

118. After completing a patient history and range-of-motion assessment, the athletic trainer is concerned that the athlete's pain may be related to glenoid labral pathology. Which of the following groups of special tests would best assist the athletic trainer in ruling out a glenoid labrum tear?

○ **A.** Clunk test and anterior drawer test

○ **B.** Apprehension test and Neer's impingement test

○ **C.** Hawkins-Kennedy test and Jobe's relocation test

○ **D.** Grind test and O'Brien's test

○ **E.** Feagin's test and posterior drawer test

119. While performing an Allen's test, the athletic trainer notes that the radial pulse has disappeared. What do these findings imply?

○ **A.** The test is indicative of thoracic outlet syndrome whereby the sternocleidomastoid is compressing the subclavian artery.

○ **B.** The test is indicative of thoracic outlet syndrome whereby the pectoralis minor is compressing the neurovascular bundle.

○ **C.** The test is indicative of brachial plexus pathology whereby the anterior and middle scalene muscles are compressing the subclavian artery.

○ **D.** The test is indicative of brachial plexus pathology whereby the sternocleidomastoid is compressing the neurovascular bundle.

○ **E.** The test is indicative of shoulder impingement whereby the costoclavicular structures of the shoulder are compressing the brachial artery.

120. Based on outcome data, which of the following statements regarding knee special tests is the *most* accurate?

○ **A.** The anterior drawer test is the best indicator of an isolated anterior cruciate ligament tear.

○ **B.** Lachman's test is the best indicator of anterior cruciate ligament injury, especially the posterolateral band.

○ **C.** The active drawer test is a better indicator of anterior cruciate insufficiency than of posterior cruciate insufficiency.

○ **D.** The pivot shift test may be the most sensitive and accurate test for assessing posterior tibiofemoral instability.

○ **E.** The jerk test is more sensitive and accurate than the pivot shift test.

121. When using a Balance Error Scoring System test to assess an athlete following a concussion, for which of the following criteria would the athlete be assigned 0 points?

○ **A.** Moving hip into greater than 10° of abduction

○ **B.** Lifting hands off iliac crests

○ **C.** Opening eyes

○ **D.** Remaining out of test position more than 5 seconds

○ **E.** Lifting forefoot or heel

122. Which of the following statements best describes the way in which a manual muscle test differs from a break test?

○ **A.** Manual muscle tests are used to provide objective measures of the strength of muscle groups, whereas break tests grade an isolated muscle.

○ **B.** Manual muscle tests are used to isolate muscles within their functional planes of motion, whereas break tests assess strength of muscle groups within the cardinal planes.

○ **C.** Manual muscle tests are performed in the horizontal plane, whereas break tests are performed in the frontal plane.

○ **D.** Manual muscle tests provide more accurate information when the patient is unable to perform active range of motion, whereas break tests are used when the patient is pain-free through the full range of motion.

○ **E.** Manual muscle tests are used more commonly to assess muscular strength, whereas break tests are used more commonly to make return-to-play decisions.

123. An athletic trainer performs Apley's compression test for the knee joint. The test is positive for pain. The athletic trainer then performs Apley's distraction test. What information is obtained from this test?

○ **A.** Pain elicited with the test indicates possible collateral ligament involvement.

○ **B.** No pain elicited with the test indicates possible cruciate ligament involvement.

○ **C.** Pain elicited with the test indicates possible meniscus pathology.

○ **D.** No pain elicited with the test indicates guarding by the hamstring tendons.

○ **E.** No pain elicited with the test indicates possible osteochondral lesion or loose body.

124. Which of the following tests cranial nerve II?

○ **A.** Lateral and vertical gaze

○ **B.** Double simultaneous stimulation of the trigeminal nerve

○ **C.** Symmetric smile

○ **D.** Visual acuity

○ **E.** Pupil reaction to light

125. An athlete is seated with his leg hanging off the edge of the table and the knee flexed to 90° and the ankle in neutral dorsiflexion. The athletic trainer stabilizes the distal tibia and fibula with one hand and, while holding the calcaneus with the other hand, applies an externally rotated force on the calcaneus. A positive test indicates possible injury to which of the following structures?

○ **A.** Anterior tibialis tendon

○ **B.** Calcaneofibular ligament

○ **C.** Deltoid ligament

○ **D.** Anterior tibiofibular ligament

○ **E.** Tibialis posterior tendon

126. A varus stress test for the elbow tests the integrity of which of the following ligaments?

○ **A.** Radial collateral and annular

○ **B.** Accessory lateral collateral and radioulnar

○ **C.** Lateral ulnar collateral and ulnar collateral

○ **D.** Radial collateral and radioulnar

○ **E.** Annular and ulnar capitellar

127. Which of the following statements is most accurate regarding the apprehension test for anterior glenohumeral laxity?

○ **A.** The glenohumeral joint is abducted to 90°, and the elbow is flexed at 10°.

○ **B.** The test should be considered positive if the subject looks apprehensive during the test.

○ **C.** The athlete admitting apprehension about completing the movement indicates a glenohumeral joint dislocation.

○ **D.** The test should be performed within the first 30 minutes following injury to confirm that a glenohumeral joint dislocation has occurred.

○ **E.** The test should be performed at the beginning of the evaluation to minimize the risk of guarding.

128. During a wrist evaluation, an athletic trainer completes Tinel's sign test. The athlete complains of tingling and paresthesia in the area of the nerve distribution. What should the athletic trainer do?

○ **A.** Inspect the area for neurovascular deficits to rule out other pathologies.

○ **B.** Assess the strength of the wrist flexor and extensor muscles.

○ **C.** Assess the strength of the muscles of the hypothenar eminence.

○ **D.** Assess the integrity of the ulnar nerve at the elbow to rule out other pathologies.

○ **E.** Assess the integrity of the median nerve at the elbow, shoulder, and neck to rule out other pathologies.

129. An athlete reports a hyperextension mechanism injury to her knee. Which of the following special tests are most appropriate to be included in the evaluation of this injury?

○ **A.** McMurray's test

○ **B.** Yergason's test

○ **C.** Reduction click test

○ **D.** Apley's compression distraction test

○ **E.** Tinel's sign

130. An athlete recovering from an ankle ligament reconstruction is suspected of having a deep vein thrombosis. Which of the following imaging techniques would be most helpful in diagnosing this condition?

○ **A.** Electromyography

○ **B.** Echocardiogram

○ **C.** Electrocardiogram

○ **D.** Doppler ultrasonography

○ **E.** Dual-energy x-ray absorptiometry scan

131. When completing an evaluation of the abdomen/thorax, in what order should the components of the evaluation be completed?

○ **A.** Auscultation, palpation, percussion

○ **B.** Urinalysis, history, auscultation

○ **C.** Percussion, palpation, auscultation

○ **D.** Palpation, observation of breathing patterns, auscultation of breathing patterns

○ **E.** Blood pressure, history, palpation

132. A high-school freshman athlete presents with polydipsia, polyuria, and polyphagia, along with a recent loss in body weight. What condition do you suspect, and what tests would assist in confirming your initial impression?

○ **A.** Type 2 diabetes mellitus; complete blood count and thyroid-stimulating hormone

○ **B.** Type 1 diabetes mellitus; fasting blood glucose level assessment

○ **C.** Kidney stones; urinalysis

○ **D.** Urinary tract infection; urinalysis

○ **E.** Chlamydia; Papanicolaou's smear

133. An athlete is hit in the head with a baseball. He is unable to smile on that side of his face. What nerve do you suspect is involved?

○ **A.** Trigeminal

○ **B.** Oculomotor

○ **C.** Facial

○ **D.** Hypoglossal

○ **E.** Optic

134. Following a severe head injury, a downed football player is having difficulty breathing and is demonstrating an irregular heartbeat. Which center of the brain is responsible for regulating these vital functions?

○ **A.** Pons

○ **B.** Medulla

○ **C.** Cerebellum

○ **D.** Spinal cord

○ **E.** Frontal lobe

135. Which of the following functional areas of the cerebral cortex deals with complex problems and abstract thought?

○ **A.** Parietal lobe

○ **B.** Temporal lobe

○ **C.** Frontal lobe

○ **D.** Occipital lobe

○ **E.** Medulla

136. During evaluation of an athlete with abdominal pain, rebound tenderness is noted in the right lower quadrant halfway between the umbilicus and the anterior superior iliac spine. Inflammation of which organ is *most* associated with this symptom?

○ **A.** Liver

○ **B.** Spleen

○ **C.** Bladder

○ **D.** Gallbladder

○ **E.** Appendix

137. Conduction velocity in the atrioventricular (AV) bundle, bundle branches, and Purkinje's fibers is much greater than it is in other nodal tissues. How is this significant to heart function?

○ **A.** The delay in conduction at the AV node must be compensated to keep the heart in time.

○ **B.** It rapidly spreads electrical activity over the entire ventricular musculature to produce unified contraction, which results in greater pressure development.

○ **C.** The inherently low discharge rates of these structures must be overcome.

○ **D.** The ventricles have more mass, and velocity must be increased to complete all activities within 0.86 second.

○ **E.** It can compensate for the low velocity produced by the ventricles.

138. The peroneal muscle group is often strained in conjunction with which of the following injury mechanisms?

○ **A.** Eversion and rotation of the ankle

○ **B.** Inversion and plantar flexion of the ankle

○ **C.** Dorsiflexion and rotation of the ankle

○ **D.** Eversion of the ankle

○ **E.** Eversion and dorsiflexion of the ankle

139. Winging of the scapula could result from injury to which nerve?

○ **A.** Median

○ **B.** Axillary

○ **C.** Long thoracic

○ **D.** Suprascapular

○ **E.** Spinal accessory

140. A patient presents with a flexion contracture of the wrist and fingers subsequent to an ulnar fracture. Which of the following pathological postures is most associated with this presentation?

○ **A.** Bishop's or benediction deformity

○ **B.** Volkmann's ischemic contracture

○ **C.** Ape hand

○ **D.** Swan neck deformity

○ **E.** Dupuytren's contracture

141. A baseball player is struck in the face by the ball. Which of the following signs or symptoms would suggest a fracture of the maxilla?

○ **A.** Depression of the cheekbone and blurring of vision

○ **B.** Facial pain and epistaxis

○ **C.** Inability to open the mouth fully and move the jaw laterally

○ **D.** Malocclusion of the teeth and numbness of the cheek

○ **E.** Hyphema and inability of the athlete to look upward

142. A soccer player has sustained a traumatic blow to the lower leg in the absence of a shin guard. He is unable to dorsiflex and invert the ankle. Which of the following conclusions would you make?

○ **A.** An injury to the lateral compartment; integrity of the peroneal artery should be assessed

○ **B.** An injury to the anterior compartment; integrity of the peroneal artery should be assessed

○ **C.** An injury to the superficial posterior compartment; integrity of the posterior tibial artery should be assessed

○ **D.** An injury to the anterior compartment; integrity of the anterior tibial artery should be assessed

○ **E.** An injury to the superficial posterior compartment; integrity of the dorsalis pedis artery should be assessed

143. An athlete has been diagnosed with stenosing tenosynovitis of the first dorsal carpal tunnel. What is another name for this condition?

○ **A.** Guyon's disease

○ **B.** Gamekeeper's thumb

○ **C.** de Quervain's disease

○ **D.** Swan neck deformity

○ **E.** Johnson's disease

144. While not wearing a helmet, a baseball player is hit in the head with a baseball. The player is stunned but walks off the field without assistance. After getting to the dugout, the player experiences a severe headache and deterioration to unconsciousness. What condition is this athlete most likely experiencing?

○ **A.** Epidural hematoma

○ **B.** Subarachnoid hematoma

○ **C.** Post-concussive symptom

○ **D.** Subdural hematoma

○ **E.** Chronic brain injuries

145. During a football game, an athlete experiences a right lateral flexion of the cervical spine while the left shoulder is thrust inferiorly. The athlete comes off the field holding the injured arm and complaining of an extreme burning sensation, numbness, and weakness of the arm. When should you allow this athlete to return to the game?

○ **A.** The athlete must wait a minimum of 20 minutes and then express confidence in returning to play.

○ **B.** The athlete must demonstrate normal sensation and strength bilaterally, be cleared for any associated injuries, and express confidence in returning to play.

○ **C.** The athlete must demonstrate full shoulder and neck range of motion and be able to complete functional activities.

○ **D.** The athlete must have his shoulder pads and helmet refitted, demonstrate full range of motion, and be able to complete functional activities.

○ **E.** The athlete must ice for 20 minutes, demonstrate normal sensation and strength bilaterally, and complete neuropsychological testing within 90% of baseline.

146. Why is horizontal adduction limited when an athlete has sustained an acromioclavicular separation?

○ **A.** It approximates the joint surfaces, creating pressure and pain.

○ **B.** It distracts the joint surfaces, stretching damaged tissue and creating pain.

○ **C.** Horizontal adduction is not limited.

○ **D.** It causes impingement of the rotator cuff in the subacromial space, creating pain.

○ **E.** It causes the biceps tendon to create a traction force at the joint, creating pain.

147. A 14-year-old skateboarder falls while performing a trick and externally rotates his foot. The anterior tibiofibular ligament is intact, but you suspect he may have sustained a fracture. Which fracture is most likely based on this information?

○ **A.** Salter-Harris V fracture of the distal tibia

○ **B.** Talar dome fracture

○ **C.** Tillaux's fracture

○ **D.** Fibular avulsion fracture

○ **E.** Jones' fracture

148. An athlete presents with flu-like symptoms and a cluster of cutaneous vesicles on an erythematous base. The vesicles are tightly clustered and appear to have developed into pustules and ulcers. Several of the vesicles have ruptured, releasing a serous material that has formed a yellowish crust. How is this condition best treated pharmacologically?

○ **A.** An oral antiviral medication such as acyclovir

○ **B.** An oral antiviral medication such as erythromycin

○ **C.** An antibiotic medication such as amoxicillin

○ **D.** An antifungal medication such as terbinafine hydrochloride (Lamisil)

○ **E.** An antifungal medication such as zanamivir (Relenza)

149. A cheerleader who has been casted for a few days for an ulnar fracture reports to the athletic training room complaining of redness, increased pain, swelling, and extreme sensitivity to touch in her hand. What condition should the athletic trainer be most concerned about?

○ **A.** Reflex sympathetic dystrophy

○ **B.** Deep vein thrombosis

○ **C.** Neurapraxia

○ **D.** Amyotrophic lateral sclerosis

○ **E.** Cellulitis

150. A female athlete presents complaining of left lower quadrant tenderness and pain and referred pain in the shoulders. The athlete reports amenorrhea for the past 3 months attributed to an increase in training intensity. Which of the following conditions should be ruled out?

○ **A.** Diverticulitis, gallstones, and ovarian cyst

○ **B.** Ectopic pregnancy, urinary tract infection, and hepatitis

○ **C.** Cholecystitis, spleen injury, and irritable bowel syndrome

○ **D.** Colitis, sexually transmitted disease, and pancreatitis

○ **E.** Spleen injury, ovarian cyst, and ectopic pregnancy

151. Which of the following is a vector-borne disease?

○ **A.** *Escherichia coli*

○ **B.** Rabies

○ **C.** AIDS

○ **D.** Lyme disease

○ **E.** Impetigo

152. An athlete who recently completed a course of antibiotics and oral steroids complains of white, cheesy, curd-like patches on the tongue and buccal mucosa. What condition is most commonly associated with this presentation, and how is it best treated?

○ **A.** Oral candidiasis; oral rinse of nystatin and oral antifungal medication

○ **B.** Oral candidiasis; oral peroxide rinse and oral antibiotic medication

○ **C.** Leukoplakia; oral rinse of nystatin and manual scraping

○ **D.** Leukoplakia; oral peroxide rinse and oral antifungal medication

○ **E.** Gingivitis; oral antibiotic rinse and fluoride supplements

153. An athlete complains of pain, numbness, and paresthesia along the medial aspect of the foot following an acute hyper–plantar flexion ankle injury. Evaluative findings are as follows: pes planus bilaterally, palpable tenderness over the tibial nerve and its branches, passive plantar flexion and eversion increase symptoms, active and resisted range of motion are within normal limits, Tinel's sign (+) inferior and distal to the medial malleolus, and sensory discrimination is decreased along medial and plantar aspect of the foot. Which of the following injuries is most associated with this presentation?

○ **A.** Tarsal tunnel syndrome

○ **B.** Os trigonum syndrome

○ **C.** Flexor tendon impingement

○ **D.** Plantar fasciitis

○ **E.** Accessory navicular

154. An athlete returns from the physician with a diagnosis of an "unhappy triad." Why was the definition of this condition recently revised?

○ **A.** The medial meniscus is involved in this type of injury more frequently than the lateral meniscus.

○ **B.** The lateral meniscus is involved in this type of injury more frequently than the medial meniscus.

○ **C.** The lateral collateral ligament is involved in this type of injury more frequently than the medial collateral ligament.

○ **D.** The lateral collateral ligament was added because it is injured as frequently as the medial collateral ligament.

○ **E.** The posterior cruciate ligament was added because it is injured as frequently as the anterior cruciate ligament.

155. In performing Renne's test, an athlete squats, flexing the knee to 30°. As the athlete returns to star position with knees in full extension, how does the function of the iliotibial band change?

○ **A.** The iliotibial band is now able to assist in hip abduction.

○ **B.** The iliotibial band acts to internally rotate the tibia.

○ **C.** The iliotibial band creates posterior tibial translation.

○ **D.** The iliotibial band assists in superior patellar glide.

○ **E.** The iliotibial band goes from being a knee flexor to being a knee extensor.

156. During a pre-participation physical examination, the athletic trainer uses a tape to measure from the umbilicus to the most distal point of the medial malleolus of one limb and compares to the other. A difference of 2 cm is appreciated. What conclusions can the athletic trainer draw?

○ **A.** The femur or tibia of one leg is longer than the contralateral limb.

○ **B.** The angle of femoral neck inclination is greater on one leg compared with the contralateral leg.

○ **C.** The athlete is demonstrating abnormal pelvic positioning.

○ **D.** The athlete is demonstrating a positive test for the presence of a true leg length discrepancy.

○ **E.** The athlete is demonstrating femoral retroversion on one leg compared with the contralateral leg.

157. A resisted range-of-motion evaluation reveals weakness in the absence of pain. What are the clinical indications of these findings?

○ **A.** Neurological deficit or chronic contractile soft-tissue injury

○ **B.** Normal findings for contractile tissue

○ **C.** Minor contractile soft-tissue injury

○ **D.** Significant contractile-tissue injury or chronic noncontractile soft-tissue injury

○ **E.** Minor contractile soft-tissue injury or chronic contractile soft-tissue injury

158. An athlete reports experiencing a minor seizure over the weekend. The team physician orders an electroencephalogram to assist in ruling out the presence of epilepsy and asks you to explain the purpose of the test to the athlete. How would you best explain the purpose of this test?

○ **A.** Records electrical activity of the heart

○ **B.** Records electrical activity in the brain

○ **C.** Measures electrical activity in peripheral nerve tissue

○ **D.** Measures electrical activity in contracting muscle tissue

○ **E.** Measures electrical activity in autonomic nerve tissue

159. An athlete recently diagnosed with deep vein thrombosis has been prescribed warfarin (Coumadin). How will you explain the pharmacological goal of this drug?

○ **A.** Antibiotic

○ **B.** Analgesic

○ **C.** Beta blocker

○ **D.** Anticoagulant

○ **E.** Beta agonist

160. During a visit to the physician's office, an athlete is diagnosed with myositis ossificans of the biceps. By what other name is this condition often referred?

○ **A.** Burner

○ **B.** Blocker's exostosis

○ **C.** Thrower's shoulder

○ **D.** Tennis elbow

○ **E.** Speed's syndrome

161. An athlete sustains an uncomplicated crown fracture. There is obvious tooth deformity and bleeding but not pain. How would you explain the absence of pain to the athlete?

○ **A.** The dentin is not affected by this fracture, and it is the primary site of nerve endings in the tooth.

○ **B.** The fracture affects only the enamel portion of the tooth, and the enamel contains no nerve endings.

○ **C.** This type of fracture exposes the pulp cavity; after the pulp cavity is exposed to air, the nerve endings cease to fire.

○ **D.** The fracture is through the gum, which causes bleeding but not pain.

○ **E.** The fracture line is through the root, which results in significant bleeding but no pain because the area is not innervated.

162. When counseling an athlete with jumper's knee, which of the following activities should you recommend be minimized?

○ **A.** Concentric closed kinetic-chain exercises

○ **B.** Eccentric open kinetic-chain exercises

○ **C.** Plyometric-type exercises

○ **D.** Aquatic conditioning exercises

○ **E.** Elliptical or cycling cardiovascular training

163. An athlete with repeated herpes type 2 eruptions should be counseled to avoid which of the following contributing factors?

○ **A.** Fatigue, psychological stress, and poor nutrition

○ **B.** Overexposure to the sun, decreased body fat percentage, and sharing water bottles

○ **C.** Sexual activity, contact with others, and dehydration

○ **D.** Contact with others, fatigue, and a high carbohydrate diet

○ **E.** Poor nutrition, overexposure to the sun, and sexual activity

164. Before releasing an athlete, who has sustained a cerebral concussion, to the responsible adult who will be monitoring him overnight, which of the following signs and symptoms require immediate referral to the emergency department?

○ **A.** Headache

○ **B.** Lethargy

○ **C.** Inability to concentrate

○ **D.** Vomiting

○ **E.** Irritability

165. During discussions with an athlete who is contemplating undergoing lateral ankle reconstruction for chronic ankle instability, which of the following is the most important long-term implication that should be brought to the athlete's attention if surgery is not chosen?

○ **A.** Osteoarthritis

○ **B.** Talar fracture

○ **C.** Joint contracture

○ **D.** Tendinosis

○ **E.** Subluxing peroneal tendon

166. An adolescent athlete has been told she has chondromalacia patellae. Which of the following best describes this condition?

○ **A.** An inflammation and bony outgrowth from the attachment of the thigh muscles to the lower leg

○ **B.** An abnormal softening of the cartilage on the underside of the patella or kneecap

○ **C.** Pain and swelling of the tendon between the kneecap and the lower leg

○ **D.** Abnormal movement of the kneecap in its groove when you bend and straighten your leg

○ **E.** Tearing of the cartilage cushions inside the knee joint

167. An athlete who recently sustained a concussion and remains symptomatic is anxious to return for tomorrow's game. As his athletic trainer you are receiving pressure from the athlete, his parents, and the coaching staff to clear him for full participation. Which of the following is the best reason for withholding this athlete from participation?

○ **A.** The athlete is at increased risk for cerebral blood clots.

○ **B.** The athlete is at increased risk for sustaining second-impact syndrome.

○ **C.** The athlete is at increased risk for sustaining a stroke.

○ **D.** The athlete is at increased risk for sustaining a brain aneurysm.

○ **E.** The athlete is at increased risk for post-concussive syndrome.

168. An athlete complains of a collection of a thick fluid within a tendinous sheath of her wrist extensor tendons. What is the most appropriate advice to give the athlete to manage this condition?

○ **A.** Seek evaluation from a wrist/hand surgeon regarding excision.

○ **B.** Treat the condition symptomatically, and play as tolerated.

○ **C.** Initiate a comprehensive rehabilitation program focusing on wrist flexion range-of-motion strength of the wrist extensors.

○ **D.** Tape to limit wrist flexion, and avoid repetitive wrist flexion exercises.

○ **E.** Utilize paraffin bath and cross-friction massage daily to break up the fluid.

169. From which secondary injury should a wrestler who has sustained repetitive severe anterior thigh trauma be protected during subsequent practices and matches?

○ **A.** Osteomyelitis

○ **B.** Osteochondritis dissecans

○ **C.** Rhabdomyolysis

○ **D.** Myokymia

○ **E.** Myositis ossificans

170. You refer an 8-year-old camper who has tenderness over the base of the fifth metatarsal to the emergency department for evaluation. The camper returns to camp the next day on crutches with paperwork indicating he should follow up with an orthopedist in 1 week for a repeat x-ray to rule out an occult fracture. The camper's mother inquires about the diagnosis. How would you best respond?

○ **A.** An occult fracture means a hidden fracture, which is common in young athletes.

○ **B.** An occult fracture is a rapidly healing fracture, which is common in young athletes because of their constant growth.

○ **C.** An occult fracture is a fracture of the fifth metatarsal that is often confused with a Jones fracture.

○ **D.** An occult fracture is an avulsion fracture; repeat x-ray is required to determine fragment displacement.

○ **E.** An occult fracture is a growth plate injury common to young athletes participating in lower-extremity sports.

171. An athlete with a 3-week history of knee pain and mild joint effusion develops Baker's cyst. After discussions with the team physician, which test would best reveal the cause of the cyst?

○ **A.** X-ray

○ **B.** Magnetic resonance imaging

○ **C.** Bone scan

○ **D.** Diagnostic ultrasound

○ **E.** Complete blood count

172. An athlete is being seen by the team physician because she is unable to bear weight due to pain and complains of swelling and tenderness localized over the dorsum of the foot. Based on this presentation, which of the following would be included in the physician's differential diagnosis?

○ **A.** Lisfranc's injury

○ **B.** Tarsal tunnel syndrome

○ **C.** Plantar fasciitis

○ **D.** Extensor tendinosis

○ **E.** Sesamoiditis

173. The physician is presenting a staff in-service on head injuries. The physician states that when the brain loses autoregulation of its blood supply, vascular engorgement within the cranium results. This engorgement leads to herniation either of the medial surface of the temporal lobe or lobes below the tentorium or of the cerebellar tonsils through the foramen magnum. This condition leads to rapid brainstem failure within 2 to 5 minutes. What injury is being discussed?

○ **A.** Antegrade amnesia

○ **B.** Transient ischemic attack

○ **C.** Skull fracture

○ **D.** Cerebral concussion

○ **E.** Second impact syndrome

174. In your role as a physician extender, you evaluate a 50-year-old male tennis player complaining of bilateral sacroiliac pain. Your differential diagnosis includes ankylosing spondylitis and sacroiliac arthritis. Which of the following evaluation techniques will provide the best information for differentiating the two conditions?

○ **A.** Sensation and reflex testing

○ **B.** Sacral stress tests

○ **C.** Palpation of sacroiliac joint

○ **D.** Active and passive movements

○ **E.** History of morning stiffness

175. An adolescent athlete sustains a fall on an outstretched hand and is seen by his pediatrician. He returns the next day and reports that the x-ray in the pediatrician's office was negative, and he can play as tolerated; however, he still presents with exquisite pain in the anatomical snuff box. You are hesitant to allow him to return to play because you feel he may have a fracture. How would you best communicate to the athlete's physician your concern that yesterday's x-ray may be a false-negative?

○ **A.** The navicular bone is too dense for x-rays to pass through.

○ **B.** A fracture line may not show on x-rays for several weeks.

○ **C.** The wrist cannot be stabilized because of a chronic or acute irritation of the proximal radial condyle.

○ **D.** It may take several months for a fracture line to show on x-rays.

○ **E.** The navicular bone is too small to be seen by x-ray.

176. You refer an athlete to the team physician for evaluation of jumper's knee. She returns with a diagnosis of bipartite patella. What does this diagnosis imply?

○ **A.** The athlete has a congenital abnormality in which the patella has developed from two centers rather than one, resulting in two parts that are connected by fibrocartilage.

○ **B.** The athlete has an avulsion fracture of the inferior pole of the patella by the patellar tendon.

○ **C.** The athlete has a stress fracture of the patella due to the pull of the quadriceps musculature.

○ **D.** The athlete has progressive degeneration of the patella that has developed from excessive maltracking and chronic tendonitis.

○ **E.** The athlete has early onset of osteoarthritis of the patella that has developed from excessive maltracking and chronic tendonitis.

177. You refer an athlete to the team orthopedist to rule out a Jones fracture. The physician calls you to confirm that the athlete has a fifth metatarsal fracture but not a Jones fracture. In what case would a fifth metatarsal fracture not be a Jones fracture?

○ **A.** The fracture is more than 1 cm from the proximal diaphysis of the fifth metatarsal.

○ **B.** The fracture is a transverse fracture.

○ **C.** The fracture is an avulsion fracture.

○ **D.** The fracture is non-displaced.

○ **E.** The fracture is where the bone changes shape and direction.

178. An athlete returns from a visit to an optometrist with a diagnosis of astigmatism. If a normal eye is shaped like a basketball, which of the following best describes the presentation of astigmatism?

○ **A.** The eye is shaped more like a boomerang.

○ **B.** The eye is shaped more like a football.

○ **C.** The eye is shaped more like a teardrop.

○ **D.** The eye is shaped more like a hockey puck.

○ **E.** The eye is shaped more like a flying disc.

179. A college student athlete visits student health services when the athletic training room is closed because he feels he has a sinus infection. He receives a prescription for an antibiotic. Which of the following health-care professionals are legally permitted to write this prescription?

○ **A.** Osteopath, physician's assistant, and registered nurse

○ **B.** Physician's assistant, nurse practitioner, and family medicine resident

○ **C.** Nurse practitioner, certified counselor, and physician

○ **D.** Registered nurse, dentist, and pulmonologist

○ **E.** Family medicine resident, licensed practical nurse, and physician

180. As a high school athletic trainer you receive a phone call from a local physician's office requesting copies of your pre-participation physical and evaluation notes from a 16-year-old football player's recent knee injury. How should you best respond to this request?

○ **A.** A release of records must be signed by the athlete, and then they can be faxed to the requesting physician.

○ **B.** The requested records may be faxed or mailed to the requesting physician's office.

○ **C.** The athlete's mother may call and request the records be sent, and then the records can be faxed to the requesting physician.

○ **D.** The coach requests the records be sent on behalf of the athlete, and then the records can be faxed to the requesting physician.

○ **E.** The athlete and a parent may come by the athletic training room and pick up copies of his records to take to the physician.

Answers for Domain II: Clinical Evaluation and Diagnosis

Role A: Obtain a history through observation, interview, and/or review of relevant records to assess current or potential injury, illness, or condition.

1. B
2. B
3. C
4. B
5. D
6. C
7. D
8. D
9. C
10. C
11. E
12. A
13. C
14. D
15. A
16. A
17. B
18. D
19. B
20. B
21. C
22. A
23. C
24. A
25. D
26. C
27. D
28. D
29. C
30. E
31. B
32. A
33. B
34. B
35. B
36. C
37. E
38. C

Role B: Inspect the involved area(s) visually to assess the injury, illness, or health-related condition.

39. D
40. C
41. A
42. D

43. C

44. A

45. A

46. B

47. C

48. E

49. B

50. C

51. C

52. B

53. C

54. A

55. A

56. A

57. D

58. E

59. A

60. B

61. C

62. A

63. E

64. B

65. D

66. A

67. C

Role C: Palpate the involved area(s) using standard techniques to assess the injury, illness, or health-related condition.

68. A

69. E

70. E

71. C

72. E

73. C

74. A

75. C

76. D

77. D

78. E

79. C

80. B

81. D

82. A

83. A

84. D

85. A

86. A

87. E

88. B

89. A

90. C

91. B

92. B

93. A

94. E

95. E

96. B

97. A

Role D: Perform specific tests in accordance with accepted procedures to assess the injury, illness, or health-related condition.

98. C

99. C

100. A

101. B

102. B

103. C

104. E

105. C

106. B

107. E

108. C

109. D

110. A

111. D

112. B

113. B

114. D

115. C

116. A

117. A

118. D

119. B

120. B

121. A

122. B

123. A

124. D

125. C

126. A

127. B

128. E

129. D

130. D

131. A

Role E: Formulate a clinical impression by interpreting the signs, symptoms, and predisposing factors of the injury, illness, or condition to determine the appropriate course of action.

132. B

133. C

134. B

135. C

136. E

137. B

138. B

139. C

140. B

141. D

142. D

143. C

144. A

145. B

146. A

147. C

148. A

149. A

150. E

151. D

152. A

153. A

154. B

155. E

156. C

157. A

Role F: Educate the appropriate patient(s) regarding the assessment by communicating information about the current or potential injury, illness, or health-related condition to encourage compliance with recommended care.

158. B

159. D

160. B

161. B

162. C

163. A

164. D

165. A

166. B

167. B

168. B

169. E

Role G: Share assessment findings with other health-care professionals using effective means of communication to coordinate appropriate care.

170. A

171. B

172. A

173. E

174. D

175. B

176. A

177. A

178. B

179. B

180. E

Domain III: Immediate Care

1. Where is cyanosis best observed in a dark-skinned person?

○ **A.** Eyes

○ **B.** Lips and abdomen

○ **C.** Tongue and nailbeds

○ **D.** Earlobes

○ **E.** Pupils

2. Which of the following signs and symptoms best characterize hypovolemic shock?

○ **A.** Slow, deep breathing; agitation; and cold, pale clammy skin

○ **B.** Dilated pupils, excessive urine output, and bluish lips and fingernails

○ **C.** Very low blood pressure; rapid weak pulse; and cold, pale clammy skin

○ **D.** Profuse sweating; hot, dry skin; and rapid, shallow breathing

○ **E.** Hyperventilation; lightheadedness; and slow, thready pulse

3. Which of the following signs is associated with insulin shock?

○ **A.** Dry mucous lining of the mouth

○ **B.** Labored breathing

○ **C.** Fruity-smelling breath

○ **D.** Physical weakness

○ **E.** Nausea and vomiting

4. What is the best way to distinguish arterial from venous bleeding?

○ **A.** Arterial blood produces a more steady flow of blood.

○ **B.** Arterial blood spurts from the wound.

○ **C.** Arterial blood produces a flow of dark red blood.

○ **D.** Arterial blood slowly oozes from the tissues.

○ **E.** Arterial blood clots rapidly.

5. A middle-aged coach falls unconscious on the sideline. Her skin is cool and dry, and she is gasping. Her face is flushed, her lips are cherry red, and there is a sweet odor on her breath. What do you suspect?

○ **A.** Cerebral hemorrhage

○ **B.** Stroke

○ **C.** Diabetic coma

○ **D.** Insulin shock

○ **E.** Anaphylactic shock

6. Which of the following physiological processes results in diabetic coma?

○ **A.** Depressed fat metabolism that cannot supply energy when glucose is scarce

○ **B.** The accumulation of insulin in the bloodstream without carbohydrate on which it can act

○ **C.** The increased concentration of hydrogen cations in the blood arising from ketone bodies

○ **D.** Poor circulation to the brain because of the buildup of fatty deposits (arteriosclerosis) in the arterial tree

○ **E.** Oversecretion of insulin

7. Which of the following statements regarding skin color assessment is correct?

○ **A.** In dark-skinned persons, fever is noted by redness of the tongue, lips, ears, and the inside of the mouth.

○ **B.** In dark-skinned persons, shock results in the nailbeds having a bluish cast.

○ **C.** In Caucasians, high blood pressure is indicated by bluish skin.

○ **D.** In Caucasians, shock in the skin around the nose, tongue and mouth has a grayish cast.

○ **E.** In dark-skinned persons, bluish color of the lips and fingernails indicates high blood pressure.

8. Which of the following best characterizes a simple partial epileptic seizure?

○ **A.** Impairment of consciousness alone or in association with purposeful movements such as automatism

○ **B.** A brief bout of uncontrolled shaking of the limbs on one side of the body and no loss of consciousness

○ **C.** A brief bout of uncontrolled shaking of the limbs bilaterally and no loss of consciousness

○ **D.** A brief bout of uncontrolled shaking of the limbs with a loss of consciousness

○ **E.** Total body convulsions with a loss of consciousness

9. What is the best location to determine the pulse rate of an athlete who has a weak radial pulse?

○ **A.** Dorsal pedal

○ **B.** Popliteal

○ **C.** Brachial

○ **D.** Carotid

○ **E.** Femoral

10. You are performing one-person cardiopulmonary respiration on an unconscious victim. What is the proper compression-to-breath ratio?

○ **A.** 5:1

○ **B.** 5:2

○ **C.** 30:1

○ **D.** 15:2

○ **E.** 30:2

11. An athlete sustains a head injury that results in no loss of consciousness. He initially exhibits dilation of one pupil and reports a headache, dizziness, nausea, and sleepiness. Upon reevaluation, you note a rapid deterioration of symptoms. Which of the following conditions is most associated with these signs and symptoms?

○ **A.** Post-concussion syndrome

○ **B.** Second impact syndrome

○ **C.** Migraine headache

○ **D.** Subdural hematoma

○ **E.** Epidural hematoma

12. Which stage of a grand mal seizure may alert an individual with epilepsy to an oncoming attack?

○ **A.** Aura

○ **B.** Clonic

○ **C.** Postictal

○ **D.** Status

○ **E.** Tonic-clonic

13. Which of the following signs is inconsistent with the diagnosis of internal bleeding?

○ **A.** Increased blood pressure

○ **B.** Weak, rapid pulse

○ **C.** Abdominal rigidity

○ **D.** Blood in the urine, stool, or vomit

○ **E.** Bleeding from the ears

14. Which of the following mechanisms would most likely cause a spontaneous pneumothorax?

○ **A.** Acute bacterial pneumonia

○ **B.** Rupture of a bleb

○ **C.** Costochondral separation

○ **D.** Posterior displaced sternoclavicular joint separation

○ **E.** Hyperventilation

15. Athletes who have completed the swimming leg of a triathlon go on to the biking segment. The ambient air temperature is 55°F, and the wind is steady at 15 mph. An athlete has difficulty and cannot continue riding. During your evaluation, you notice the following: the athlete is disoriented and lethargic, has garbled speech, and has a core temperature of 95°F. The athlete's respirations are shallow, and the heart rate is notably slow. What would be the appropriate initial treatment for this athlete?

○ **A.** Cover the athlete with cool, damp towels, and send for emergency assistance.

○ **B.** Administer a warm IV saline solution, and prepare for immediate transport.

○ **C.** Move the athlete to a sheltered area, remove wet clothing, wrap the athlete in a warm blanket, and administer warm fluids.

○ **D.** Position the athlete on a table with feet elevated, cover with a blanket, and monitor for shock.

○ **E.** Move the athlete to a sheltered area, administer cool fluids, and prepare the athlete for transportation.

16. What should be the primary goal of treatment when caring for an athlete with suspected heat illness?

○ **A.** Have the athlete transported to the hospital.

○ **B.** Rehydrate the athlete.

○ **C.** Move the athlete to a cooler environment.

○ **D.** Lower the victim's body temperature.

○ **E.** Replenish blood glucose levels.

17. A male referee running down the sidelines during a punt return suddenly grasps at his chest and collapses. His face becomes ashen, and his breathing is difficult. Because you are trained in first aid, you suspect a heart attack. What should you do?

○ **A.** Treat for shock, and send someone to get an automated external defibrillator.

○ **B.** Begin artificial respirations, monitor pulse, and activate emergency medical services.

○ **C.** Monitor the patient's vital signs, send someone to get an automated external defibrillator, and activate emergency medical services.

○ **D.** Administer cardiopulmonary resuscitation, monitor vital signs, and activate emergency medical services using your cell phone.

○ **E.** Place the patient in a semireclining position, provide electrolyte fluids along with low-dose aspirin, send someone to get an automated external defibrillator, and activate emergency medical services.

18. When providing primary emergency care to an unconscious athlete with a suspected cervical spine injury, what is the first action that should be taken?

○ **A.** Apply a rigid cervical collar to stabilize the spine.

○ **B.** Place a towel in the posterior curve of the neck to establish normal lordotic curve.

○ **C.** Treat the athlete for shock by elevating the lower extremity.

○ **D.** Assess heart rate via the carotid pulse.

○ **E.** Establish and maintain an open airway.

19. Which of the following actions should you take when treating a person who is in shock?

○ **A.** Administer oral fluids.

○ **B.** Elevate the legs.

○ **C.** Elevate the head and trunk.

○ **D.** Induce vomiting.

○ **E.** Assist the patient in taking shock medications.

20. What is the primary goal when providing emergency care?

○ **A.** Maintain cardiovascular function and, indirectly, central nervous system function

○ **B.** Maintain central nervous system function and, indirectly, respiratory system integrity

○ **C.** Maintain adequate blood supply and, indirectly, brain function

○ **D.** Maintain breathing and, indirectly, central nervous system function

○ **E.** Maintain visceral organs and, indirectly, peripheral function

21. Which of the following descriptions best defines an emergency action plan?

○ **A.** A written document that defines the standard of care required in every conceivable event during an emergency situation

○ **B.** Procedures that are specific to the needs of each institution and athletic facility during an emergency situation

○ **C.** A statement that will drive the institution's functional goals, which in turn formulate all medical operating procedures

○ **D.** A detailed plan that describes the roles of involved personnel during an emergency situation

○ **E.** A written, site-specific plan for transporting injured athletes in an emergency situation

22. Which of the following components should be addressed in a comprehensive emergency action plan?

○ **A.** Emergency personnel, modes of communication, and venue or site maps

○ **B.** Roles of first responders, list of emergency numbers, and emergency contact information for the athlete

○ **C.** List of athlete's allergies, directions to the venue, and roles of involved personnel

○ **D.** Activation of medical services, injury-specific treatment protocols, and emergency equipment

○ **E.** Documentation of emergency action plan practice sessions, qualifications of all personnel, and location of personal protective equipment

23. A goalie hits her head against the post while making a save. The athlete is unconscious and unresponsive. The athlete's parent is not in attendance, and no written consent-to-treat form exists. Which of the following statements best reflects the athletic trainer's ability to treat this athlete?

○ **A.** Actual consent can be obtained from the parent via phone prior to the athletic trainer administering any treatment.

○ **B.** The coach can act as the parent and provide consent for treatment.

○ **C.** The athletic trainer may not provide direct treatment to the athlete but may activate emergency medical services and communicate findings.

○ **D.** Consent to treat is provided through the Good Samaritan Law.

○ **E.** Consent to treat is implied on the part of the athlete and the parents because this is a potentially life-threatening injury.

24. An athlete presents with sudden onset of complete unconsciousness. Her pulse is fast and weak, and respirations are quick and shallow. Her pupils are equal and dilated, and her skin is pale, cold, and clammy. Which of the following conditions is most associated with this presentation?

○ **A.** Diabetic coma

○ **B.** Syncope

○ **C.** Heatstroke

○ **D.** Insulin shock

○ **E.** Brain injury

25. When completing a primary survey, what is the first component that should be assessed?

○ **A.** Airway, breathing, and circulation

○ **B.** Presence of spinal cord involvement

○ **C.** Athlete's position and presence of deformities

○ **D.** Level of consciousness

○ **E.** Profuse bleeding

26. In which of the following situations would it be appropriate for the athletic trainer to progress from the primary survey to the secondary survey when completing an on-field assessment?

○ **A.** Airway, breathing, and circulation have been established, and the athlete is bleeding profusely from an open leg wound.

○ **B.** The athlete has been stabilized, bleeding has been controlled, and you are ready to make an emergency transport decision once the secondary survey is completed.

○ **C.** The athlete is conscious, stable, and is being treated for shock.

○ **D.** The athlete is unconscious, supine, and breathing, and vital signs are stable.

○ **E.** The patient is conscious with an obvious closed tibia-fibula fracture and is exhibiting nervousness, nausea, and chills and appears pale.

27. In 1992, what piece of equipment did the Occupational Safety and Health Administration mandate athletic trainers use while performing cardiopulmonary resuscitation?

○ **A.** Bag-valve mask to provide standard quantity of oxygen delivery

○ **B.** Barrier device or pocket mask to minimize transmission of bloodborne pathogens

○ **C.** Gloves to minimize transmission of bloodborne pathogens

○ **D.** Supplemental oxygen to increase oxygen saturation

○ **E.** Watch with a second hand to more accurately perform compressions at the recommended rate

28. According to the NATA position statement on Management of the Cervical Spine Injured Athlete, which of the following statements is correct regarding face mask removal?

○ **A.** If the face mask cannot be removed in a reasonable amount of time, the helmet should be removed in the safest manner possible.

○ **B.** If the face mask cannot be removed in a reasonable amount of time, a pocket mask should be inserted under the face mask while ensuring cervical stabilization.

○ **C.** If the face mask must be removed, cutting tools are generally faster and produce less head movement than powered (cordless) screwdrivers.

○ **D.** Once the decision to immobilize and transport has been made, the athletic trainer should allow the paramedics to determine whether the face mask should be removed.

○ **E.** The face mask should be removed prior to a primary assessment to ensure the most accurate evaluation of the airway.

29. Which of the following statements regarding administration of supplemental oxygen is most correct?

○ **A.** Supplemental oxygen provides 90% oxygen as compared with a bag-valve mask, which provides 21% oxygen, and rescue breathing, which only provides 16% oxygen.

○ **B.** An athletic trainer who has completed a cardiopulmonary resuscitation class at the professional rescuer level may provide supplemental oxygen to a victim who is having trouble breathing.

○ **C.** Supplemental oxygen cylinders are easily identified because they are red in color and bear a yellow diamond that clearly states oxygen.

○ **D.** Supplemental oxygen should be delivered at a rate of 5 to 10 liters per minute as indicated by a flow rate meter.

○ **E.** An athletic trainer must have physician's prescription on file in all states to administer supplemental oxygen.

30. Why are automated external defibrillators effective in preventing sudden death from a cardiac emergency during sport activity?

○ **A.** Most cardiac emergencies in sport involve atrial fibrillation.

○ **B.** Most cardiac emergencies in sport involve cardiac arrest.

○ **C.** Most cardiac emergencies in sport involve ventricular fibrillation and cardiac arrest.

○ **D.** Most cardiac emergencies in sport involve cardiac arrhythmia and congestive heart failure.

○ **E.** Most cardiac emergencies in sport involve valve dysfunction.

31. An adolescent lacrosse crease defender is struck in the chest directly over the area of the left ventricle with a shot on goal. He collapses immediately to the turf. What condition would you suspect and what is the most appropriate immediate treatment?

○ **A.** Fractured sternum; activate emergency medical services

○ **B.** Spontaneous pneumothorax; rescue breathing

○ **C.** Hypertrophic cardiomyopathy; cardiopulmonary resuscitation and automated external defibrillator use

○ **D.** Ruptured aortic aneurysm; cardiopulmonary resuscitation and automated external defibrillator use

○ **E.** Commotio cordis; cardiopulmonary resuscitation and automated external defibrillator use

32. Axial loading is the primary mechanism for cervical spine injury. What is the only technique that results in axial loading?

○ **A.** Head-down contact

○ **B.** Face mask–to–face mask contact

○ **C.** Shoulder pad–to–face mask contact

○ **D.** Shoulder pad–to–posterior helmet contact

○ **E.** Face-forward contact

33. During practice, a member of your softball team approaches you complaining of intensely itchy erythematous areas on her body. As you begin to question her about this condition, you note some facial edema and that she is beginning to have difficulty breathing and talking because her tongue is swelling. What is the most appropriate immediate treatment for this athlete's condition?

○ **A.** Apply ice bags over the throat and mouth areas.

○ **B.** Use an epinephrine auto-injector.

○ **C.** Give the athlete two doses of an oral antihistamine.

○ **D.** Use a rapid-acting beta-agonist inhaler.

○ **E.** Apply topical anesthetic over erythematous areas.

34. Which type of shock is caused by general dilation of blood vessels within the cardiovascular system?

○ **A.** Cardiogenic

○ **B.** Hypovolemic

○ **C.** Respiratory

○ **D.** Psychogenic

○ **E.** Neurogenic

35. A soccer player collides with an opponent and walks off the field in a partially flexed position with the contralateral arm splinted against his body. During your evaluation you suspect a rib fracture with possible lung involvement. Which of the following signs would confirm your suspicion?

○ **A.** The athlete's respiration rate is 20 breaths per minute.

○ **B.** The athlete reports increased pain on inspiration.

○ **C.** The athlete's breathing is asymmetrical in appearance.

○ **D.** The athlete begins hyperventilating.

○ **E.** The athlete begins coughing up frothy red blood.

36. You are assessing an injured athlete's level of consciousness. The athlete responds to your voice but is not fully oriented to person, time, or place. How would this be categorized employing the AVPU scale?

○ **A.** V

○ **B.** A-1

○ **C.** P

○ **D.** U

○ **E.** P-2

37. While assessing an athlete's blood pressure, you initially inflate the cuff to 150 mm Hg. When you release the pressure, the first sound you hear is a swooshing sound or soft murmur. What does this sound indicate?

○ **A.** The cuff was inflated too high initially, and you are hearing the brachial artery blood flow occlusion.

○ **B.** The cuff was inflated to a correct pressure, and you are hearing the first Korotkoff sound, which should be recorded as systolic pressure.

○ **C.** The cuff was not inflated to a high-enough initial pressure, and you are hearing the second Korotkoff sound instead of the first.

○ **D.** The cuff was inflated to a correct pressure, and you are hearing the fifth Korotkoff sound, which should be recorded as diastolic pressure.

○ **E.** The cuff was inflated to a correct pressure, and you are hearing the first Korotkoff sound, which should be recorded as diastolic pressure.

38. Your soccer team is practicing on a recently mowed and fertilized field. One of the athletes, who has asthma, begins to wheeze uncontrollably. What is the first action you should take to manage this athlete?

○ **A.** Send another athlete to get an inhaled corticosteroid from the athlete's locker.

○ **B.** Give the athlete oral fluids, and encourage her to relax and slow her breathing.

○ **C.** Position the athlete in a semi-recumbent position to open the airway.

○ **D.** Send another athlete to get a fast-acting beta$_2$ agonist inhaler from your kit.

○ **E.** Have the athlete put her hands over her head and breathe in through her nose and out through her mouth.

39. The NATA position statement on Acute Management of the Cervical Spine Injured Athlete recommends considering the removal of the helmet and shoulder pads to be an all-or-nothing endeavor for which sport in addition to American football?

○ **A.** Men's lacrosse

○ **B.** Men's ice hockey

○ **C.** Field hockey

○ **D.** Women's lacrosse

○ **E.** Australian rules football

40. During assessment of the vital signs of an 8-year-old baseball player, you note the following: respirations: 25/minute, pulse: 108 beats/minute, temperature: 98°F, pink skin. What should you conclude?

○ **A.** The athlete is hyperventilating.

○ **B.** The athlete is tachycardic.

○ **C.** The athlete is exhibiting normal vital signs.

○ **D.** The athlete is hyperventilating and tachycardic.

○ **E.** The athlete is erythremic and tachycardic.

41. You have been caring for an athlete who is unconscious, but his vital signs are stable, and you do not suspect a cervical spine injury. Prior to arriving on the scene, emergency medical services request that you position the athlete in the recovery position and monitor vital signs. Which of the following best describes this position?

○ **A.** Side-lying on the left side with the left arm moved aside and the right arm draped across the body as support and the right leg crossed over the left

○ **B.** Side-lying on the right side with right arm moved aside and the left arm draped across the body as support and the right leg crossed over the left

○ **C.** Side-lying on the right side with right arm moved aside and the left arm draped across the body as support and the left leg crossed over the right

○ **D.** Side-lying on the left side with the left arm moved aside and the right arm draped across the body as support and the left leg crossed over the right

○ **E.** Side-lying on the right side with both arms overhead, next to the ears and the left leg crossed over the right

42. Which of the following situations is *least* likely to require the need to activate the emergency transport system?

○ **A.** The athlete has lost consciousness.

○ **B.** The athlete has suffered a posterior glenohumeral joint dislocation.

○ **C.** The athlete is unresponsive.

○ **D.** Cardiopulmonary resuscitation is being performed on the athlete.

○ **E.** Bleeding from an open fracture cannot be controlled.

43. Which technique should be used to remove the most common airway obstruction in an unconscious victim?

○ **A.** Head tilt–chin lift

○ **B.** Heimlich's maneuver

○ **C.** Abdominal thrusts

○ **D.** Chest compressions

○ **E.** Back blows

44. During the pre-game meal a volleyball player begins choking. Heimlich's maneuver is utilized unsuccessfully, and the athlete becomes unconscious. After you help the athlete to the ground and place her in a supine position, what is the next step you should take to care for this athlete?

○ **A.** Perform a finger sweep.

○ **B.** Begin abdominal thrusts.

○ **C.** Begin chest compressions.

○ **D.** Position the athlete in the recovery position.

○ **E.** Open the airway and attempt to ventilate.

45. During a thunderstorm, lightning strikes a power pole, resulting in a live power line falling onto an outfield chain-link fence. After the storm passes, the coaches go out to assess the damage. One of the coaches inadvertently touches the fence, receives an electrical shock, and collapses several feet away from the fence. What is first step you should take to care for the injured coach?

○ **A.** Perform a primary survey.

○ **B.** Call the power company to have the electricity shut off.

○ **C.** Move the coach off the wet grass and onto a dry blanket.

○ **D.** Activate emergency medical services, and do not touch the victim to protect yourself.

○ **E.** Use a wooden bat to see if the coach is still carrying a charge.

46. To what pressure point should digital pressure be applied to control bleeding from a wound in the lower leg?

○ **A.** Brachial

○ **B.** Femoral

○ **C.** Subclavian

○ **D.** Bicipital

○ **E.** Carotid

47. Which of the following statements best describes how a sling should be fitted for an athlete with a shoulder injury?

○ **A.** The elbow is positioned half the distance of the bottom of the sling.

○ **B.** The end of the sling is positioned at the wrist joint to allow free movement of the entire hand.

○ **C.** The hand should be positioned slightly higher than the elbow.

○ **D.** The forearm should be positioned in a fully pronated position.

○ **E.** The sling should be fitted while the patient is standing in a functional position.

48. During a gymnastics meet, an athlete falls from the balance beam, injuring her right shoulder. Palpation reveals a posterior displacement of the head of the humerus. The athlete's arm is abducted approximately 45°, and any movement results in severe pain. The decision is made to splint the arm as it was found using pillows and cravats. Which of the following parameters should be assessed before and after the splint is applied?

○ **A.** Blood pressure in the injured arm

○ **B.** Heart rate, rhythm, and strength

○ **C.** Distal neurovascular and circulatory functions

○ **D.** Respiratory rate, rhythm, and depth

○ **E.** Strength of the forearm muscles

49. Which of the following statements regarding caring for a blister is the most correct?

○ **A.** Drain the blister using a needle and syringe to pull the fluid out, and then inject a drying agent into the blister space.

○ **B.** After the fluid has been drained via a small incision, disinfect the area with alcohol, ensuring the alcohol penetrates the open blister.

○ **C.** Apply a skin lubricant to the blister, and cover it with gauze and tape until the blister ruptures on its own.

○ **D.** With the blister intact, apply a protective skin or film, and then apply a skin lubricant prior to applying a doughnut pad.

○ **E.** When the blister has been drained via a small incision, the roof of the blister should remain intact to provide a natural bandage.

50. Which of the following is the best method for managing a traumatic hyphema?

○ **A.** Irrigate the eye with copious amounts of sterile eyewash.

○ **B.** Cover the eye with a functional eye patch, and allow the athlete to return to competition.

○ **C.** Instruct the athlete to lie supine with the eyes closed for the next 48 to 72 hours.

○ **D.** Perform an eyelid flip using a cotton-tipped applicator, and inspect the eye for foreign materials.

○ **E.** Immediately refer the athlete to an ophthalmologist for further evaluation.

51. Which method is recommended to preserve an avulsed tooth until the athlete can see a dentist?

○ **A.** Wrap the tooth as is in moist gauze, and take the tooth and athlete to the dentist.

○ **B.** Place the tooth in a 10% hydrogen peroxide solution to preserve it, and take the athlete to the dentist within the next 24 hours.

○ **C.** Scrub the tooth vigorously, then place it in milk, and take the athlete to the dentist within the next 3 days.

○ **D.** Apply a topical dental anesthetic (such as Orajel) to the tooth, and take the tooth and the athlete to the dentist.

○ **E.** Place the tooth in a commercially prepared preservation solution, and take the tooth and the athlete to the dentist.

52. A golfer reports to the athletic training room complaining of sharp pain in the ball of her foot. She states that it feels like there is a piece of glass stuck in her foot. The athletic trainer observes callus formation embedded with tiny black or dark red dots on the ball of the foot. What is this condition, and how should it best be managed?

○ **A.** Tinea pedis; apply an over-the-counter antifungal cream, and educate the athlete on proper foot hygiene and drying techniques

○ **B.** Chronic eczema; apply topical steroids, use oral antihistamines to reduce itching, and educate the athlete about proper foot hygiene and drying techniques

○ **C.** Plantar warts; shave excessive callus, apply over-the-counter chemicals designed to dissolve the warts, and use doughnut padding for pressure relief

○ **D.** Tinea pedis; use oral antibiotics, shave excessive callus, and instruct the athlete on proper footwear selection

○ **E.** Plantar warts; use an oral antiviral medication, and educate the athlete on proper foot hygiene and drying techniques

53. What should an athletic trainer do when splinting any body part?

○ **A.** Immobilize the joints above and below the fracture site

○ **B.** Remove all clothing from the extremity

○ **C.** Secure the splint in a fashion that decreases nerve conduction velocity

○ **D.** Spray the splint with a disinfecting solution prior to application

○ **E.** Manually test the muscle in the distal extremity

54. Which of the following actions should be included in the treatment of an ingrown toenail?

○ **A.** Cut out the ingrown part of the nail, and soak the foot in Epsom salts.

○ **B.** Soak the nail in a warm povidone-iodine solution bath, cut a "V" in the nail, and place cotton under the corner of the nail.

○ **C.** Shave the top of the nail, and spread the toes apart with cotton.

○ **D.** Remove excess dirt from the nail, and soak it in hot water with antibiotic soap.

○ **E.** Surgically remove the entire toenail, and allow it to grow back properly.

55. What is the first step that should be taken when providing immediate care for a chemical burn of the eye?

○ **A.** Irrigate the eye with a solution of sodium bicarbonate.

○ **B.** Clean the eye with a sterile cloth.

○ **C.** Cover the eye with a moist sterile cloth.

○ **D.** Irrigate the eye with copious amounts of clear water.

○ **E.** Irrigate the eye with a hypertonic glucose solution.

56. An athlete has ruptured the extensor tendon of the distal interphalangeal (DIP) joint of the ring finger. What is the recommended supportive technique during the first 4 to 6 weeks of healing?

○ **A.** Splint the DIP joint in flexion.

○ **B.** Splint the DIP joint in extension.

○ **C.** Tape to the longest adjacent finger.

○ **D.** Tape to the most lateral finger.

○ **E.** Splint the proximal interphalangeal and DIP joints in flexion.

57. An athlete suffers a compound fracture of the middle third of the right tibia. In an initial attempt to control the bleeding, which of the following techniques would be the most effective and appropriate?

○ **A.** Elevate the leg above the level of the heart to slow the bleeding.

○ **B.** Gently apply sterile gauze over the wound, and apply digital pressure over the femoral artery.

○ **C.** Apply sterile gauze and direct pressure over the fracture site.

○ **D.** Apply a tourniquet just above the knee.

○ **E.** Gently apply sterile gauze over the wound, and apply pressure at the dorsal pedal pressure point.

58. What is the first step in administering first aid to a victim with an open fracture?

○ **A.** Splint the involved limb.

○ **B.** Position the patient to treat for shock.

○ **C.** Control hemorrhage.

○ **D.** Apply a dressing to the wound.

○ **E.** Take vital signs.

59. An athlete with which of the following injuries should be instructed to refrain from blowing the nose?

○ **A.** Corneal abrasion

○ **B.** Ruptured globe

○ **C.** Conjunctivitis

○ **D.** Blow-out fracture

○ **E.** Traumatic anisocoria

60. When treating an athlete suffering from chilblains, which of the following treatments should be avoided?

○ **A.** Applying friction massage to re-warm the tissue

○ **B.** Removing wet or constrictive clothing

○ **C.** Washing or drying the area

○ **D.** Covering the affected area

○ **E.** Placing a space heater near the patient

61. Which of the following conditions associated with training at high altitudes is self-limiting and will resolve with supplemental oxygen use as needed and acclimatization?

○ **A.** Acute mountain sickness

○ **B.** High-altitude pulmonary edema

○ **C.** High-altitude cerebral edema

○ **D.** Splenomegaly associated with sickle cell trait

○ **E.** High-altitude asthma exacerbation

62. Which of the following over-the-counter medications should be recommended for pain management of an acute musculoskeletal injury in the first 48 hours following an acute injury?

○ **A.** Ibuprofen

○ **B.** Acetaminophen

○ **C.** Aspirin

○ **D.** Naproxen sodium

○ **E.** Acetylsalicylic acid

63. When caring for an adolescent running a fever and who has a suspected viral infection, which antipyretic medication should be avoided based on epidemiological studies?

○ **A.** Acetaminophen

○ **B.** Ibuprofen

○ **C.** Naproxen sodium

○ **D.** Diphenhydramine

○ **E.** Acetylsalicylic acid

64. An athlete's blood work comes back from the lab indicating (+) Epstein-Barr virus. What care is dictated by this laboratory result?

○ **A.** The athlete should be started on an antiviral medication and be instructed on increasing protein and fluid intake.

○ **B.** The athlete should be inspected for the presence of any herpetic lesions, which should be covered to prevent transmission.

○ **C.** Mononucleosis should be ruled out using a monospot test, and appropriate precautions should be taken in the interim.

○ **D.** The athlete should be started on an antibiotic medication for strep throat and treated symptomatically for headache, fever, and malaise.

○ **E.** Acute hepatitis should be ruled out using an abdominal ultrasound, and the athlete should be withheld from all activity pending test results.

65. An athlete with exercise-induced asthma uses his short-acting beta$_2$ agonist metered-dose inhaler (MDI) with spacer 10 to 15 minutes before practice. During the practice session, the athlete repeats MDI use three times. How should you best manage this athlete?

○ **A.** The athlete should be instructed to drink more water than his teammates because this medication can cause dehydration.

○ **B.** The athlete should be reinstructed in proper usage of his inhaler.

○ **C.** The athlete should be instructed to take an over-the-counter antihistamine before practice to minimize the effects of environmental triggers.

○ **D.** The athlete should be referred to the team physician for evaluation of current asthma treatment plan.

○ **E.** The athlete should be encouraged to continue to use this medication as needed because usage will decrease as his fitness level increases.

66. An equestrian athlete with cystic fibrosis must be treated with consistent postural drainage. How is postural drainage best accomplished?

○ **A.** Cupping or hacking massage techniques followed by deep breathing and coughing

○ **B.** Repeated prone to supine positioning exercises followed by recumbent seating

○ **C.** Inverted prone positioning combined with moist heat application

○ **D.** Inhalation of menthol and eucalyptus steam followed by inverted prone positioning

○ **E.** Deep breathing, breath holding, and simple yoga posturing combined with high fluid intake

67. After returning from a road trip, a member of your swim team is diagnosed with bacterial meningitis. Which of the following is the most appropriate management approach for this condition?

- ○ **A.** Individuals who have been in close contact with the sick athlete should be placed on prophylactic antibiotics.

- ○ **B.** Individuals who have been in close contact with the sick athlete should be tested for the disease using a nasal swab.

- ○ **C.** Everyone in the travel party should be quarantined and monitored for 48 hours to ensure no one else has contracted the disease.

- ○ **D.** Everyone in the travel party is tested for the presence of the condition using a lumbar puncture.

- ○ **E.** Everyone in the travel party should be encouraged to eat well, get plenty of rest and fluids, and report to the athletic training room immediately if they begin to experience any symptoms.

68. An athlete reports to the athletic training room with itchy, watery eyes; a runny nose, and postnasal drip. Which of the following classifications of medications is most appropriate for the relief of these symptoms?

- ○ **A.** Antitussive
- ○ **B.** Analgesic
- ○ **C.** Expectorant
- ○ **D.** Antipyretic
- ○ **E.** Antihistamine

69. Which of the following classifications of medications is most appropriate for the relief of headache?

- ○ **A.** Anesthetic
- ○ **B.** Analgesic
- ○ **C.** Anti-inflammatory
- ○ **D.** Antipruritic
- ○ **E.** Antipyretic

70. While grooming her horse after practice, an equestrian athlete is kicked by her horse in the anterior lower leg. She presents to the athletic training room later that evening with significant swelling, pain, and tenderness of the anterior lower leg. You assess the injury and note decreased sensation between her first and second toes and a decreased ability to dorsiflex. What is the best way to manage this athlete?

- ○ **A.** Activate emergency medical services for transport to emergency facility.

- ○ **B.** Provide ice and elevation for 20 minutes, and then reassess.

- ○ **C.** Provide RICE for 20 minutes, and then reassess.

- ○ **D.** Apply a compression wrap and instruct the athlete in RICE technique for home care.

- ○ **E.** Submerge the leg in an ice bath, apply a compression wrap from toes to knee, and fit the athlete for crutches.

71. A 40-year-old male tennis pro grabs his calf and falls to the court. He states it felt like someone kicked him in the calf and he is unable to plantar-flex his ankle. You observe a soft mass in the superior posterior lower leg. What is the best treatment plan for this condition?

- ○ **A.** Provide RICE, fit for crutches, and refer the athlete to the orthopedist for probable surgical repair.

- ○ **B.** Provide RICE, fit for a walking boot, and instruct the athlete to return the next day for reassessment and treatment.

- ○ **C.** Activate emergency medical services for transport to an emergency facility.

- ○ **D.** Provide ice massage for 10 minutes followed by gentle stretching and massage.

- ○ **E.** Apply an over-the-counter counterirritant to increase blood flow, and follow with gentle stretching and massage.

72. A suspected fracture of which of the following bones requires assistance from emergency medical services to properly splint?

- ○ **A.** Tibia
- ○ **B.** Humerus
- ○ **C.** Mandible
- ○ **D.** Femur
- ○ **E.** Sacrum

73. A field hockey player sustains a noncontact lateral patellar dislocation during play. What is the accepted method for on-field reduction of this dislocation?

○ **A.** With the athlete supine, apply gentle pressure to the patella in the medial direction while the athlete actively flexes the knee.

○ **B.** With the athlete seated, apply gentle pressure to the patella in an inferior and lateral direction while the athlete actively extends the knee.

○ **C.** With the athlete seated, apply gentle pressure to the patella in the medial direction while the athlete actively extends the knee.

○ **D.** With the athlete side-lying, apply gentle pressure to the patella in the medial direction while the athlete actively flexes the knee to the chest.

○ **E.** With the athlete seated, apply gentle pressure to the patella in the superior and lateral direction while the athlete actively flexes the knee.

74. An athlete ruptures the extensor tendon dorsal to the middle phalanx of the index finger of his right hand. How should this best be splinted?

○ **A.** With the proximal interphalangeal joint in flexion and the distal interphalangeal joint in extension without restricting movement of the metacarpophalangeal joint

○ **B.** With the distal interphalangeal joint in extension without restricting movement of the adjacent joints

○ **C.** With the proximal interphalangeal joint in extension without restricting movement of the adjacent joints

○ **D.** With the distal interphalangeal and proximal interphalangeal joints in extension without restricting movement of the metacarpophalangeal joint

○ **E.** With the metacarpophalangeal joint, proximal interphalangeal joint, and distal interphalangeal joint in full extension

75. What treatment is recommended for a 15-year-old female soccer player who has been diagnosed with mittelschmerz?

○ **A.** Anti-inflammatory medications and ice packs

○ **B.** Analgesic medications and moist hot packs

○ **C.** Antidiarrheal medications and electrolyte fluids

○ **D.** Antiemetics and a bland diet

○ **E.** Antihistamines and nebulizer treatments

76. While traveling with your softball team, one of your pitchers exhibits symptoms consistent with a migraine headache. She has prescription medication, but she left it in her dorm room. What suggestions can you give this athlete for managing this condition?

○ **A.** Recommend that the athlete call her physician to phone in a duplicate prescription, take a hot shower, and get out in the sunshine.

○ **B.** Recommend that the athlete focus on the team activities, go for a run or swim in the hotel pool, and consume high-carbohydrate sports drinks.

○ **C.** Recommend that the athlete lie supine with her head off the end of the bed to promote blood flow, apply a warm towel to the back of her neck, and rest quietly.

○ **D.** Recommend that the athlete get a workout in the hotel fitness center, take a hot shower, and ensure adequate hydration.

○ **E.** Recommend that the athlete take an over-the-counter migraine analgesic medication, rest in a quiet room with the lights off, and consume caffeinated beverages.

77. You are traveling with your high school ice hockey team to an away game approximately 2 hours from your home town. One of the players sustains a facial laceration in the first period. You apply adhesive skin closures to the wound and allow him to return to play but believe he will require sutures following the game. Because his parents are not at the game, you must decide whether to have the athlete treated at the nearby emergency department or treated by his physician when he returns home. Which of the following factors will have the biggest impact on your decision?

○ **A.** Ability to have the athlete treated within 12 hours

○ **B.** Athlete's preference for treatment location

○ **C.** Coach's travel schedule

○ **D.** Parents' presence during treatment

○ **E.** Insurance coverage restrictions

78. A young athlete suffers epistaxis. The bleeding has been controlled. What instructions should you give the athlete regarding continued care?

○ **A.** The athlete should be cautioned to refrain from blowing the nose for several hours and should avoid taking aspirin or nonsteroidal anti-inflammatory drugs.

○ **B.** The athlete should be instructed to apply antibiotic ointment over the scab and to keep the area dry and covered.

○ **C.** The athlete can return to full activity but is required to wear a protective face guard.

○ **D.** The athlete should sit out for the remainder of the day's practices and use ice and analgesic medication as needed.

○ **E.** The athlete should rinse the mouth with an antibacterial rinse three times daily for the next 5 days.

79. Which type of immobilization device is used in the immediate treatment of hematoma auris?

○ **A.** Orthoplast splint

○ **B.** Therafoam splint

○ **C.** Collodion cast

○ **D.** Fiberglass cast

○ **E.** Traction splint

80. A male soccer player is struck in the scrotum by the ball. You have the athlete lie supine and flex his hips and knees to 90° and then perform a Valsalva maneuver. What is the purpose of this management technique?

○ **A.** To distract the athlete from the pain by completing a psychomotor skill

○ **B.** To maintain the player's privacy regarding the nature of the injury

○ **C.** To increase blood flow to the area

○ **D.** To reduce associated muscle spasm

○ **E.** To reduce possible spermatic cord torsion

81. An athlete sustains a blow to the solar plexus. What is the best way to manage this condition?

○ **A.** Provide back blows, and encourage the athlete to cough forcefully.

○ **B.** Encourage the athlete to take short inspirations and long expirations as if trying to whistle.

○ **C.** Position the athlete supine with hands over head to maximally open the air passages.

○ **D.** Encourage the athlete to rebreathe using a paper bag.

○ **E.** Position the athlete seated at the end of a table with the head between the knees.

82. Which of the following supplies would be most important to have in a field kit to manage an athlete with a displaced contact lens?

○ **A.** Penlight, mirror, and sterile gauze pads

○ **B.** A blue light, fluorescein strips, and eye patch

○ **C.** Sterile eyewash, tweezers, and cotton-tipped applicators

○ **D.** Contact lens case, eye patch, and sterile saline solution

○ **E.** Sterile saline solution, mirror, and contact lens case

83. An athlete presents to the athletic training room with a chief complaint of unilateral ankle swelling. When you palpate the ankle, you note your fingerprints are embedding in the tissue. What is the best treatment plan for managing this condition?

○ **A.** RICE

○ **B.** Contrast bath using a cold whirlpool and a warm whirlpool

○ **C.** Intermittent compression combined with elevation

○ **D.** Continuous ultrasound followed by ice massage

○ **E.** Transcutaneous electrical nerve stimulation combined with ice and elevation

84. When treating an athlete who is recovering from an acute musculoskeletal injury, what clinical criteria best assist the athletic trainer in determining that the athlete is transitioning from the acute inflammatory phase to the fibroblastic repair phase?

○ **A.** Swelling is resolving.

○ **B.** Ecchymosis is transitioning from purple to yellow.

○ **C.** Subjective pain is replaced by soreness.

○ **D.** Elevated tissue temperature remains constant.

○ **E.** Red color of skin becomes blue and purple.

85. For which of the following injuries would a manual conveyance method for transporting a mildly injured athlete be used?

○ **A.** An athlete sitting in the middle of the track and exhibiting signs of heat illness

○ **B.** An athlete kneeling by the sideline with a lateral ankle sprain

○ **C.** An athlete sitting in front of the goal with a suspected anterior cruciate ligament sprain

○ **D.** An athlete lying in the middle of the football field with a hip pointer

○ **E.** An athlete exhibiting signs of an acute asthma attack on the bench during a baseball game

86. Which of the following statements best describes correct fitting of crutches?

○ **A.** Crutch tips should be placed 6″ from the outer margin of the shoe and 2″ in front of the shoe.

○ **B.** The underarm crutch brace is positioned 3″ below the anterior fold of the axilla.

○ **C.** The hand brace is adjusted so that it is even with the patient's hand when the elbow is flexed 5°.

○ **D.** The patient should wear running sneakers and stand with one foot in front of the other when being fitted.

○ **E.** Approximate crutch length can be estimated by measuring the hand-to-hand distance of the patient's outstretched arms.

87. Which of the following statements is correct regarding crutch and cane ambulation?

○ **A.** When ambulating with a cane, the cane should be placed on the ipsilateral side.

○ **B.** When ambulating with a single crutch, the ambulatory aid should be placed on the contralateral side.

○ **C.** When ambulating using the tripod gait, the athlete should be instructed to place the crutch tips 3″ to 4″ ahead of the feet before leaning forward on the crutches.

○ **D.** When ambulating using a four-point gait, the right crutch should be placed 12″ to 15″ ahead of the right foot at heel strike and then repeated with the left.

○ **E.** When ascending stairs with two crutches, the crutches should move up followed by the injured limb.

88. An athlete has been prescribed amoxicillin to treat an acute bronchial infection. What is the mechanism of action of this drug?

○ **A.** It inhibits bacterial protein synthesis.

○ **B.** It inhibits bacterial DNA synthesis.

○ **C.** It inhibits bacterial folic acid synthesis.

○ **D.** It inhibits bacterial mitochondrial synthesis.

○ **E.** It inhibits bacterial cell wall synthesis.

89. An athlete has sustained an abrasion that has developed into a yellow or honey-colored crusted lesion on an erythematous base. Small pea-shaped lesions have erupted, leaving purulent discharge on the skin. The lesions are painless yet pruritic. What is the best treatment for this condition?

○ **A.** Topical antifungal medication and removal from activity for 48 hours

○ **B.** Oral antiviral medication and cover lesions for all contact activity

○ **C.** Topical or oral antibiotics and removal from contact activities until lesions have cleared

○ **D.** Topical antihistamine medication and an oral antiviral medication and remove from activity for 24 hours

○ **E.** Oral steroid medication and cover lesions for all contact activity

90. A volleyball player sustains an acute eversion ankle sprain. What taping technique should be applied to best control swelling and provide limited support?

○ **A.** Open basket weave

○ **B.** Gibney

○ **C.** Low-Dye

○ **D.** Kinesio taping

○ **E.** McConnell taping

91. A male basketball player complains to the athletic trainer that he is experiencing intense itching around his wrist, between his fingers, and on the back of his hands, which is keeping him from sleeping. Upon examination you note small, red bumps arranged in a linear fashion focused in the web spaces of the fingers. What is the most appropriate treatment plan for this condition?

○ **A.** Instruct the athlete to review his past close and sexual contacts in the past 30 days and to notify those individuals because treatment may be necessary.

○ **B.** Apply a topical antibiotic cream, and instruct the athlete to sleep with socks on his hands.

○ **C.** Apply a topical antifungal cream, and instruct the athlete on proper hand washing and drying.

○ **D.** Apply an aloe lotion, and instruct the athlete to avoid extreme hot water and soap and reapply lotion frequently.

○ **E.** Apply zinc oxide, and instruct the athlete on proper hand washing and drying.

92. Under most circumstances, after how many minutes of oxygen deprivation will brain damage occur in the nonbreathing victim?

○ **A.** Less than 1 minute

○ **B.** 1 to 2 minutes

○ **C.** 2 to 3 minutes

○ **D.** 3 to 4 minutes

○ **E.** 4 to 6 minutes

93. An athlete initially presents with generalized viral illness symptoms, including fever, body aches, nausea, vomiting, diarrhea, and mild fatigue. Upon follow-up, he presents with increased fatigue, dyspnea, palpitations, and exercise intolerance. Based on these symptoms, which cardiac condition should be ruled out?

○ **A.** Myocarditis

○ **B.** Wolff-Parkinson-White syndrome

○ **C.** Hypertrophic cardiomyopathy

○ **D.** Long QT syndrome

○ **E.** Aortic valve stenosis

94. When performing cardiac auscultations, which of the following findings would necessitate referral to a physician for further evaluation?

○ **A.** During inspiration, the S_2 sound is split into two components.

○ **B.** While taking the carotid pulse during auscultation, you note that the "lubb" sound is synchronous with the carotid pulse.

○ **C.** When auscultating over the fourth intercostal space along the lower left sternal border, you fail to hear a bruit sound.

○ **D.** When auscultating over the mitral valve, you note turbulent blood flow or valvular vibration during systole and diastole.

○ **E.** When auscultating over the second right intercostal space at the right sternal border, you note a loud "lubb-dupp" sound.

95. Following a chest wall contusion, an athlete presents with shallow, slow breathing. Which breathing term should you use when communicating this to the physician?

○ **A.** Tachypnea

○ **B.** Hyperpnea

○ **C.** Bradypnea

○ **D.** Hypopnea

○ **E.** Orthopnea

96. During a practice, an athlete with diabetes walks over to the athletic trainer exhibiting Kussmaul's breathing. What is the immediate treatment you should provide for this athlete?

○ **A.** Provide the athlete with a glucose beverage, and monitor for possible referral.

○ **B.** Provide the athlete with a paper bag to slow his breathing.

○ **C.** Encourage the athlete to take deep breaths while sitting in a comfortable position.

○ **D.** Assist the athlete in administering an insulin injection, and monitor for possible referral.

○ **E.** Activate emergency medical services for immediate transport to an emergency facility.

97. Which of the following adventitious breath sounds would require referral to a physician for further evaluation?

○ **A.** Scratching, high-pitched vesicular sounds

○ **B.** Coarse, loud bronchial sounds

○ **C.** Coarse bronchovesicular sounds

○ **D.** High-pitched, breezy vesicular sounds

○ **E.** Whistling bronchovesicular sounds

98. An athlete reports to the athletic training room with an erythema migrans that has enlarged over the last few days. She is experiencing mild headache, some muscle aches, joint aches, and fatigue. Which condition is most associated with this presentation, and how is it best managed?

○ **A.** Lyme disease; referral to a physician for serological testing and antibiotic therapy

○ **B.** Syphilis; referral to a physician for cerebrospinal fluid screening

○ **C.** Tinea corporis; treat with antifungal cream

○ **D.** Allergic reaction to over-the-counter cold medication; treat with antihistamine

○ **E.** Mononucleosis; referral to physician for complete blood count and monospot

99. An incoming freshmen on your basketball team presents for orthopedic screening prior to being seen by the physician during the pre-participation examination. The athlete exhibits elongated metacarpals and metatarsals, kyphoscoliosis, and laxity in multiple joints. What concern should you raise to the physician?

○ **A.** This athlete is exhibiting postural findings typical of the basketball player this school normally recruits.

○ **B.** This athlete is exhibiting postural findings consistent with Marfan's syndrome.

○ **C.** This athlete is exhibiting postural findings that put him at increased risk for stress fractures.

○ **D.** This athlete is exhibiting postural findings, indicating the need for postural stabilization and proprioception training.

○ **E.** The athlete is exhibiting postural findings consistent with connective tissue disorder.

100. An athlete reports to the athletic training room for evaluation of a blister that is open, red, and markedly swollen, and the skin around the blister is tight and shiny. No outward leakage of pus is noted. The athlete complains of overall feeling of malaise and a low-grade fever for the past 12 hours. How would this condition best be treated?

○ **A.** Apply an antibacterial ointment, and give the athlete an over-the-counter antipyretic for fever and malaise.

○ **B.** Soak the blister in a povidone-iodine bath, apply a triple antibiotic ointment, and cover the blister.

○ **C.** Apply zinc oxide to dry the blister, cover with a bandage, and use a doughnut pad to disperse force.

○ **D.** Treat the blister with ice for 20 minutes, and recommend the athlete take an over-the-counter analgesic medication.

○ **E.** Refer the athlete immediately to a physician.

101. An athletic trainer is concerned that one of her college athletes may have an eating disorder. How should this condition best be managed?

○ **A.** The athlete should be confronted by the athletic trainer, and concerns should be discussed.

○ **B.** The athletic trainer should speak with the athlete and recommend the athlete speak with a counselor or psychiatrist.

○ **C.** The athletic trainer should notify the coach of her concerns and ask that the coach handle the situation.

○ **D.** The athletic trainer should notify the athlete's parents and ask that they take her to see a psychiatrist.

○ **E.** The athletic trainer should speak with other athletes on the team to determine whether concerns are founded.

102. An athlete sustains a head injury. During the evaluation of the athlete, the Halo test is positive. What does this indicate, and what steps should be taken to manage this injury?

○ **A.** The athlete is leaking cerebrospinal fluid and should be referred immediately for evaluation of possible skull fracture.

○ **B.** The athlete is bleeding from a skull fracture and should be referred immediately.

○ **C.** The athlete has an epidural hematoma, and emergency medical services should be called for immediate transport.

○ **D.** The athlete has a concussion and should be monitored and reassessed every 20 minutes.

○ **E.** The athlete has sustained a nasal fracture that involves the sinuses and should be referred to an ear, nose, and throat specialist.

103. Following a head injury, an athlete is unable to recall events that happened since the time of injury. Which type of amnesia is the athlete experiencing, and what steps should be taken based on this information?

○ **A.** Anterograde amnesia; refer the athlete for further evaluation to rule out intracranial bleeding

○ **B.** Retrograde amnesia; continue to monitor the athlete's condition and vital signs serially

○ **C.** Global amnesia; refer the athlete to a neurologist to rule out possible brain tumor

○ **D.** Stable amnesia; continue to monitor the athlete's condition and vital signs serially

○ **E.** Progressive amnesia; refer the athlete to team physician to rule out a degenerative dementia

104. An athlete sustains a laceration to the forearm that is producing significant bleeding. Underlying tissue, including fat, tendon, and vessels, is exposed. What is the most appropriate immediate care for this injury?

○ **A.** The wound should be cleaned and closed with adhesive skin closures.

○ **B.** The wound should be abraded with mild soap and water and débrided with a brush.

○ **C.** The wound should be closed with sutures.

○ **D.** The wound should be irrigated with hydrogen peroxide and closed with butterfly bandages.

○ **E.** The wound should be cleaned and covered with a nonstick pad.

105. What is indicated by an EMT-D classification?

○ **A.** Trained in basic ambulance services

○ **B.** Trained in basic ambulance services, defibrillator use, and endotracheal intubation

○ **C.** Trained in defibrillator use and intravenous infusion administration

○ **D.** Trained in basic ambulance services along with defibrillator use

○ **E.** Trained as a paramedic

106. Which branch of dentistry specializes in the care of the pulp of the tooth?

○ **A.** Orthodontics

○ **B.** Endodontics

○ **C.** Periodontics

○ **D.** Family dentistry

○ **E.** Oral and maxillofacial surgery

107. Which branch of medicine specializes in physical medicine?

○ **A.** Physiatry

○ **B.** Osteopathy

○ **C.** Pathology

○ **D.** Chiropractic

○ **E.** Internal medicine

108. An athlete with an 8-year history of epilepsy has incurred a generalized tonic-clonic seizure. Which of the following situations requires you to call 911, local police, or an ambulance?

○ **A.** The athlete does not start breathing within 15 seconds after the seizure has ended.

○ **B.** The athlete has one seizure right after another.

○ **C.** You are unable to insert a jaw stabilization device into the seizing athlete's mouth during the seizure.

○ **D.** The athlete refuses to drink fluids once the seizure has ended.

○ **E.** You are unable to restrain the athlete during the seizure.

109. You observe a 10-year-old pitcher drop to the mound after sustaining a line drive to the posterior lateral aspect of his head. When you reach the mound, the player is seated, alert, crying, and rubbing his head. From your off-field evaluation of this athlete, you determine that he must be transported to a health-care facility to be evaluated by a physician. What is the most appropriate method for transporting this athlete?

○ **A.** Call emergency medical services, and request an ambulance transport the athlete to a health-care facility.

○ **B.** Ask the assistant coach to drive the athlete to the health-care facility.

○ **C.** Ask the athlete's parent to take him to the health-care facility.

○ **D.** Ask the parent of the athlete's teammate to take the injured athlete to the health-care facility.

○ **E.** Ask the athletic training student to take the athlete to the health-care facility.

110. According to the National Association of EMS Physicians, which of the following is an accepted criterion for cessation of cardiopulmonary resuscitation procedures?

○ **A.** A non-hypothermic athlete is in cardiac arrest for more than 30 minutes.

○ **B.** An emergency medical technician instructs you to discontinue treatment of the athlete.

○ **C.** The arresting athlete regains normal breathing pattern.

○ **D.** Another rescuer arrives on the scene and offers assistance.

○ **E.** The automated external defibrillator has provided at least one shock.

111. An offensive lineman sustains a low chop block while he also incurs a posteriorly directed blow to his upper body, resulting in a posterior-superior tibiofibular dislocation of the femur. What is the most appropriate immediate care for this knee injury?

○ **A.** Apply a vacuum splint, use a manual conveyance technique to transport the athlete to the sidelines, and perform a complete lower extremity evaluation.

○ **B.** Apply a padded, long board splint; assess the athlete for shock; and activate emergency medical services.

○ **C.** Perform a lower-extremity evaluation, use a manual conveyance technique to transport the athlete to the sidelines, and activate emergency medical services.

○ **D.** Activate emergency medical services, apply a traction splint, and monitor for shock.

○ **E.** Assess circulation and neurological status of the leg, assess the athlete for shock, and activate emergency medical services.

112. In the last 2 minutes of a soccer game, a forward charging toward the goal collides with the sweeper from the opposing team and sustains a compound mid-shaft tibiofibular fracture. What is the most appropriate immediate care for this injury?

○ **A.** Activate emergency medical services, splint the injury in correct alignment, elevate the distal extremity, and monitor for shock.

○ **B.** Apply dressing to the wound, splint the injury in the position it was initially found, continually check neurovascular status, and activate emergency medical services.

○ **C.** Monitor the patient's vital signs, activate emergency medical services, and remain with the athlete until assistance arrives.

○ **D.** Apply dressing to the wound, splint the injury in correct alignment, transport the athlete to the sideline using ambulatory aid techniques, and reassess.

○ **E.** Apply an antibiotic dressing to the wound, apply a half-ring splint ensuring correct alignment, activate emergency medical services, and monitor for shock.

113. When should emergency medical services be activated when managing an athlete with an acute airway obstruction?

○ **A.** If the athlete complains of throat irritation following dislodgment of the obstruction

○ **B.** On initiation of cardiopulmonary resuscitation

○ **C.** When the athlete cannot cough, speak, or breathe

○ **D.** If the athlete cannot be stopped from coughing forcefully and continually

○ **E.** If the athlete has sickle cell trait

114. While assisting athletes in the emergency care tent at a local marathon, you observe a physician begin an IV treatment on a recently collapsed runner. Which of the following is most likely the purpose of this treatment?

○ **A.** To minimize the risk of hyponatremia

○ **B.** To achieve rapid hydration

○ **C.** To minimize the risk of exertional sickling

○ **D.** To decrease core body temperature

○ **E.** To restore blood glucose levels

115. A football player conditioning during a summer workout collapses. Which of the following factors aids in determining a sickling collapse?

○ **A.** The collapse occurs early in the workout, and the athlete's core temperature is not greatly elevated.

○ **B.** The collapse is associated with visible, rock-hard muscle contractions.

○ **C.** The athlete's rectally assessed core temperature is above 106°F at collapse.

○ **D.** The collapse is associated with excruciating pain and occurs late in the conditioning session.

○ **E.** The athlete is of African-American descent with a history of hypertension.

116. What is the most appropriate immediate treatment for an athlete with exertional heat illness?

○ **A.** Use ice bags and wet towels to cool the athlete, and then transport to a health-care facility.

○ **B.** Immediately transport the athlete to a health-care facility.

○ **C.** Move the athlete into an air-conditioned room, and provide fluids.

○ **D.** Provide IV fluids along with oral fluids, and transport to a health care facility.

○ **E.** Use full-body ice immersion to cool the athlete, and transport to a health-care facility.

117. Following a yelling and screaming episode, a basketball coach appears confused. He drops the pen from his clipboard, begins to slur his speech, and complains of numbness and weakness on the right side of his face. What conditions should be suspected, and how is this condition best treated?

○ **A.** Cerebrovascular accident; activate emergency medical services, and encourage the coach to remain calm

○ **B.** Myocardial infarction; activate emergency medical services, and provide a low-dose aspirin to the coach

○ **C.** Transient ischemic attack; provide a low-dose aspirin, and instruct him to call his physician

○ **D.** Supraventricular tachycardia; instruct the coach to lie supine and monitor him for shock

○ **E.** Deep vein thrombosis; provide a glucose beverage, and reassess vital signs every 10 minutes

118. A young club lacrosse player sustains a severe blow to the right flank area during a game. He is unable to continue playing, so you conduct an evaluation and treat this athlete. Before releasing this athlete to his parents' care for the evening, what instructions should you provide?

○ **A.** Instruct the parents to encourage the athlete to drink copious amounts of water and other fluids over the next 8 hours.

○ **B.** Instruct the parents to wake the athlete every hour during the night and encourage him to urinate as much as possible.

○ **C.** Instruct the parents to check for hematuria during the athlete's next two to three voiding episodes.

○ **D.** Instruct the parents to check for occult blood in the stool for each bowel movement over the next 3 days.

○ **E.** Instruct the parents to take the athlete immediately to the emergency department at the nearby hospital.

119. A freshmen women's basketball player who is struggling with balancing schoolwork, roommate issues, and the demands of the team arrives at practice in tears. Midway through practice, she walks off the court. When you approach her in the hallway, she is visibly upset and she tells you she just wants to put an end to all the pain and hurting. You are concerned that she may attempt suicide. What is the most appropriate immediate management for this situation?

○ **A.** Notify Public Safety of your suspicions, and request that they transport her to the emergency department for a psychiatric evaluation.

○ **B.** Comfort the athlete, and then escort her to the campus counseling center.

○ **C.** Call the athlete's parents and request that they take her home for treatment.

○ **D.** Ask the coach to get her involved in practice to get her mind off her worries, and make an appointment at the campus counseling center for the next morning.

○ **E.** Ask the coach to assign a teammate to stay with her at all times until you can arrange an appointment with your team physician the next day.

120. A wrestler is visibly uncomfortable and complains of scrotal swelling, abdominal pain, nausea, and unilateral testicular tenderness. He reports no trauma, tells you he woke up with the symptoms this morning, and feels like his left testicle is not in the right place. You ask him to elevate the involved testicle, but no relief is noted. What condition should you suspect, and what is the most appropriate immediate care?

○ **A.** Testicular torsion; refer immediately to the team physician or emergency department

○ **B.** Testicular torsion; apply ice and attempt manual reduction after area is numb

○ **C.** Epididymitis; refer to the team physician for antibiotic prescription

○ **D.** Epididymitis; apply ice and notify coach that he will be unable to practice today

○ **E.** Hydrocele; athlete should be scheduled to see the team physician later in the day

121. A tennis player moves up to the net to volley a hard return but misses and sustains an orbital blowout fracture. How should you best coordinate care for this athlete?

○ **A.** Ask the assistant coach to transport the athlete to the local emergency facility.

○ **B.** Activate emergency medical services, and transport the athlete to the local emergency facility.

○ **C.** Call a local ophthalmologist, and request the next available appointment.

○ **D.** Transport the athlete to the team physician's office for evaluation.

○ **E.** Call a local optometrist to evaluate the athlete immediately.

122. An athlete reports to the athletic training room complaining of nausea, slight fever, mild diarrhea, and nonspecific discomfort located around the umbilicus and the right lower quadrant. The athlete is able to manage pain only by staying in the fetal position. The pain has been steadily increasing over the past several hours. Which acute condition do you suspect, and how should this best be managed?

○ **A.** Acute pelvic inflammatory disease; instruct the athlete to call her gynecologist

○ **B.** Irritable bowel syndrome; schedule the athlete to see the team physician later in the day

○ **C.** Cholecystitis; schedule an appointment with a gastroenterologist for the athlete

○ **D.** Appendicitis; refer the athlete to the local emergency facility

○ **E.** Kidney stone; refer the athlete to the local emergency facility

123. An athlete has sustained a crown fracture. Referral to which health-care provider is most appropriate for this condition?

○ **A.** Oral surgeon

○ **B.** Oral and maxillofacial surgeon

○ **C.** Endodontist

○ **D.** Periodontist

○ **E.** Dentist

124. Which of the following acute conditions would be most appropriately referred to a primary care sports medicine physician for evaluation and treatment?

○ **A.** Nondisplaced nasal fracture

○ **B.** Traumatic hyphema

○ **C.** Avulsed tooth

○ **D.** Scapholunate dislocation

○ **E.** Acute appendicitis

125. You are concerned that an athlete may have a symptomatic ovarian cyst? Referral to which health-care provider is most appropriate for this condition?

○ **A.** Obstetrician

○ **B.** Gynecologist

○ **C.** Gastroenterologist

○ **D.** General surgeon

○ **E.** Internist

126. As the forward on your high school girls soccer team runs toward the goal, she plants her right foot and rotates toward midfield to receive a pass. Suddenly, she is hit by the opposing team's defender. She falls to the ground writhing in pain and holding her knee. On evaluation you suspect the athlete has sustained a severe knee ligament injury. When you share this information with the athlete and her parents, they are upset. What should be the role of the athlete in this situation?

○ **A.** The athlete should know and understand the risks associated with participation in this sport.

○ **B.** The athlete should get the name of the defender who tackled her so she can retaliate in a future match.

○ **C.** The athlete should encourage her parents to pursue litigation against the school to cover medical costs.

○ **D.** The athlete should schedule a meeting with the school's athletic director to discuss coaching and conditioning techniques used by the team coach.

○ **E.** The athlete should encourage her parents to meet with the athletic trainer to determine why she was not screened for this injury during the pre-participation physical examination.

127. After completing a first down, you notice that the running back on your football team is still lying face down on the field as the other players return to the huddle. As you watch from the sideline, a teammate jogs over to the down player before you can get to him. What is the most helpful action this teammate could take to assist in the care of this injured athlete?

○ **A.** Help the player to get up by grabbing his shoulder pads and lifting superiorly so he can get his feet under him.

○ **B.** Take the player by one shoulder and arm and gently roll him over onto his back to improve airflow.

○ **C.** Ask the down player if he is injured and instruct him to lie still until the athletic trainer comes out.

○ **D.** Tell the player that because he cannot move his legs he is probably paralyzed and should not move until the athletic trainer comes out.

○ **E.** Tell his teammates in the huddle to stay where they are because the down player is seriously hurt.

128. Which roles are considered appropriate for an athlete who has sustained an acute ankle sprain?

○ **A.** Comply with nighttime care instructions, report any changes in signs or symptoms, and use prescribed ambulatory aids.

○ **B.** Ensure adequate nutritional intake, apply RICE when at home as instructed, and select therapeutic modalities that best addresses his healing process.

○ **C.** Communicate extent of injury to coaches, schedule an x-ray to rule out a fracture, and increase fluid intake.

○ **D.** Protect the injured ankle, tell weight room staff he refuses to lift, and use an Epsom salt bath.

○ **E.** Take an anti-inflammatory medication, inform teachers he will not be in class, and keep a compression wrap on the ankle.

129. After a big win, the members of your soccer team throw a party where alcohol is served. In the early morning hours, a player calls you because he is unable to wake his teammate. You ask the player what the teammate actually did. What is the role of the player in the immediate care of the ill teammate?

○ **A.** The player should relate information only about the teammate's current condition.

○ **B.** The player should be completely honest about the evening's activities.

○ **C.** The player should avoid providing details without the teammate's permission.

○ **D.** The player should request that the athletic trainer keep all provided information strictly between them.

○ **E.** The player should convene a team meeting to make sure all players provide the same story.

130. An athlete suspects that her teammate has an eating disorder. She has come to you seeking advice on the best way to handle this situation. What should you recommend?

○ **A.** The athlete should meet with the coach to share her concern.

○ **B.** The athlete should call the teammate's parents and share her concerns by providing specific examples.

○ **C.** The athlete should schedule a team meeting without the coaching staff or involved athlete to plan an intervention.

○ **D.** If comfortable, the athlete should share her concern with the teammate who may have the eating disorder.

○ **E.** The athlete should use deception to get her teammate to a meeting at the campus counseling center.

131. A sophomore on your university tennis team confides in you that she is 3 months pregnant. She asks you to abstain from sharing this information with anyone, especially her coach and her parents. What should you tell this athlete?

○ **A.** Encourage the athlete to continue prenatal care with her physician and to wait until she can no longer hide the pregnancy to share the information with others.

○ **B.** Encourage the athlete to keep this information from the coach as long as possible because such information affects her scholarship.

○ **C.** Encourage the athlete to meet with the team physician to determine a plan for participation and then share this plan with her coach and parents.

○ **D.** Encourage the athlete to take care of herself and to let you know if there is anything that she needs.

○ **E.** Encourage the athlete to meet with the coach immediately before he receives the e-mail notice you are obligated to send within 24 hours.

132. As the athletic trainer for a high school football team, you hold a team meeting before the start of each season to discuss emergency management protocols with the players. What is the most important information the athletes should receive?

○ **A.** If an injury occurs, they should not remove any of their equipment until instructed to do so by the athletic trainer.

○ **B.** If an injury occurs, the players should form a protective circle around the injured player and then signal the athletic trainer to come onto the field.

○ **C.** If an injury occurs, every effort should be made to get the injured player to the sideline, where care can be provided.

○ **D.** If an injury occurs, the team captain should signal the ambulance staff to come onto the field to transport the athlete.

○ **E.** If an injury occurs, four players should remain at the athletic trainer's shoulder during the entire evaluation to assist the athletic trainer with transport.

133. A football player incurs an axial load mechanism injury. During your neurological assessment of this athlete, you note bilateral sensation deficits in the lower extremity. The athlete becomes anxious at this time and tells you he cannot feel his legs. What is the most appropriate response to this injured athlete?

○ **A.** Encourage the athlete to relax, and assure him that you are going to get him the best possible care.

○ **B.** Indicate to the athlete that your findings are consistent with his sensations, and tell him he needs to go to the emergency department.

○ **C.** Encourage the athlete to take deep breaths and to try not to think about the seriousness of this injury.

○ **D.** Ask the athlete if his parents are in the stands and how they handle bad news.

○ **E.** Tell the athlete that you have handled other serious neck injuries and that your team physicians are the best in the area, so he will be perfectly fine.

134. You are assisting in the transfer into the waiting ambulance of a lacrosse player who has sustained a non-reducible anterior glenohumeral joint dislocation. The athlete is extremely anxious about the injury and worried that he will never play again. What is the most appropriate response to the injured athlete?

○ **A.** Encourage the athlete to think of other things he can do with his time when his lacrosse career is over.

○ **B.** Tell the athlete that you have seen other athletes come back from this injury very quickly.

○ **C.** Tell the athlete that this injury could be much worse than just a dislocation.

○ **D.** Tell the athlete his neurovascular status was intact and a simple closed reduction should be easily achieved.

○ **E.** Encourage the athlete to relax and not to draw any conclusions until the physicians have completed their evaluation.

135. During a practice session, while running a post pattern, a wide receiver dives for a ball that was underthrown and sustains an axial load when his head hits a metal post just past the sideline. The athlete sustains a cervical fracture/dislocation resulting in paralysis. Later, the quarterback who threw the pass expresses guilt and responsibility for his teammate's paralysis. What is the most appropriate response to this distraught athlete?

○ **A.** Tell the athlete there is no reason for him to feel guilty or responsible. Explain to him that the wide receiver should have been aware of the post and taken actions to avoid it.

○ **B.** Tell the athlete if anyone should feel guilty, it should be the coach who designed a drill that put his teammate at risk. Tell him that you are planning to meet with coaches about designing future drills to avoid a similar situation.

○ **C.** Sympathize with the athlete by telling him you cannot imagine how horrible it must feel to carry that guilt around. Explain to him that he will work through these emotions and that time will help him heal.

○ **D.** Validate his guilt and sense of responsibility. Explain to him that everyone who steps on the field assumes some risk of injury and that when he threw the pass he did not intend for his teammate to be injured.

○ **E.** Tell the athlete that you are unable to discuss the situation with him as there is a lawsuit pending. Recommend he seek professional help by visiting the campus counseling center.

136. A field hockey player sustains a direct blow to her right anterior lower leg from an opponent's stick. Following your evaluation, you are concerned that the athlete may develop acute compartment syndrome. What instructions should you give the athlete before allowing her to return to her dorm for the evening?

○ **A.** Keep her leg elevated, ice the injury as much as possible, and call you if she experiences any numbness, tingling, or increased pain overnight.

○ **B.** Keep the compression wrap on until she returns for reevaluation the next morning, and take ibuprofen as needed for pain.

○ **C.** Use crutches if walking is painful, soak in a hot bath with Epsom salt, and wear a neoprene compression sleeve while sleeping.

○ **D.** Use the transcutaneous electrical nerve stimulation unit as instructed for pain control, take acetaminophen only as needed for pain, and go to the emergency department if these two modalities do not manage her pain.

○ **E.** Schedule an appointment with the massage therapist, use topical thermal cream to relieve pain and spasm, and call the athletic trainer if she experiences an increase in symptoms.

137. What is the consequence of failing to have an emergency action plan?

○ **A.** Fails to comply with the NATA Code of Ethics

○ **B.** May breach the institution's legal responsibility to conduct safe athletic programs

○ **C.** Potentially invalidates assumption of risk waiver

○ **D.** Extends the statute of limitations for each athletic program

○ **E.** Negates any protections provided by governmental immunity

138. Which of the following best describes a catastrophic incident?

○ **A.** An injury that is so severe that activities of daily living are permanently compromised

○ **B.** An injury that results in the death or paralysis of an athlete

○ **C.** An injury that ends a career

○ **D.** An injury that results in legal ramifications

○ **E.** An injury that permanently compromises the central nervous system

139. Which individuals would comprise the Catastrophic Injury Management Team at a college or university?

○ **A.** Emergency medical technician, head athletic trainer, and the university lawyer

○ **B.** Director of public safety, director of campus health center, and team coach

○ **C.** Director of student housing, university provost, and team physician

○ **D.** Athletic administrator, school media liaison, and director of campus counseling center

○ **E.** University president, university chaplain, and team sports psychologist

140. What is the role of the athletic trainer when a catastrophic injury occurs during an out-of-state match?

○ **A.** Notify the athletic director of the incident, and identify the person most qualified to remain with the athlete when the team returns to campus.

○ **B.** Notify the athlete's parents, transfer care of the team to the host athletic trainer, and accompany the athlete to the hospital.

○ **C.** Request that officials cancel the remainder of the game to allow staff and teammates to accompany the athlete to the hospital.

○ **D.** Notify the university president of the incident and request mobilization of the Catastrophic Injury Management Team.

○ **E.** Provide media relations with accurate information for press release, and assist the athlete's parents with flight and travel plans.

141. What information should be provided to the 911 dispatcher by an athletic trainer?

○ **A.** Time the injury occurred, directions to the injury site, and name of your team physician

○ **B.** Exact location of the emergency, location of the person reporting the emergency, and summary of last vital signs taken

○ **C.** Description of the emergency, level of consciousness of the injured athlete, and name of injured athlete's emergency contact person

○ **D.** Telephone number from which you are calling, name of person who will meet the ambulance, and qualifications of person providing care

○ **E.** Location of the injured athlete, current care being rendered, and the athletic trainer's name and position

142. When creating your emergency action plan, what information should be included on each facility map?

○ **A.** Gates, windows, and fire escapes

○ **B.** Driveways, doors, and telephone locations

○ **C.** Elevators, fire extinguishers, and stairwells

○ **D.** Fire doors, roof access, and ramps

○ **E.** Automated doors, sprinkler locations, and service elevators

143. What is the purpose of writing a chronology of events following a catastrophic injury?

○ **A.** It assists the injured party's legal team in developing legal action against the medical staff and the institution.

○ **B.** It allows the management team to critique the process while providing a basis for reviewing the efficacy of the procedures.

○ **C.** It assists the counseling team by providing a comprehensive background of events from which they can formulate a care plan.

○ **D.** It aids the administration in making decisions regarding the employment status of involved personnel.

○ **E.** It forms a document that can be provided to the media via the institution's Web site.

144. While providing medical coverage at a high school football game, the athletic trainer is called onto the field to attend to a downed athlete. During the evaluation, a physician comes onto the field from the stands and takes over. What must the athletic trainer do in this situation?

○ **A.** The athletic trainer must allow the physician to assume care.

○ **B.** The athletic trainer must inform the physician that the physician is acting outside the scope of practice.

○ **C.** The athletic trainer must immediately summon security to remove the physician.

○ **D.** The athletic trainer must return to the sideline.

○ **E.** The athletic trainer must request the athletic director to explain the role of the athletic trainer to the physician.

145. A gymnast dismounting into a pit misses the pit and sustains a severe head injury. The athletic trainer activates emergency medical services (EMS), but the arrival of the ambulance is delayed because it has difficulty finding the gymnastics room in the athletic complex. This delay results in irreversible brain damage to the gymnast. Which component of the emergency action plan (EAP) was poorly executed?

○ **A.** Identifying qualified personnel

○ **B.** Ensuring presence of emergency care equipment

○ **C.** Assignment of duties and responsibilities

○ **D.** Activation of EMS

○ **E.** Writing a facility-specific EAP

Answers for Domain III: Immediate Care

Role A: Employ life-saving techniques through the use of standard emergency procedures in order to reduce morbidity and the incidence of mortality.

1. C
2. C
3. D
4. B
5. C
6. C
7. B
8. B
9. D
10. E
11. D
12. A
13. A
14. B
15. C
16. D
17. C
18. E
19. B
20. A
21. A
22. A
23. E
24. B
25. D
26. C
27. B
28. A
29. A
30. C
31. E
32. A
33. B
34. E
35. E
36. A
37. C
38. D
39. B
40. C
41. A
42. B
43. A
44. E
45. A

Role B: Prevent exacerbation of non–life-threatening condition(s) through the use of standard procedures in order to reduce morbidity.

46. B
47. C
48. C
49. E
50. E
51. E
52. C
53. A
54. B
55. D
56. B
57. B
58. C
59. D
60. A
61. A
62. B
63. E
64. C
65. D
66. A
67. A
68. E
69. B
70. B

71. A

72. D

73. C

74. C

75. B

76. E

77. A

78. A

79. C

80. D

81. B

82. E

83. C

84. C

85. A

86. A

87. B

88. E

89. C

90. A

91. A

Role C: Facilitate the timely transfer of care for conditions beyond the scope of practice of the athletic trainer by implementing appropriate referral strategies to stabilize and/or prevent exacerbation of the condition(s).

92. E

93. A

94. D

95. D

96. D

97. A

98. A

99. B

100. E

101. B

102. A

103. A

104. C

105. D

106. B

107. A

108. B

109. C

110. A

111. E

112. B

113. C

114. B

115. A

116. E

117. A

118. C

119. B

120. A

121. B

122. D

123. E

124. A

125. B

Role D: Direct the appropriate patient(s) in standard immediate care procedures using formal and informal methods to facilitate immediate care.

126. A

127. C

128. A

129. B

130. D

131. C

132. A

133. A

134. E

135. D

136. A

Role E: Execute the established emergency action plan using effective communication and administrative practices to facilitate efficient immediate care.

137. B

138. A

139. D

140. A

141. E

142. B

143. B

144. A

145. C

Domain IV: Treatment, Rehabilitation, and Reconditioning

1. Prior to applying joint mobilization techniques, the clinician must consider the relative position of the articulating joint surfaces. In what anatomical position is the glenohumeral joint considered to be in a close-packed position?

○ **A.** The humerus is in anatomical position.

○ **B.** The humerus is abducted to 90° and externally rotated.

○ **C.** The humerus is abducted to 90° and internally rotated.

○ **D.** The humerus is flexed to 180° and externally rotated.

○ **E.** The humerus is flexed to 180° and internally rotated

2. Prior to applying joint mobilization for the talocrural joint, the joint must be placed in the resting position. What best defines the resting position for this joint?

○ **A.** 10° of plantar flexion

○ **B.** 10° of dorsiflexion

○ **C.** Full dorsiflexion

○ **D.** Full plantar flexion

○ **E.** 20° of plantar flexion

3. To use joint mobilization to increase an athlete's glenohumeral abduction, in which direction should you perform the glides?

○ **A.** Glide the glenoid in an inferior direction.

○ **B.** Glide the humerus in a superior direction.

○ **C.** Glide the humerus in an inferior direction.

○ **D.** Glide the glenoid and clavicle superiorly.

○ **E.** Glide the humerus anteriorly.

4. To improve an athlete's knee extension, limited due to pain and spasm at the end of the range, you perform joint mobilization on the tibiofemoral joint. Which of the following application techniques is most appropriate for treating this athlete?

○ **A.** Grade III anterior tibial glide with the knee in 25° of flexion

○ **B.** Grade IV anterior tibial glide with the knee in 20° of flexion

○ **C.** Grade II anterior femoral glide with the knee in 25° of flexion

○ **D.** Grade III posterior tibial glide with the knee in 90° of flexion

○ **E.** Grade II posterior femoral glide with the knee in 30° of flexion

5. A middle-aged recreational softball player has been diagnosed with a lumbar disc injury. On which types of therapeutic exercises should your initial rehabilitation program focus?

○ **A.** Bent knee sit-ups to increase abdominal strength

○ **B.** Proprioceptive neuromuscular facilitation to increase hamstring flexibility normal posture

○ **C.** Resistive hamstring curls to increase hamstring strength

○ **D.** Lumbar flexion exercises to increase strength and core stabilization

○ **E.** Lumbar extension exercises to reduce protrusion and restore normal posture

6. What is the role of active assistive exercises in a comprehensive rehabilitation program?

○ **A.** To promote strengthening when the athlete can work only against resistance through a partial range of motion

○ **B.** To increase strength when the athlete can produce maximum force against a resistance through the full range of motion

○ **C.** To improve joint kinesthesia when the athlete can move through the full range of motion without resistance

○ **D.** To improve range of motion when the athlete lacks more than 50% of joint range of motion compared with the uninvolved side

○ **E.** To improve range of motion when the strength of muscles is not sufficient to move the joint through a full unrestricted range of motion

7. While completing a rehabilitation program, a baseball player performs resistive glenohumeral internal rotation exercises using an exercise band. As the athlete returns to the start position of the exercise and allows the exercise band to recoil, which muscle is the athlete using?

○ **A.** Subscapularis

○ **B.** Deltoid

○ **C.** Supraspinatus

○ **D.** Infraspinatus

○ **E.** Biceps brachii

8. An Amateur Athletic Union basketball player is completing a rehabilitation program to address his bilateral Osgood-Schlatter disease. What exercises should this athlete avoid because they will exacerbate his symptoms?

○ **A.** Resisted terminal knee extension

○ **B.** Closed kinetic chain knee flexion beyond 90° of flexion

○ **C.** Prone full-range hamstring curls

○ **D.** Quadriceps setting

○ **E.** Proprioceptive neuromuscular facilitation stretching

9. On what should the initial phase of a rehabilitation program focus?

○ **A.** Restoring passive range of motion

○ **C.** Restoring active range of motion

○ **C.** Protecting injured tissues

○ **D.** Facilitating muscular strength

○ **E.** Restoring proprioceptive function

10. For an athlete to safely resume full sport participation and normal pre-injury activities, in what order should the specific parameters of therapeutic rehabilitation programs be completed?

○ **A.** Range of motion and muscular strength; flexibility and functional progression; coordination and agility

○ **B.** Isometric exercises and flexibility; proprioception and coordination; functional progression and agility

○ **C.** Active assistive exercises and proprioception; coordination and muscular strength; muscular endurance and functional activities

○ **D.** Muscular strength and endurance; proprioception and range of motion; isokinetic exercises and cardiovascular conditioning

○ **E.** Flexibility and range of motion; muscular strength and endurance; proprioception, coordination, and agility

11. You are developing a hand rehabilitation program for a professional billiards player. Which of the following therapeutic exercises would most effectively strengthen the palmar and dorsal interosseous muscles?

○ **A.** Abduction/flexion of the digits using a resistance web

○ **B.** Abduction/adduction of the digits using resistance provided by rubber bands

○ **C.** Wrist flexion exercises holding a dumbbell weight

○ **D.** Wrist extension exercises using resistance provided by an exercise band

○ **E.** Extension of the digits using resistance provided by surgical tubing

12. In setting a goal for lower-extremity rehabilitation, what is the accepted relationship between the quadriceps and hamstring muscle groups?

○ **A.** The hamstrings should be equally strong.

○ **B.** The hamstrings should be more flexible than the quadriceps.

○ **C.** The hamstrings should demonstrate more proprioception than the quadriceps.

○ **D.** The hamstrings should be two-thirds as strong as the quadriceps.

○ **E.** The hamstrings should demonstrate an endurance factor 1.5 times that of the quadriceps.

13. When rehabilitating an athlete with an excessive Q-angle who is suffering from a laterally subluxating patella, the strength and neuromuscular control of which muscle should be emphasized?

○ **A.** Tensor fascia latae

○ **B.** Gracilis

○ **C.** Rectus femoris

○ **D.** Semimembranosus

○ **E.** Vastus medialis oblique

14. Which of the following exercises demonstrates the appropriate application of cryokinetics?

○ **A.** The athlete performs active pain-free dorsiflexion exercises immediately following immersion of the ankle in ice water until it is numb.

○ **B.** The athlete performs passive Achilles tendon stretching while immersed in an ice-water bath.

○ **C.** The athlete performs resisted inversion and eversion exercises immediately following ice massage.

○ **D.** The athlete performs therapist-assisted joint mobilization exercises and then immerses the ankle in ice water to control the pain.

○ **E.** The athlete performs active assisted inversion and dorsiflexion exercises through the complete range of motion regardless of pain while immersed in an ice-water bath.

15. A women's basketball player has a history of lateral ankle sprains resulting in ligamentous laxity. On which muscles should a program to reestablish proprioception and neuromuscular control focus?

○ **A.** Tibialis anterior and tibialis posterior

○ **B.** Tibialis anterior and flexor hallucis longus

○ **C.** Gastrocnemius and tibialis posterior

○ **D.** Peroneus longus and peroneus brevis

○ **E.** Extensor hallucis longus and posterior tibialis

16. Which of the following exercises should be avoided during the initial stages of a rehabilitation program for an athlete with an acute subluxation of the glenohumeral joint?

○ **A.** Rhythmic stabilization

○ **B.** Isometric muscle strengthening

○ **C.** Passive range of motion within a nonprovocative range

○ **D.** Joint mobilization

○ **E.** Gentle active range of motion

17. Which of the following is a major advantage of isokinetic resistance exercise for rehabilitating an injured athlete?

○ **A.** A constant amount of resistance delivered through the full range of motion

○ **B.** The ability to work through a full unrestricted range of motion

○ **C.** Enhanced hyperplasia of muscle fibers compared with other types of resistance training

○ **D.** Decreased lactic acid accumulation during exercise bout

○ **E.** The safety of the exercise because the resistance will not exceed the amount of force that can be produced

18. Following a knee injury, an athlete is unable to move from a seated to a standing position in the usual efficient and pain-free manner. Which of the following elements of the disablement model is this athlete exhibiting?

○ **A.** Functional limitation

○ **B.** Impairment

○ **C.** Pathology

○ **D.** Disability

○ **E.** Kinesthetic dysfunction

19. A soccer player is recovering from a knee ligamentous injury. At this point in his rehabilitation protocol, you initiate on-field cone drills with a ball. In which phase of the healing process is this athlete?

○ **A.** Remodeling phase

○ **B.** Repair phase

○ **C.** Acute inflammatory phase

○ **D.** Subacute inflammatory phase

○ **E.** Pre-repair phase

20. Following an acute quadriceps contusion, an athlete demonstrates the following: swelling has plateaued completely; the area is still tender to the touch; and active and passive motions are less painful. Which phase of the healing process is most associated with this presentation?

○ **A.** Acute inflammatory

○ **B.** Repair

○ **C.** Pre-remodeling

○ **D.** Remodeling

○ **E.** Functional

21. An athlete has an acute ulnar collateral ligament injury. Which of the following physiological responses is most associated with the inflammatory phase of the healing process?

○ **A.** Histamines are released from the leukocytes causing vasodilation and decreased cell permeability.

○ **B.** Cytokines are responsible for margination of the leukocytes along the cell walls.

○ **C.** Fibroblasts synthesize an intercellular matrix.

○ **D.** Leukocytes phagocytize most of the foreign debris in the area subsequent to clot formation.

○ **E.** Granulation tissue occurs with the breakdown of the fibrin clot.

22. You are progressing an athlete who is recovering from a femoral stress fracture by transitioning him from non–weight-bearing activities to partial weight-bearing activities. The basis of your progression is to place controlled stresses on the bone and soft tissue, causing them to remodel and realign along the lines of tensile force. Which principle of rehabilitation are you applying to this athlete?

○ **A.** Wolff's law

○ **B.** SAID principle

○ **C.** Watkins' progression

○ **D.** Oxford technique

○ **E.** DAPRE principle

23. An athlete is completing a leg extension exercise as part of a rehabilitation program for his knee injury. In the first set, he performs 10 repetitions at 50% of working weight. In the second set, he performs six repetitions at 75% of working weight. In the third set, he performs four repetitions at 100% of working weight. Based on his performance in the third set, he performs as many repetitions as possible in the fourth set at a weight that is 5 lb more than the working weight. Which of the following commonly used progressive overload systems is the athlete employing?

○ **A.** MacQueen's technique

○ **B.** DeLorme's system

○ **C.** DAPRE technique

○ **D.** Watkins' system

○ **E.** Oxford technique

24. An athlete is completing a core stabilization program. You instruct the athlete to complete three sets of 10 pelvic tilts with a 10-second hold and 45 seconds between sets. How would you properly note the 45-second period in your documentation of the rehabilitation session?

○ **A.** Rest period: 45 sec

○ **B.** Recovery period: 45 sec

○ **C.** Total rest time: 90 sec

○ **D.** Refractory period: 45 sec

○ **E.** Relaxation period: 45 sec

25. Which of the following statements best describes an athlete's macrocycle?

○ **A.** Preseason training period

○ **B.** Complete training period

○ **C.** Transition period

○ **D.** Competition season

○ **E.** Strength phase

26. During a depth jump drill, the athletic trainer encourages the athlete to minimize the time his feet are in contract with the floor. The athletic trainer is encouraging minimization of which plyometric exercise phase?

○ **A.** Eccentric

○ **B.** Concentric

○ **C.** Pre-load

○ **D.** Absorption

○ **E.** Amortization

27. In which population is the use of maximal isometric contractions for strength gains contraindicated?

○ **A.** A college-age football player with hypertension

○ **B.** A 14-year-old baseball pitcher with open epiphyseal plates

○ **C.** A 65-year-old golfer with history of low back pain

○ **D.** A 35-year-old tennis player with type 1 diabetes

○ **E.** A college-age women's basketball player with sickle cell trait

28. The design of which type of resistance equipment aims at achieving accommodating resistance?

○ **A.** Pulley-based machines such as the Universal weight system

○ **B.** Functional movement equipment such as surgical tubing or exercise bands

○ **C.** Attenuable polymer band-based equipment such as Bowflex

○ **D.** Cam-based machines such as Nautilus

○ **E.** Freely moveable weights and iron plates such as dumbbells and barbells

29. A physician's rehabilitation prescription states the following: Dx: 4wks s/p ACL recon US 100% qod. LE: CKC exs qd. Which of the following best illustrates correct application of the prescription?

○ **A.** The athlete should receive ultrasound at 100% intensity every day and complete concentric knee contractions every day.

○ **B.** The athlete should receive continuous ultrasound every other day and complete mini-squat exercises every day.

○ **C.** The athlete should receive ultrasound before each rehabilitation session and complete terminal knee extensions every other day.

○ **D.** The athlete should complete concentric knee co-contractions while receiving continuous ultrasound daily.

○ **E.** The athlete should receive 100% intensity ultrasound every other day and complete BAPS board exercises twice a day for the next 4 weeks.

30. Which of the following statements most accurately reflects the adverse effects of immobilization on body systems and tissues?

○ **A.** Joints demonstrate an increased production of lubricating fluids.

○ **B.** Bones increase in stiffness and lose pliability proportionally to time immobilized.

○ **C.** Resting heart rate increases approximately ½ beat per minute each day of immobilization.

○ **D.** Motor nerves become hypersensitive, increasing recruitment and stimulation of muscle fibers.

○ **E.** With extended immobilization, fast-twitch muscle fibers develop slow-twitch muscle fiber characteristics.

31. A physician's rehabilitation protocol recommends that at this stage of the athlete's rehabilitation program, you begin upper-extremity closed kinetic chain exercises. Which of the following exercises is considered a closed kinetic chain exercise?

○ **A.** Catching a ball tossed into a pitch-back machine or vertical trampoline

○ **B.** Internal and external rotation with exercise bands

○ **C.** Supine medicine ball toss and catch

○ **D.** Push-up on a Swiss ball

○ **E.** Supine rhythmic stabilization

32. As the athletic trainer at a small, rural high school, your budget does not provide for heart rate monitors. Which of the following would best assist you in ensuring that an athlete who is completing a cardiovascular training program on a bicycle is staying within the aerobic training zone?

○ **A.** Rating of perceived exertion

○ **B.** Sweat rate

○ **C.** Fluid consumption

○ **D.** Peak flow

○ **E.** Respiratory exchange ratio

33. During your evaluation before initiating a rehabilitation program for a baseball player's shoulder, you determine an internal rotation deficit of the throwing shoulder. What anatomic factor is most likely limiting this athlete's flexibility?

○ **A.** Bony structure

○ **B.** Connective tissue

○ **C.** Fat

○ **D.** Skin

○ **E.** Cartilage

34. An athletic trainer is using a contract-relax proprioceptive neuromuscular facilitation stretching technique to improve flexibility of an athlete's hamstrings. The hip is passively moved into flexion, and then the athlete is asked to contract the hamstrings against resistance provided by the athletic trainer. In this example, what role are the hamstrings playing?

○ **A.** Antagonist

○ **B.** Agonist

○ **C.** Synergist

○ **D.** Initiator

○ **E.** Inhibitor

35. An athletic trainer is using proprioceptive neuromuscular facilitation (PNF) stretching techniques to improve an athlete's glenohumeral joint motion. The athletic trainer positions the athlete in a supine position with the glenohumeral joint in 90° of abduction and the elbow flexed to 90°. The athlete performs a concentric contraction of the internal rotators until the end of the range is reached. The athlete then performs an isometric contraction of the external rotators. This is followed by relaxation of the shoulder musculature and then a contraction of the internal rotators concentrically to achieve a stretch. Which of the following PNF techniques is being employed?

○ **A.** Slow reversal-hold-relax technique to increase glenohumeral external rotation

○ **B.** Slow reversal-hold-relax technique to increase glenohumeral internal rotation

○ **C.** Contract-relax technique to increase glenohumeral internal rotation

○ **D.** Contract-relax technique to increase glenohumeral external rotation

○ **E.** Hold-relax technique to increase glenohumeral internal rotation

36. An athlete is completing a contract-relax proprioceptive neuromuscular facilitation stretching technique. The athlete is instructed to push maximally against the therapist's resistance for at least 10 seconds and then relax while the therapist passively stretches further into the range. What neurophysiological basis of stretching is employed during the "push" phase of this technique?

○ **A.** Contraction of the agonist results in a reflex relaxation of the antagonist via reciprocal inhibition.

○ **B.** Changes in length and tension of the muscle result in muscle relaxation via the stretch reflex.

○ **C.** Increased length in the muscle stimulates the muscle spindles, resulting in relaxation via autogenic inhibition.

○ **D.** Contraction of the antagonist results in a reflex relaxation of the agonist via reciprocal inhibition.

○ **E.** Increased tension in the muscle stimulates the Golgi tendon organ, resulting in relaxation via autogenic inhibition.

37. When incorporating neuromuscular training into a rehabilitation protocol, which of the following exercises would be considered a multiplanar exercise for the lower extremity?

○ **A.** Mini-squats on a foam roller

○ **B.** Hip adduction using an exercise band for resistance

○ **C.** Forward step-up onto an unstable surface

○ **D.** Carioca drill through an agility ladder

○ **E.** Backward walking on an incline treadmill

38. What three systems contribute to the body's ability to maintain equilibrium by controlling the body's center of gravity over its base of support?

○ **A.** Cerebellar response, sensory, and visual

○ **B.** Auditory, circulatory, and integumentary

○ **C.** Vestibular, oculomotor, and somatosensory

○ **D.** Vestibulocochlear, neuromuscular, and spinal accessory

○ **E.** Reflex arc, mechanoreceptor, and kinesthetic

39. An athlete with a functionally unstable ankle is completing a neuromuscular control rehabilitation program. The athlete has completed the bilateral balancing exercises on an unstable surface with visual input. Which of the following is most appropriate to follow this exercise in the progression?

○ **A.** Two-foot balance on a foam pad with eyes closed

○ **B.** One-foot balance on a rocker board with eyes open

○ **C.** One-foot balance on hard floor with eyes closed

○ **D.** One-foot balance on hard floor with eyes open and therapist providing perturbation

○ **E.** Two-foot balance on a foam pad with eyes closed and therapist providing perturbation

40. Which of the following best defines hysteresis as it relates to stretching?

○ **A.** The inability of tissue to completely respond to successive load application forces, resulting in tissue elongation

○ **B.** The ability of tissue to return to its normal length following application of successive load forces

○ **C.** The inability of tissue to resist a load, resulting in the tissue's yield point being exceeded

○ **D.** The ability of tissue to receive and respond to successive stimuli, resulting in tissue and joint stabilization

○ **E.** The inability of tissue mechanoreceptors to sense and respond to changes in tissue length and tension

41. Which therapeutic technique would best be used in the treatment of joint malalignments and complex kinetic chain dysfunction?

○ **A.** Proprioceptive neuromuscular facilitation

○ **B.** Joint mobilization techniques

○ **C.** Core stabilization training

○ **D.** Continuous passive motion

○ **E.** Muscle energy techniques

42. During a phase of an athlete's rehabilitation program, you are emphasizing strength gains for the lower extremity. The athlete is completing a leg press exercise. Which of the following exercise protocols is most effective in increasing muscular strength?

○ **A.** 6 to 12 repetitions at a weight that is 70% to 90% of his one rep max

○ **B.** 20 repetitions at a weight that is 70% of his one rep max

○ **C.** Three to nine repetitions at a weight that is at least 90% of his one rep max

○ **D.** 12 to 15 repetitions at a weight that is 66% of his one rep max

○ **E.** 10 repetitions at a weight that is 80% of his one rep max

43. A wheelchair basketball athlete has been diagnosed with acute carpal tunnel syndrome. In your initial rehabilitation evaluation, how should you best objectively assess strength of the involved musculature?

○ **A.** Use a pinch dynamometer to assess strength of the thumb-finger flexion.

○ **B.** Use a grip dynamometer to assess strength of finger extensors.

○ **C.** Use a handheld dynamometer to assess strength of the wrist flexors.

○ **D.** Use a manual muscle test to assess the strength of the flexor digitorum supercilia and flexor digitorum profundus.

○ **E.** Use an isokinetic dynamometer to assess the strength of the wrist flexors concentrically and eccentrically.

44. A tennis player is in the late stages of rehabilitation for impingement syndrome and has returned to practice drills. The player reports feeling weakness at ball contact during the serve. Which of the following rehabilitation exercises would be most appropriate to address this weakness?

○ **A.** D1 proprioceptive neuromuscular facilitation pattern emphasizing the flexion portion of the pattern

○ **B.** D2 proprioceptive neuromuscular facilitation pattern emphasizing the extension portion of the pattern

○ **C.** Internal and external rotation with an exercise band at 90° of shoulder abduction

○ **D.** Closed kinetic chain weight shifting on a Swiss ball

○ **E.** Closed kinetic chain multiplanar slide board exercises

45. You are completing a D2 lower extremity proprioceptive neuromuscular facilitation strengthening pattern moving into flexion. As the athlete reaches the end of the pattern, what verbal cues should you provide?

○ **A.** Pull the top of your foot toward your nose, push your foot out against my hand, and extend your toes.

○ **B.** Push the gas pedal, turn your foot in against my hand, and curl your toes.

○ **C.** Pull the top of your foot toward your nose, turn the bottom of your foot inward against my hand, and extend your toes.

○ **D.** Push the gas pedal, turn your foot out against my hand, and curl your toes.

○ **E.** Push the gas pedal, turn your foot out against my hand, and extend your toes.

46. An athlete has undergone anterior cruciate ligament reconstruction and is progressing to active concentric quadriceps contractions by using an isokinetic dynamometer. Which of the following parameters should be employed to protect the healing graft?

○ **A.** Flexion stop should be set at 100 degrees of knee flexion, speeds of 180 to 300 degrees/sec should be used, and the tibial pad should be placed mid-shaft.

○ **B.** Extension stop should be set at 10 degrees of knee flexion, speeds of 60 to 90 degrees/sec should be used, and the tibial pad should be placed in a proximal position.

○ **C.** Flexion stop should be set at 90 degrees of knee flexion, speeds of 60 to 90 degrees/sec should be used, and the tibial pad should be placed in a distal position.

○ **D.** Extension stop should be set below 30 degrees of knee flexion, speeds of 180 to 300 degrees/sec should be used, and the tibial pad should be placed in a proximal position.

○ **E.** Extension stop should be set at the point of pain-free motion, speeds of 180 to 300 degrees/sec should be used, and the tibial pad should be placed mid-shaft.

47. When initiating a lower extremity plyometric training program during the rehabilitation of an athlete with patellar tendonitis, which of the following exercises should be completed in the first week of the program?

○ **A.** Two-legged one-box side jump

○ **B.** Two-legged side-to-side line jumping

○ **C.** Single-leg plyo leg press

○ **D.** Lateral step-overs

○ **E.** Side-to-side bounding

48. You are rehabilitating a basketball player following an anterior cruciate ligament reconstruction. You have just initiated plyometric training in preparation for the season, which is 6 weeks away. Which of the following plyometric training schedules will be most effective in preparing this athlete for the upcoming season?

○ **A.** One session per day with at least 48 hours between sessions

○ **B.** Two sessions per day with at least 48 hours between sessions

○ **C.** One session per day with 24 hours between the first two sessions and 48 hours between the next two sessions

○ **D.** Two sessions per day with at least 24 hours between sessions

○ **E.** One session per day with 48 hours between the first two sessions and 24 hours between the next two sessions

49. You are treating a swimmer for impingement syndrome. When initiating the rehabilitation program, the flexibility of which muscle groups should be assessed and emphasized because they are prone to develop tightness?

○ **A.** Rhomboids and levator scapulae

○ **B.** Serratus anterior and supraspinatus

○ **C.** Sternocleidomastoid and teres minor

○ **D.** Upper trapezius and triceps

○ **E.** Pectoralis minor and scalenes

50. You are initiating a comprehensive core stabilization program for an athlete with chronic low back pain attributed to muscle imbalances and overall kinetic chain dysfunction. A comprehensive evaluation has been conducted on this athlete. Which of the following best describes the suggested guidelines for this core stabilization program?

○ **A.** The program should emphasize dynamic stabilization while minimizing force production and force reduction.

○ **B.** Program exercises should progress from high forces to low forces as well as specific to general.

○ **C.** The program should begin in the most challenging environment the athlete can control.

○ **D.** Program variables of range of motion and body position should be altered while the amount of control and speed of execution should remain constant.

○ **E.** The quantity of exercises the athlete can complete should be considered over the quality of the exercises when progressing the athlete.

51. You are treating an athlete who is postoperative for a metal screw placement in the shoulder. Your primary treatment goal is to increase blood flow to the tissue to assist in increasing tissue extensibility. Which of the following available modalities would be contraindicated for the athlete?

○ **A.** Short-wave diathermy

○ **B.** Hydrocollator packs

○ **C.** Ultrasound

○ **D.** Muscle stimulation

○ **E.** Paraffin bath

52. You have chosen to use ultrasound treatment to increase tissue temperature and increase tissue extensibility on an athlete with jumper's knee. To most effectively reach the target tissue, which treatment parameters should be selected?

○ **A.** Select a 20% duty cycle, 1-MHz frequency, and a ketoprofen-based coupling medium.

○ **B.** Select a 50% duty cycle, 2-w/cm² frequency, and a bladder coupling medium.

○ **C.** Select a 75% duty cycle, 1.5-w/cm² frequency, and an underwater coupling medium.

○ **D.** Select a 100% duty cycle, 1-MHz frequency, and a direct coupling medium.

○ **E.** Select a 100% duty cycle, 3-MHz frequency, and a gel-based coupling medium.

53. During diathermy application, which mechanism of heat transfer results in an increase in body tissue temperature?

○ **A.** Radiation

○ **B.** Polarization

○ **C.** Conversion

○ **D.** Convection

○ **E.** Conduction.

54. An athletic trainer is treating an athlete with electrical stimulation by applying the following treatment protocol: bipolar electrode placement, frequency set at 80 to 150 pps, and intensity set at sensory-level stimulation. By which theory of pain management is the athletic trainer attempting to control this athlete's pain?

○ **A.** Ascending A-Beta input

○ **B.** Descending A-Delta and C-fiber input

○ **C.** Beta-endorphin release

○ **D.** Motor pain modulation

○ **E.** Noxious pain modulation

55. You are testing an athlete to determine the minimal erythemal dose prior to performing an ultraviolet treatment. You have followed the five-window test protocol. When the athlete returns 24 hours later, the 75-second window is faintly erythematous. Based on your baseline testing, what are the first and second treatment exposure times that should occur on consecutive days?

○ **A.** 75 seconds and 101 seconds, respectively

○ **B.** 75 seconds and 75 seconds, respectively

○ **C.** 75 seconds and 150 seconds, respectively

○ **D.** 37 seconds and 75 seconds, respectively

○ **E.** 37 seconds and 37 seconds, respectively

56. You are testing an athlete to determine minimal erythemal dose prior to performing an ultraviolet treatment. You have followed the five-window test protocol. When the athlete returns 24 hours post exposure, the 45-, 60-, and 75-second windows are erythematous. At 48 hours post exposure, the 60- and 75-second windows are erythematous, and at 72 hours post exposure, the 75-second window is erythematous. Which of the following represents a first-degree erythemal dose?

○ **A.** 30 seconds

○ **B.** 45 seconds

○ **C.** 60 seconds

○ **D.** 75 seconds

○ **E.** 150 seconds

57. Which of the following are commonly accepted physiological responses to superficial heat application?

○ **A.** Decreased viscosity, increased tissue elasticity, and decreased inflammation

○ **B.** Anesthetic effects, increased phagocytosis, and increased lymphatic drainage

○ **C.** Analgesia, increased metabolic activity, and increased inflammation

○ **D.** Decreased antibodies, increased axon reflex, and decreased muscle spasm

○ **E.** Increased capillary permeability, increased edema formation, and decreased metabolic wastes

58. For which of the following athletes would massage be contraindicated?

○ **A.** An athlete with chronic biceps tendonitis who presents with limited range of motion

○ **B.** An athlete who is 2 weeks status post anterior cruciate ligament reconstruction who presents with normally healing scar tissue

○ **C.** An athlete who is 2 days post forearm cast removal who presents with muscle atrophy

○ **D.** An athlete with chronic bilateral paraspinal muscle spasm secondary to a partially herniated vertebral disc

○ **E.** An athlete who is 4 days status post second-degree ankle sprain who presents with tight, red, shiny skin

59. Which nonthermal effect of ultrasound is most associated with low-frequency, high-intensity sound waves and is believed to result in tissue damage?

○ **A.** Stable cavitation

○ **B.** Unstable cavitation

○ **C.** Stable acoustical streaming

○ **D.** Unstable acoustical streaming

○ **E.** Acoustical microstreaming

60. When equipment manufacturers of electrical stimulation units determine preset pulse durations, they are based on the phase duration required to depolarize a nerve fiber when the amplitude is two times rheobase. What is the term associated with this phase duration?

○ **A.** Chronaxie

○ **B.** Motor depolarization potential

○ **C.** Resting potential

○ **D.** Electropiezo activity

○ **E.** Interpulse interval

61. In which of the following ways does cold application best address the inflammatory phase of the healing process?

○ **A.** Decreases swelling in the injured area

○ **B.** Decreases the cell's metabolic need for oxygen

○ **C.** Decreases the viscosity of fluids in the injured area

○ **D.** Decreases the amount of hemorrhage that occurs

○ **E.** Decreases the extensibility of associated tissues to enhance stability

62. For which of the following treatment goals is transcutaneous electrical nerve stimulation an acceptable modality?

○ **A.** Enhance movement from inflammatory to repair phase of healing

○ **B.** Decrease pitting edema and enhance lymphatic drainage

○ **C.** Manage athlete's chronic pain

○ **D.** Minimize excess scar-tissue formation

○ **E.** Increase range of motion and tissue extensibility

63. Which of the following responses are associated with the reflexive effects of therapeutic massage?

○ **A.** Elimination of toxins, sedation, and shift in acid-base equilibrium of blood

○ **B.** Increased capillary permeability, pain control, and no significant alterations in general metabolism

○ **C.** Decreased cellular metabolism, increased dispersion of waste products, and release of B-endorphins and enkephalins

○ **D.** Increased fibroplasia, increase in blood volume and blood flow, and increase in tissue temperature

○ **E.** Central pooling of blood, decreased resting heart rate, and retardation of muscle atrophy

64. Which of the following theories of pain management is most likely employed when an athletic trainer utilizes massage to stimulate myofascial trigger points?

○ **A.** Gate control theory

○ **B.** Gate control theory with endogenous opioid analogue

○ **C.** Central biasing

○ **D.** Cognitive influence

○ **E.** B-endorphin and enkephalin release

65. Following a superficial heat application, the athlete demonstrates spotty reddening of the treated area. What is the correct term for this physiological response?

○ **A.** Allergic reaction to the modality equipment contacting the skin

○ **B.** Tissue ischemia secondary to Hunting's response

○ **C.** Heat urticaria secondary to increased blood flow

○ **D.** Tissue hyperhydrosis secondary to increased metabolism

○ **E.** Tissue mottling secondary to an excessive local histamine release

66. You are treating an athlete with a subacute ankle sprain who has been receiving only cryotherapy. You choose to employ a contrast bath as a transitional modality. Which of the following is a physiological effect of a contrast bath?

○ **A.** Only a superficial capillary response

○ **B.** Constriction of deep blood vessels with ice immersion

○ **C.** Dilation of deep blood vessels in response to heating

○ **D.** A vascular pumping action to effectively remove swelling

○ **E.** A cumulative tissue temperature increase is achieved

67. When treating a wrist injury with a warm whirlpool, what is the maximum recommended water temperature in degrees Fahrenheit?

○ **A.** 98°F

○ **B.** 106°F

○ **C.** 110°F

○ **D.** 112°F

○ **E.** 120°F

68. An athletic trainer is treating an athlete with shortwave diathermy using a drum electrode. The drum electrode has been placed 6 inches from the athlete's low back. Based on the inverse square law, how would the intensity alter if the drum is moved to a position 3 inches from the treatment area?

○ **A.** Intensity at the new position will be ⅑ of full intensity.

○ **B.** The intensity of the original position will be ¹⁄₁₂ of full intensity.

○ **C.** The intensity will decrease by ½ as the drum is moved from the original position to the new position.

○ **D.** The intensity will increase by ½ as the drum is moved from the original position to the new position.

○ **E.** The intensity will increase by ⅑ as the drum is moved from the original position to the new position.

69. Which of the following athletes would benefit from ultraviolet therapy?

○ **A.** A sprinter with diabetes

○ **B.** A wrestler with herpes simplex

○ **C.** A field hockey player with chronic psoriasis

○ **D.** A linebacker taking tetracycline

○ **E.** A swimmer with lupus erythematosus

70. An athletic trainer is utilizing motor level stimulation to promote muscle reeducation. Where should the active electrode be placed to facilitate this treatment?

○ **A.** At least 6 inches from the dispersive electrode and over the muscle belly

○ **B.** Over the motor point

○ **C.** Over an active trigger point

○ **D.** No more than 6 inches from the dispersive electrode

○ **E.** Any soft-tissue area outside the electrical field

71. Prior to completing grade IV joint mobilizations, an athletic trainer chooses to use ultrasound to create vigorous tissue heating to stretch collagen. What degree of tissue temperature increase is required to achieve this treatment goal?

○ **A.** 1°C

○ **B.** 2°C

○ **C.** 3°C

○ **D.** 4°C

○ **E.** 5°C

72. What causes the ultrasound transducer crystal to vibrate and create sound waves?

○ **A.** It is mechanically oscillated by the electrical current.

○ **B.** It is chemically stimulated by the electrical current.

○ **C.** It expands and contracts due to the alternating polarity of the electrical current.

○ **D.** It becomes part of the athlete's electrical field.

○ **E.** It utilizes mechanical deformation to produce electrical voltage.

73. Your treatment goal is to increase tissue temperature by 2°C in the piriformis muscle. Which therapeutic modality, whose wavelengths are within the electromagnetic spectrum, is capable of achieving this treatment goal?

○ **A.** Microwave diathermy

○ **B.** Ultrasound

○ **C.** Moist hot pack

○ **D.** Warm whirlpool

○ **E.** Ultraviolet

74. Based on wavelength and frequency, which infrared modality is capable of achieving the greatest effective depth of penetration?

○ **A.** Cold packs

○ **B.** Hot whirlpool

○ **C.** Paraffin bath

○ **D.** Moist heat

○ **E.** Cold whirlpool

75. Which of the following statements best illustrates the relationship between wavelength, frequency, and depth of penetration as it applies to modalities?

○ **A.** There is a direct relationship between frequency and depth of penetration.

○ **B.** There is a direct relationship between wavelength and frequency.

○ **C.** There is an inverse relationship between wavelength and frequency.

○ **D.** There is an inverse relationship between wavelength and depth of penetration.

○ **E.** There is an equal relationship between wavelength and frequency.

76. With respect to therapeutic ultrasound, what is the stretching window?

○ **A.** Minimal number of minutes that tissue should be stretched following an ultrasound treatment

○ **B.** Theoretical time interval between cessation of an ultrasound treatment and initiation of a stretching protocol

○ **C.** Minimal number of minutes between onset of ultrasound treatment and achievement of maximal tissue heating

○ **D.** Theoretical period following a stretching session before a second ultrasound treatment can be initiated

○ **E.** Theoretical period of vigorous heating when tissues will undergo the greatest extensibility and elongation

77. What factors should be considered when calculating ultrasound treatment time?

○ **A.** Intensity, coupling medium, frequency, and fat percentage of treated tissue

○ **B.** Effective radiating area of the sound head, duty cycle, and desired tissue temperature change

○ **C.** Resting tissue temperature, size of treatment area, output, and coupling medium

○ **D.** Frequency, output, duty cycle, and desired tissue temperature change

○ **E.** Density of treatment tissue, hydration status of athlete, duty cycle, and speed of transducer movement

78. You are treating a hamstring muscle belly strain. Your treatment goal is to increase tissue temperature of the affected muscle. The treatment area is approximately 8″ × 20″. Which of the following methods would best assist in achieving this treatment goal?

○ **A.** Two hot packs side by side to effectively cover the area

○ **B.** Dividing the area in half and doing two identical continuous ultrasound treatments

○ **C.** Continuous ultrasound treatment at an intensity twice that used for a smaller treatment area

○ **D.** Warm whirlpool at a temperature of 98°F to 108°F

○ **E.** Two hot packs one on top of the other placed over the belly of the muscle

79. What is the purpose of a coupling medium when completing an ultrasound treatment?

○ **A.** To provide a conduit for the sound waves

○ **B.** To minimize the athlete's potential adverse reaction to sound-wave transmission

○ **C.** To reduce the uncomfortable sensation associated with sound-wave absorption

○ **D.** To minimizes risk of accumulating harmful rebound waves

○ **E.** To minimize deflection of the energy by the skin

80. A clinician is using Hoffa massage to treat a musculoskeletal disorder. Which stroke type should be utilized if the goal is to accustom the athlete to the physical contact of the clinician?

○ **A.** Pétrissage

○ **B.** Tapotement

○ **C.** Effleurage

○ **D.** Vibration

○ **E.** Percussion

81. Which method of heat transfer is applied when an athlete uses a warm whirlpool to heat the lower extremity?

○ **A.** Conduction

○ **B.** Convection

○ **C.** Radiation

○ **D.** Conversion

○ **E.** Evaporation

82. Which therapeutic modality's wavelength places it between infrared and ultraviolet on the electromagnetic spectrum?

○ **A.** Microwave diathermy

○ **B.** Shortwave diathermy

○ **C.** Electromyographic biofeedback

○ **D.** Laser

○ **E.** Electrical stimulation

83. The physiological effects of which of the following therapeutic modalities would assist in overcoming the method by which oxygen tension impedes healing?

○ **A.** Cryotherapy

○ **B.** Pulsed ultrasound

○ **C.** Transcutaneous electrical nerve stimulation

○ **D.** Iontophoresis

○ **E.** Thermotherapy

84. Which of the following statements best describes a typical mechanical cervical traction protocol?

○ **A.** The athlete is supine or long-sitting with the neck flexed between 20° and 30°, and a traction force greater than 20 lb is applied intermittently.

○ **B.** The athlete is prone with the neck in a neutral position, and a traction force of 20 lb is applied continuously.

○ **C.** The athlete is long-sitting with the neck extended 20°, and a traction force of 15 lb is applied intermittently.

○ **D.** The athlete is supine with the neck in a neutral position, and a traction force of 5% of body weight is applied continuously.

○ **E.** The athlete is prone with the neck flexed 10° to 20°, and a traction force greater than 10 lb is applied continuously.

85. An athlete presents to the athletic training room complaining of left-sided low back pain and left leg radicular pain. The athlete is assuming a right lateral flexed posture. In which position should the athlete be placed to treat with positional traction?

○ **A.** Side-lying on a towel roll with left side up

○ **B.** Side-lying on a towel roll with right side up

○ **C.** Supine with both knees held tightly to the chest

○ **D.** Supine with hips and knees supported in a 90/90 position

○ **E.** Prone with bolster placed bilaterally under the ASISs

86. During the course of treating an athlete using lumbar positional traction, you note that the athlete is receiving only partial relief of symptoms. What steps can you take to improve the athlete's outcome for this treatment?

○ **A.** While lying supine, bring the athlete's left knee to the opposite shoulder; repeat on the opposite side.

○ **B.** While side-lying, flex the athlete's hips maximally, and rotate the top shoulder posteriorly.

○ **C.** While lying prone, press the athlete up onto forearms, and rotate torso, lifting one hand toward the ceiling.

○ **D.** While side-lying, flex the athlete's knee, and maximally extend hips.

○ **E.** While lying prone, extend the athlete's opposite arm and leg while the athlete is looking upward toward the ceiling.

87. You are using a bipolar electrode placement technique for muscle reeducation of the quadriceps muscle group. Two equally sized electrodes are placed in series along the direction of the muscle fibers. If this setup fails to achieve a maximal muscle contraction, what is the most appropriate alteration?

○ **A.** Place one large electrode over the muscle fibers and a small electrode out of the treatment area.

○ **B.** Increase the current frequency.

○ **C.** Increase the intensity.

○ **D.** Increase the space between the electrodes.

○ **E.** Use a more aqueous conduction medium under the electrodes.

88. A tennis player reports to the athletic training room with palpable pain over the common origin of the wrist extensors. There is no obvious swelling or redness, although the area is warm to the touch. Passive wrist flexion and resisted wrist extension increase pain. Which therapeutic modality is contraindicated in the treatment of this athlete?

○ **A.** Ice bag

○ **B.** Moist hot pack

○ **C.** Iontophoresis

○ **D.** Electrical stimulation

○ **E.** Pulsed ultrasound

89. What is the recommended frequency for cleaning and disinfecting a whirlpool?

○ **A.** Daily

○ **B.** Weekly

○ **C.** Before and after an athlete with an open wound uses it

○ **D.** Twice daily

○ **E.** After every athlete's use

90. An athlete has been told to be completely non–weight-bearing on his lower extremity and has been instructed on the proper use of crutches. Which of the following statements about this use of crutches is correct?

○ **A.** The athlete should maintain normal gait pattern by making contact with the crutch and the opposite limb simultaneously.

○ **B.** The athlete should contact the floor with the two crutches and the injured limb simultaneously.

○ **C.** When descending stairs, the crutches and the injured limb should touch down on the step simultaneously.

○ **D.** The uninvolved limb leads, and crutches stay on the riser below when ascending a flight of stairs.

○ **E.** The knee of the involved limb should remain extended during the swing phase of gait.

91. Which of the following would be the most effective way to protect an anterior thigh contusion on a basketball player?

○ **A.** A neoprene sleeve

○ **B.** A doughnut pad with a thermoplastic dome

○ **C.** A ½″ solid closed cell pad

○ **D.** A compression elastic wrap

○ **E.** A ½″ felt doughnut pad under a compression wrap

92. A distance runner has developed plantar fasciitis. Which of the following methods would best support this injury?

○ **A.** A medial longitudinal arch pad

○ **B.** A lateral heel wedge

○ **C.** A heel cup

○ **D.** An adhesive metatarsal pad

○ **E.** A dorsal foot pad

93. What is the biomechanical rationale for the use of a forearm strap in the treatment of lateral epicondylitis of the elbow?

○ **A.** Increases the mechanical advantage of the flexor-pronator muscle groups

○ **B.** Provides improved stability to the proximal radioulnar joint

○ **C.** Reduces the range of the humeroulnar joint

○ **D.** Modifies the pull of the extensor-supinator mechanism at its origin

○ **E.** Changes the angle of pull at the origin of the flexor muscle group

94. Which of the following is considered a purpose of dynamic (mobilization) splints?

○ **A.** To correct an existing deformity

○ **B.** To prevent further deformity

○ **C.** To immobilize

○ **D.** To provide support for joint laxity and ligament injury

○ **E.** To prevent a soft-tissue contracture

95. Which of the following is considered a purpose of static splints?

○ **A.** To substitute for loss of motor function

○ **B.** To correct an existing deformity

○ **C.** To provide controlled motion

○ **D.** To aid in fracture alignment and wound healing

○ **E.** To decrease soft-tissue adherence

96. An athlete's mother contacts you following her son's knee surgery. She states that he was sent home with a machine that the physician explained would help restore range of motion. She also communicates that her son is supposed to use it as much as possible whenever resting. What type of assistive device has this athlete most likely been given?

○ **A.** Dynamic splint

○ **B.** Functional brace

○ **C.** Controlled mobility device

○ **D.** Continuous passive motion machine

○ **E.** Postoperative hinged brace

97. A soccer player is returning to limited participation drills following a medial collateral ligament and medial meniscus injuries. Which type of knee brace is most appropriate for this athlete?

○ **A.** Custom derotation brace

○ **B.** Functional medial hinge brace

○ **C.** Neoprene sleeve

○ **D.** Rehabilitation brace

○ **E.** Prophylactic hinge brace

98. A football lineman is returning to practice and competition 1 week following an ulnar collateral ligament injury in his thumb. Which material would best meet the treatment goals of immobilization and support without violating sport rules?

○ **A.** Fiberglass cast tape

○ **B.** Soft fiberglass cast tape

○ **C.** Plaster cast material

○ **D.** Thermoplastic material

○ **E.** 1 ½″ white tape

99. Which of the following orthotics would be most appropriate for an athlete with turf toe?

○ **A.** A full-length semi-rigid orthotic with a rigid forefoot extension

○ **B.** A full-length semi-rigid orthotic with a medial post

○ **C.** A ¾-length semi-rigid orthotic with a medial longitudinal arch support

○ **D.** A ¾-length semi-rigid orthotic with a Nickelplast cut for a forefoot post

○ **E.** A full-length semi-rigid orthotic with a Nickelplast teardrop pad under the second and third metatarsal heads

100. For which of the following conditions would the placement of a heel cup in the shoe be of benefit?

○ **A.** Sesamoiditis

○ **B.** Turf toe

○ **C.** Spring ligament sprain

○ **D.** Jones' fracture

○ **E.** Achilles tendonitis

101. Which characteristic of commonly used custom padding and orthotic fabrication material is defined as the ability of the material to return to its preheated or original shape, size, and thickness when reheated?

○ **A.** Elasticity

○ **B.** Drapability

○ **C.** Memory

○ **D.** Conformability

○ **E.** Rigidity

102. Which biomechanical principle is best explained by the most commonly used loading systems in orthotics: the three-point pressure system?

○ **A.** Pressure

○ **B.** Lever arm

○ **C.** Force distribution

○ **D.** Equilibrium

○ **E.** Inhibition

103. Which type of brace is the most appropriate for treating chronic infrapatellar tendonitis?

○ **A.** Counterforce

○ **B.** Neoprene with medial support

○ **C.** Prophylactic

○ **D.** Rehabilitative

○ **E.** Derotation

104. When fabricating a thumb spica splint, how should the thumb be positioned to facilitate a palmar prehension?

○ **A.** In opposition to the index and long fingers

○ **B.** In lateral opposition to the index finger

○ **C.** In slight flexion

○ **D.** In full abduction

○ **E.** In full adduction

105. When caring for a blister, what is the rationale for leaving the blister cover intact?

○ **A.** It prevents infection.

○ **B.** It prevents enlargement of the original wound.

○ **C.** It allows the wound to heal faster.

○ **D.** It disperses force.

○ **E.** It protects immature skin.

106. A physician holds a weekly clinic in your athletic training room two mornings per week. The physician has requested permission to store and dispense a few select prescription medications from the athletic training room. How would you best respond to the request?

○ **A.** You agree with the stipulation that a Drug Enforcement Agency (DEA) facility certificate be obtained and that in the signed physician agreement you be listed as an agent assigned by the DEA.

○ **B.** You agree, with the only stipulation being that the physician must install a locked cabinet for which the physician has the only key and is the only one to dispense medications.

○ **C.** You decline, stating that the athletic training rooms are not permitted to house prescription drugs because doing so would put the facility in violation of DEA laws.

○ **D.** You decline, stating you believe doing so would put the staff in violation of state pharmacology laws.

○ **E.** You decline, stating that dispensing medication is outside the scope of practice of an athletic trainer.

107. Which of the following health-care providers has authority for prescribing drugs?

○ **A.** Chiropractor

○ **B.** Nurse practitioner

○ **C.** Registered nurse

○ **D.** Psychologist

○ **E.** Paramedic

108. Following an injury, an athlete is exhibiting the characteristics of the bargaining stage of the Kübler-Ross classic model of reaction to death and dying. Which stage is this athlete most likely to enter next?

○ **A.** Acceptance

○ **B.** Denial

○ **C.** Anger

○ **D.** Depression

○ **E.** Recovery

109. Which of the following correctly describes the schedule of controlled substances, of which oxycodone is an example?

○ **A.** Drug has moderate abuse potential

○ **B.** Only moderate psychic or physical dependence liability

○ **C.** No refills without an additional prescription

○ **D.** Verbal orders from physician are permitted

○ **E.** Contains limited quantity of narcotic or non-narcotic ingredients

110. During the rehabilitation process, an athlete is exhibiting the outward signs of excessive talking, argumentativeness, inappropriate joke telling, and hyperactivity. What is the most appropriate reaction by the athletic trainer?

○ **A.** Pity the athlete, and excuse the behaviors.

○ **B.** Tell the athlete that the behavior is abnormal.

○ **C.** Allow the athlete to vent emotions.

○ **D.** Reprimand the athlete for inappropriate behavior.

○ **E.** Speak with teammates, and encourage them to counsel the athlete.

111. Which of the following statements is true regarding delivery of a drug via intra-articular injection versus the oral route?

○ **A.** The action of the drug is less predictable.

○ **B.** The drug is absorbed at more regular intervals over time.

○ **C.** The drug moves into the blood stream more quickly.

○ **D.** The drug is metabolized more readily.

○ **E.** There is a lower incidence of systemic side effects.

112. For which of the following conditions is an injectable corticosteroid indicated?

○ **A.** Acute traumatic bursitis

○ **B.** Plantar fasciitis

○ **C.** Medial hamstring strain

○ **D.** Nonunion scaphoid fracture

○ **E.** Acute contact dermatitis

113. An athlete has been prescribed tetracycline to treat acne. Which of the following foods should this athlete avoid because they will decrease the body's ability to absorb tetracycline?

○ **A.** Dairy products high in calcium

○ **B.** Alcoholic beverages

○ **C.** Coffee and caffeinated sodas

○ **D.** Grapefruit

○ **E.** Root vegetables

114. Which of the following is a potential local complication of corticosteroid injection?

○ **A.** Transient hyperglycemia

○ **B.** Hypopigmentation

○ **C.** Adrenal suppression

○ **D.** Avascular necrosis

○ **E.** Vasovagal syncope

115. Which of the following is a potential systemic complication of corticosteroid injection?

○ **A.** Peripheral nerve injury

○ **B.** Tendon or ligament rupture

○ **C.** Vasovagal syncope

○ **D.** Injection site infection

○ **E.** Subcutaneous atrophy

116. Which recommendation should you make to an athlete who is taking a narcotic analgesic prescribed for postoperative knee pain?

○ **A.** Increase fluid and fiber intake.

○ **B.** Minimize intake of dairy products.

○ **C.** Finish the entire prescription.

○ **D.** Minimize sun exposure, and use a high SPF sunscreen when in the sun.

○ **E.** Use alternative forms of contraception if currently taking birth control pills.

117. Which of the following drug classes is restricted by the NCAA but allowed by the U.S. Anti-Doping Agency?

○ **A.** Local anesthetics

○ **B.** Beta$_2$ agonists

○ **C.** Narcotics

○ **D.** Stimulants

○ **E.** Alcohol

118. Given their known side effects, which family of anti-hypertensive medications may be most appropriate for a physically active 35-year-old athlete with stage 1 hypertension?

○ **A.** Diuretics

○ **B.** Beta blockers

○ **C.** Calcium channel blockers

○ **D.** Angiotensin-converting enzyme inhibitors

○ **E.** Angiotensin II blockers

119. An athlete returns from the student health center with a prescription for cephalexin (Keflex). You immediately realize that the athlete will most likely have an allergic reaction to this drug. A history of allergy to which of the following antibiotic classes would make this athlete sensitive to this drug?

○ **A.** Fluoroquinolone

○ **B.** Tetracycline

○ **C.** Macrolide

○ **D.** Sulfonamide

○ **E.** Penicillin

120. Which of the following is considered a rescue inhaler?

○ **A.** Azmacort

○ **B.** Albuterol

○ **C.** Serevent

○ **D.** Advair

○ **E.** Singulair

121. An athlete with seasonal allergies reports to the athletic training room before practice complaining of itchy, watery eyes; runny nose; and scratchy throat. Which of the following antihistamines would be most appropriate for this athlete?

○ **A.** Tavist

○ **B.** Benadryl

○ **C.** Claritin

○ **D.** Actifed

○ **E.** Chlor-Trimeton

122. An athlete complains of a dry, irritating cough. Which of the following types of medications do you advise?

○ **A.** Expectorant

○ **B.** Decongestant

○ **C.** Antihistamine

○ **D.** Analgesic

○ **E.** Antitussive

123. An athlete complains of frontal and maxillary sinuses that are congested and preventing breathing and sleeping well. Which of the following medication combinations should be recommended to effectively manage the congestion?

○ **A.** Decongestant and mucolytics

○ **B.** Antihistamine and analgesic

○ **C.** Expectorate and antitussive

○ **D.** Saline spray and anti-inflammatory

○ **E.** Bronchodilator and corticosteroid

124. Which of the following commonly prescribed gastrointestinal drugs treat peptic ulcer disease, gastroesophageal reflux disease, and *Helicobacter pylori* through inhibition of protein-pump acid secretion?

○ **A.** Pepto-Bismol

○ **B.** Prevacid

○ **C.** Tagamet

○ **D.** Pepcid

○ **E.** Zantac

125. What recommendations would you make to an athlete who has recently been diagnosed with viral bronchitis?

○ **A.** Drink copious amounts of water, use decongestants as needed, and sleep with a heating pad.

○ **B.** Use anti-inflammatory medication as needed, get plenty of rest, and use cough suppressants as needed.

○ **C.** Use mucolytics as needed, increase protein intake, and refrain from practicing.

○ **D.** Isolate yourself from others, use antihistamines as needed, and sleep with the head elevated.

○ **E.** Use antipyretic agents as needed, avoid caffeinated beverages, and use antimicrobial soaps when showering.

126. An athlete who has been suffering with constipation has been instructed to begin taking the laxative Correctol. What is the mechanism of action of this drug?

○ **A.** It is a fecal softener that works by facilitating formation of a fat and water mixture.

○ **B.** It is a saline that draws water into the intestine.

○ **C.** It is a hyperosmotic that acts as a local irritant to increase colon fluid.

○ **D.** It is a stimulant that increases peristaltic activity.

○ **E.** It is a bulk-forming agent that absorbs water and forms emollient gel.

127. A member of your college tennis team fails to report to practice. When you finally reach this athlete by phone she tells you that she felt very ill this morning and was seen by a physician at the college's student health services. She tells you that the physician gave her a prescription for Relenza and instructed her to rest and intake plenty of fluids for the next few days. He also told her to take analgesics for any muscle soreness she may experience as well as any other over-the-counter medications needed for her symptoms. For which of the following conditions is the treatment provided this athlete most associated?

○ **A.** Strep throat

○ **B.** Sinusitis

○ **C.** Influenza

○ **D.** Pneumonia

○ **E.** Mononucleosis

128. Which of the following viral infections has an associated vaccine?

○ **A.** Influenza

○ **B.** Mononucleosis

○ **C.** Herpes simplex

○ **D.** Hepatitis C

○ **E.** Tuberculosis

129. Treatment for symptomatic Wolff-Parkinson-White syndrome typically involves which of the following?

○ **A.** Use of beta blockers

○ **B.** Use of Holter's monitor

○ **C.** Implantation of a pacemaker

○ **D.** Cardiac catheterization

○ **E.** Radiofrequency catheter ablation

130. An athlete has been diagnosed with deep vein thrombosis following a recent surgery and has been prescribed the appropriate medication to treat this condition. Given the treatment goals of the prescribed medication, which of the following recommendations would you make?

○ **A.** The athlete should increase vitamin K intake to 1000 times the recommended daily allowance.

○ **B.** The athlete should avoid intake of alcoholic beverages.

○ **C.** The athlete should increase protein intake.

○ **D.** The athlete should avoid analgesic medications.

○ **E.** The athlete should ice the involved area daily.

131. When should an athlete be referred to a physician during the treatment of suspected food poisoning?

○ **A.** When hematuria is present

○ **B.** When hematochyluria is present

○ **C.** When hematochezia is present

○ **D.** When hematocytozoon is present

○ **E.** When hematolymphangioma is present

132. A cross-country runner reports to the athletic training room complaining of seeing blood in the urine each day for the past 4 days following workouts. The runner reports no other signs or symptoms. How should this condition best be managed?

○ **A.** Immediate referral to physician for evaluation, urinalysis, and diagnostic ultrasound

○ **B.** Urinalysis to confirm hematuria, rest for 24 to 72 hours, repeat urinalysis to confirm resolution, return to play when hematuria resolves

○ **C.** Urinalysis to confirm hematuria, hyperhydrate before the next workout, repeat urinalysis following next workout

○ **D.** Referral to the physician for a diuretic prescription, increased fluid intake along with soluble vitamin intake

○ **E.** Increased intake of cranberry juice over the next 24 hours, urinalysis, clear for participation if afebrile

133. What is the recommended treatment for the most common sexually transmitted disease in the United States?

○ **A.** A one-time dose of azithromycin

○ **B.** A 7- to 10-day course of acyclovir

○ **C.** A one-time vaginal suppository of Lamisil

○ **D.** Surgical colposcopy

○ **E.** Daily application of Valtrex for 1 week

134. A swimmer with a history of migraines is traveling to the Caribbean to train over winter break. Which of the following activities would be contraindicated for this athlete?

○ **A.** Sunbathing

○ **B.** Parasailing

○ **C.** Scuba diving

○ **D.** Jet skiing

○ **E.** Surfing

135. What is the most important factor to consider when deciding to clear an athlete with a seizure disorder for participation?

○ **A.** Extent of seizure control

○ **B.** Sport type (collision, contact, or noncontact)

○ **C.** Level of supervision

○ **D.** Age at diagnosis

○ **E.** Type of seizure commonly experienced

136. An athlete presents with a 2-day history of a red, watery, itchy eye. The roommate was diagnosed 3 days ago with viral conjunctivitis. The athlete might have the same condition. Which of the following treatment recommendations would be most helpful for this athlete?

○ **A.** Refer the athlete for an antibiotic eyedrop prescription.

○ **B.** Recommend the athlete take an over-the-counter expectorant.

○ **C.** Rinse the eye with saline solution at least twice a day.

○ **D.** Apply warm compresses as frequently as possible.

○ **E.** Wash all linens, towels, and clothing in very hot water.

137. An athlete presents with a loose foreign body under the upper eyelid. You have treated this condition by removing the athlete's contact lens, rinsing the eye for several minutes with eyewash, and attempting to dislodge the foreign body by pulling the athlete's upper eyelid over the lower eyelid and instructing the patient to blink several times. Unfortunately, none of your efforts has been successful. What is your next treatment step?

○ **A.** Evert the eyelid, and attempt to remove the foreign body with tweezers.

○ **B.** Evert the eyelid, and attempt to remove the foreign body with a cotton-tipped applicator.

○ **C.** Pull the eyelid away from the eye, and use a squirt bottle to irrigate.

○ **D.** Cover the eye with a patch, put the athlete on bedrest, and tell the athlete to avoid reading and watching TV until reevaluation the next day.

○ **E.** Cover the eye with a patch, and refer the athlete to an ophthalmologist.

138. An athlete has recently been diagnosed with scabies and is undergoing treatment. Which of the following recommendations should you make to this athlete?

○ **A.** All bedding and recently worn clothing should be destroyed.

○ **B.** Exterminate all rooms of the living quarters with a commercially available fogger.

○ **C.** Avoid any skin-to-skin contact with another person until treatment is completed.

○ **D.** The athlete should notify the Centers for Disease Control and Prevention and complete an incident report.

○ **E.** The athlete should be retested every 3 months to ensure complete eradication of the parasite.

139 A basketball player is struck in the ear by the opponent's open hand. The player reports immediate, intense ear pain along with a decrement in hearing. During your evaluation, you visualize a tympanic membrane perforation. What instructions will you give this athlete until a physician can evaluate?

○ **A.** The injury will most likely need surgery; the player should contact parents regarding insurance coverage.

○ **B.** The player will miss several weeks of practice and will most likely be prescribed an antibiotic.

○ **C.** This injury will most likely heal on its own, but the player should avoid getting water in the ear.

○ **D.** The injury will permanently affect the player's hearing, and disability services on campus should be consulted.

○ **E.** The injury will slowly heal over the next 6 months, but the player will be unable to fly for at least 5 years.

140. Despite instructions, an athlete refuses to address a case of chronic gingivitis. If left untreated, what condition is this athlete at risk for developing?

○ **A.** Kaposi's sarcoma

○ **B.** Leukoplakia

○ **C.** Periodontitis

○ **D.** Squamous cell carcinoma

○ **E.** Candidiasis

141. You hear during discussions in the athletic training room that several of your freshmen women's basketball players have recently started taking birth control pills. You know that one of these women has type 1 diabetes. What information should you provide to this particular athlete?

○ **A.** Stop taking the oral contraceptive immediately because it will inhibit the insulin response.

○ **B.** Add additional carbohydrates to her diet to compensate for the effects of the oral contraceptive on blood glucose levels.

○ **C.** Have this information added to her medic alert bracelet.

○ **D.** Increase her meal frequency to compensate for the effects of the oral contraceptive on blood glucose levels.

○ **E.** Carefully monitor her blood glucose levels because the oral contraceptive can reduce the effects of insulin.

142. Which of the following conditions is treated with graded exercise, proper nutrition, improved sleep, antidepressant medication, and behavioral therapy?

○ **A.** Infectious mononucleosis

○ **B.** Chronic fatigue syndrome

○ **C.** Anemia

○ **D.** HIV

○ **E.** Systemic lupus erythematosus

143. A wrestler is being treated for a furuncle. The wound has been excised. He has been taking antibiotic medication for 72 hours, and no new lesions have appeared in the past 48 hours. The wound demonstrates mild oozing with drainage. What return to activity information will you provide to the coach?

○ **A.** The athlete may not return to activity.

○ **B.** The athlete may return to activity as long as the wound is covered.

○ **C.** The athlete may return to full activity without restriction.

○ **D.** The athlete may return to noncontact activity as long as the wound is covered.

○ **E.** The athlete may return to full activity after he has been on the antibiotics for at least another day.

144. Manual muscle testing does not attempt to quantify the amount of force generated by a muscle group precisely. Which of the following is a major purpose of manual muscle testing during the rehabilitation process?

○ **A.** Compare the injured limb's range of motion with the opposing extremity

○ **B.** Objectively measure the muscle function of the injured limb

○ **C.** Rehabilitate the muscles of the injured limb

○ **D.** Reeducate the neurological functions of the injured limb

○ **E.** Qualify the effectiveness of the rehabilitation program

145. Following a joint mobilization treatment, you measure an athlete's dorsiflexion with the knee flexed to 20°. How many degrees of normal dorsiflexion motion is this athlete lacking?

○ **A.** None; the athlete has achieved full range of motion

○ **B.** 10

○ **C.** 15

○ **D.** 5

○ **E.** 20

146. Which of the following information should be recorded in the objective portion of an athlete's SOAP note?

○ **A.** "The athlete does not want to return to athletics."

○ **B.** "The athlete will regain 10° of flexion in 2 weeks."

○ **C.** "The athlete's swelling has decreased 0.5 inch."

○ **D.** "The athlete is not putting maximal effort into the rehabilitation plan."

○ **E.** "The athlete displays 1+ instability of the MCL."

147. You have been rehabilitating an athlete for the past 4 weeks following a postoperative anterior capsular shift procedure. Using a goniometer, you have assessed the athlete's active shoulder flexion to be 80°. Which of the following rehabilitation components should be added to your athlete's rehabilitation program to address this limitation?

○ **A.** Inferior humeral glides

○ **B.** D1 extension pattern

○ **C.** Weight shifting in the quadruped position

○ **D.** Glenohumeral internal and external rotation with exercise band resistance

○ **E.** Codman's pendulum

148. An athlete has reached the last phase of an anterior cruciate ligament reconstruction rehabilitation program. You have assessed his knee extension, and the athlete is lacking 5° of terminal knee extension. Which of the following rehabilitation components should be added to address this limitation?

○ **A.** Prone extension hangs with distally positioned weight

○ **B.** Functional biofeedback

○ **C.** Posterior tibial glides

○ **D.** Plyometrics

○ **E.** Proprioception training

149. A basketball player sustained a grade I lateral ankle sprain during the first half of a game. The athlete has iced, and during halftime you tape the athlete. What criteria will you use to determine if the athlete can play in the second half?

○ **A.** Athlete demonstrates full range of motion and equal strength compared bilaterally

○ **B.** Athlete can walk on toes and heels without pain

○ **C.** Athlete can successfully balance on the injured ankle for 30 seconds with eyes closed

○ **D.** Athlete can successfully sprint, hop on the injured ankle, and perform defensive slides

○ **E.** Athlete can make a contribution to the game's outcome despite decreased performance level

150. During a rehabilitation session, an athlete completes the following: three sets of straight leg raises with 14 repetitions using a 5-lb weight; terminal knee extensions, 20 repetitions in three sets using black Thera-Bands; three sets of 12 mini-squats using body weight for resistance; and gastrocnemius stretching using an incline board for 20 seconds repeated four times. Which of the following is the most appropriate way to document this rehabilitation information in the athlete's chart?

○ **A.** SLR 3×14×5#, TKEs 3×20×black, mini-squats 3×12×BW, and gastroc stretching on angle board 4×20"

○ **B.** Straight leg raises 3×14 w/5#, terminal knee exts 3×20 w/BTB, squats (mini) 3×12 no weight, calf stretch on incline for 80 sec

○ **C.** Three sets of 14 reps for straight leg raises w/5 pounds, terminal knee extensions 20 repetitions in three sets w/black Thera-Band, 3 sets of 12 for mini-squats × BW, and calf stretching on angle board for 20 seconds repeated 4 times

○ **D.** SLR 3×14 w/5lb, TKEs 3×20 w/black TB, baby squats 3×12×150 lb, and gastroc stretching at an angle for 20 sec (repeat as needed)

○ **E.** 3×14 SLR w/5 lb, 3×20 for terminal knee exts w/black, 3×12 squats in shortened range w/o wt, 4×20 sec angle board stretch

151. An athletic trainer is employing the DeLorme and Watkins technique for strength training as part of a rehabilitation program. In the last set, the athlete is able to perform only six repetitions. How should the next day's training be altered based on this information?

○ **A.** The athlete should decrease by 50% the amount of resistance in the next training session.

○ **B.** The athlete should maintain the amount of resistance in the next training session.

○ **C.** The athlete should decrease the resistance by 5 to 10 lb in the next training session.

○ **D.** The athlete should decrease repetitions in the first two sets to 8 instead of 10.

○ **E.** The athlete should increase resistance in the first two sets and maintain resistance in the final set.

152. You are completing a D1 shoulder flexion pattern during an athlete's postoperative shoulder rehabilitation. While completing rhythmic initiation, you appreciate some weakness at a point in the range. How would you modify this exercise to address this weakness?

○ **A.** Perform a rhythmic stabilization technique at the weak point in the range.

○ **B.** Increase verbal encouragement when the athlete is at the weak point in the range.

○ **C.** Reduce manual resistance being provided at the weak point in the range until the athlete's strength improves.

○ **D.** Reverse the pattern at the weak point in the range, and move into extension.

○ **E.** Perform a slow reversal-hold technique with an isometric contraction at the weak point in the range.

153. You are completing a D2 lower extremity proprioceptive neuromuscular facilitation strengthening pattern with an athlete. While performing D2 flexion, the athlete is not completing the required ankle motion. What adjustments should you make to improve the exercise?

○ **A.** Apply more pressure to the medial longitudinal arch area, and verbally encourage inversion.

○ **B.** Stop the pattern until the athlete completes the ankle motion, and then proceed.

○ **C.** Repeatedly tap the dorsal surface of the foot to provide biofeedback, and verbally encourage plantar flexion.

○ **D.** Apply more pressure on the dorsal surface of the foot, and verbally encourage dorsiflexion.

○ **E.** Decrease pressure throughout the range to minimize muscular weakness, and verbally encourage inversion.

154. An athlete who is rehabilitating following an anterior cruciate ligament reconstruction is experiencing some patellar tendonitis. The athlete returns from a follow-up visit with the physician bearing a prescription that requests the rehabilitation program be modified to minimize shear forces. Which of the following modifications would most effectively comply with the physician's request?

○ **A.** Discontinue squats, and replace with the slide board.

○ **B.** Discontinue stationary cycling, and replace with running in the pool.

○ **C.** Discontinue leg extensions, and replace with lunges.

○ **D.** Discontinue retrowalking on the treadmill, and replace with hamstring curls

○ **E.** Discontinue plyometrics, and replace with isokinetic leg extensions.

155. How do lower extremity closed kinetic chain exercises minimize anterior tibial translation forces?

○ **A.** The shear force is negated by the compressive forces created in a closed kinetic chain posture.

○ **B.** The shear force is counteracted by a co-contraction of the hamstrings.

○ **C.** The shear force is counterweighted by the ground reaction forces created by foot contact.

○ **D.** The anterior tibial translation forces are counteracted by a co-contraction of the quadriceps and iliotibial band.

○ **E.** The anterior tibial translation forces are negated by the simultaneous rotational forces about the tibia.

156. You are using intermittent compression to treat post-acute edema following a knee injury of your starting point guard. Which of the following assessment techniques will provide the best determination of the efficacy of your treatment?

○ **A.** Volumetric measurements

○ **B.** Isokinetic strength measurements

○ **C.** Girth measurements

○ **D.** Goniometric measurements

○ **E.** Pain assessment scale

157. When collecting girth measurements on the knee of an athlete who is 2 weeks status postoperative anterior cruciate ligament reconstruction, you note the measurement taken 4″ above the joint line is 2 cm less this week than the previous week's measurement. How should this change be interpreted?

○ **A.** Inhibition of the quadriceps muscle secondary to pain

○ **B.** Decrease in joint effusion

○ **C.** Movement of swelling distally

○ **D.** Injury to the femoral nerve during surgery

○ **E.** Probable deep vein thrombosis

158. A swimmer with excessive kyphosis secondary to weak scapular musculature presents with bilateral impingement syndrome. She has been progressing through a comprehensive rehabilitation program focused on scapular stabilizers for 90 minutes each day. How can you encourage correct posture throughout the day as she performs her activities of daily living?

○ **A.** Fit the athlete with a figure-eight clavicle brace.

○ **B.** Encourage the athlete to wear her backpack on both shoulders and tighten the straps.

○ **C.** Apply a tape pattern to the upper back to provide constant proprioceptive feedback.

○ **D.** Encourage the athlete to keep both feet flat on the floor when seated.

○ **E.** Instruct the athlete to place her mattress on the floor for sleeping.

159. Why is it important to document an athlete's deficiencies and functional limitations in a discharge summary?

○ **A.** It is necessary to demonstrate the need for the athlete to return to the physician.

○ **B.** It assists the athlete in any future litigation proceedings.

○ **C.** Doing so justifies the purchase of new equipment in your clinic.

○ **D.** The athlete may need the documentation for insurance reimbursement purposes.

○ **E.** The athlete may be forced to discontinue treatment before long-term goals are achieved.

160. Why might rehabilitation goals for a 60-year-old athlete be different from those of a 30-year-old athlete with a similar injury?

○ **A.** Motivation is the key to a successful rehabilitation program and is typically low in older adults.

○ **B.** Nutritional status plays an important part in healing, and younger patients tend to have better nutritional practices.

○ **C.** Older patients have a higher rate of infection, which may result in more scar tissue.

○ **D.** Blood supply is essential for healing and is commonly impaired with increased age.

○ **E.** Swelling amounts are increased in older persons resulting in delayed progression from inflammation to proliferation.

161. Which assessment technique would best assist the clinician in determining when an athlete should be moved from cryotherapy to thermotherapy modalities?

○ **A.** Goniometric measurements

○ **B.** Visual analogue pain scale

○ **C.** Functional testing

○ **D.** Palpation to assess point tenderness

○ **E.** Ligamentous stress tests

162. An athlete with degenerative disk disease has been completing a core stabilization rehabilitation program for the past 6 months and is becoming discouraged by the lack of improvement of symptoms. What tool might help provide you with an objective means to show the athlete that progress is being made?

○ **A.** McGill's pain questionnaire

○ **B.** Activity pattern indicators pain profile

○ **C.** Visual analogue scale

○ **D.** Isokinetic strength test

○ **E.** Sit and reach test

163. In what way can a clinician best measure the effectiveness of a functional exercise progression program?

○ **A.** Use an isokinetic dynamometer to quantify strength

○ **B.** Employ a pain scale such as McGill's pain questions

○ **C.** Employ a functional scoring system such as the Knee Outcome Survey

D. Use a goniometer to quantify motion available in major joints

E. Use Cooper's test to quantify overall fitness levels

164. Which of the following is the best tool for quantifying lower extremity function following a postsurgical rehabilitation program?

A. Lysholm's scale

B. Pittsburgh functional assessment scale

C. Force plate

D. Balance platform

E. Single leg hop for distance

165. Which of the following criteria should be met by an athlete prior to progressing to the running phase of a knee rehabilitation program?

A. Quadriceps strength of ⅘ upon manual muscle testing, full knee extension and 100° of flexion, and no swelling

B. 70% of quadriceps and hamstring strength, full knee flexion, and can complete 2 miles of walking

C. 90% of quadriceps and hamstring strength, 15° of dorsiflexion, and able to do 50 side step-downs

D. Quadriceps/hamstring ratio of 60%, full knee flexion and fewer than 10° extension lag, and adequate balance

E. Able to hop on one leg, 10° of dorsiflexion, and able to bike for 30 minutes

166. Which of the following is the best example of a well-written treatment goal?

A. Regain muscular strength before progressing to the next phase of rehabilitation

B. Decrease athlete's pain from 8 to 5 on numeric pain scale

C. Keep the athlete motivated throughout the rehabilitation program

D. Use a variety of modalities and exercises during rehabilitation program design

E. Achieve full unrestricted knee range of motion by 4 weeks s/p ACL reconstruction

167. Which grade of Kaltenborn's Grade of Traction should be used in conjunction with joint mobilization techniques to treat hypomobility?

A. I

B. II

C. III

D. IV

E. V

168. You are using biofeedback to assist an athlete with patellofemoral pain syndrome in regaining neuromuscular control of the vastus medialis. The athlete has just completed a straight leg raise exercise using the biofeedback device and is ready to progress to a more challenging exercise. Which of the following exercises is the most appropriate exercise to incorporate into the rehabilitation progression next?

A. Mini-squat

B. Lateral step-up

C. Single leg squat

D. Supine quad sets

E. Slide board

169. Which of the following would be considered a long-term rehabilitation goal?

A. Four weeks from today's treatment session, the athlete will have full elbow flexion.

B. The athlete will have full strength in all elbow joint muscles at discharge.

C. At the next treatment session, the athlete's pain will decrease from a 7 to a 6 on the numeric pain scale.

D. In 6 months, the athlete will have a biceps brachii manual muscle testing grade of ⅘.

E. In 3 months, the athlete will begin functional exercises.

170. You are performing an isokinetic test for knee extension at 60° per second. You note flattening of the middle of the curve. What should you conclude?

A. Decreased torque production in the middle of the range secondary to pain

B. Normal-shaped curve for testing this muscle group at this velocity

C. Muscular fatigue noted in the middle to end of the range

D. Altered biomechanics at the beginning and end of the range resulting in excessively high torque production

E. Failure of the hamstrings to engage in reciprocal inhibition

171. You are conducting an isokinetic strength test for a baseball pitcher who is in the late stage of a rehabilitation program for a rotator cuff repair of the pitching shoulder. With what should you compare the results of your isokinetic test in order to determine the pitcher's readiness to return to play?

○ **A.** The contralateral limb

○ **B.** Normative strength data and agonist/antagonist ratio data

○ **C.** Previous isokinetic tests performed during the rehabilitation process

○ **D.** A goal database of athletes of similar gender, age, and activity level

○ **E.** A similar isokinetic test performed on the team's number one starting pitcher

172. Which of the following exercises should be incorporated into the rehabilitation program of an athlete exhibiting Trendelenburg's gait?

○ **A.** Hip adduction in 90° of hip flexion

○ **B.** Hip abduction in 45° of hip extension

○ **C.** Hip extension with the knee flexed to 90°

○ **D.** Squats with hip in 20° of external rotation

○ **E.** Hip abduction in 0° of hip flexion

173. Before beginning a continuous ultrasound treatment, what should you tell the athlete to expect to feel?

○ **A.** A mild muscle contraction

○ **B.** "Pins and needles" sensation

○ **C.** No sensation

○ **D.** A mild sensation of warmth

○ **E.** An intense sensation of warmth

174. An athlete returns from the physician with a prescription that reads "ice baths PRN." The athlete is unsure what to do. What should you tell the athlete?

○ **A.** Complete an ice bath before noon each day.

○ **B.** Complete an ice bath after each running session.

○ **C.** Complete an ice bath right before going to bed.

○ **D.** Complete an ice bath before each running session.

○ **E.** Complete an ice bath as needed for pain.

175. An athlete sustained a season-ending injury 3 weeks ago. During the subsequent week, the athlete was in denial and then had a week of acceptance of the situation. This week the athlete is demonstrating frustration and has a short temper with teammates and the athletic training staff. What should you conclude about the athlete's response to this injury?

○ **A.** Experiencing a grieving process but progression is atypical

○ **B.** Progression through the grieving process following a normal sequence

○ **C.** Having difficulty dealing with the situation and may be a risk to self

○ **D.** Used to having things go favorably and will have to get over this issue

○ **E.** May need a break from rehabilitation and teammates to find a way to accept the situation

176. An athlete with an acute lateral ankle sprain reports to the athletic training room with severe joint effusion and not wearing the compression wrap or open basket weave you applied the night before. When the athlete went home last night, the athlete soaked the injured ankle in a warm Epsom salt bath. How would you best address this situation with the athlete?

○ **A.** Explain the inflammatory phase of the healing process to the athlete and why heat should be avoided while in this phase.

○ **B.** Explain your role as a certified athletic trainer and detail your educational experiences.

○ **C.** Ask the athlete on what research the use thermotherapy was based.

○ **D.** Scold the athlete for ignoring your directions.

○ **E.** Instruct the athlete that the salt attracted fluid to the area and tonight the treatment should be completed without salt.

177. During training, a member of your soccer team refrains from eating and drinking during daylight hours as part of a religious observance. How will you best assist this athlete?

○ **A.** Explain that the athlete will have to choose between religious practices and athletic participation.

○ **B.** Disqualify the athlete from participation until the end of the religious observance.

○ **C.** Acknowledge the athlete's religious convictions, and ensure the athlete gets caloric and fluid intake during the evening hours.

○ **D.** Arrange with the team physician to provide IV fluids and glucose during the religious observance.

○ **E.** Work with the coach to schedule training sessions after sundown.

178. An athlete undergoing a rehabilitation program has become noncompliant, missing appointments and not completing the home exercise program. What action can you take to improve this athlete's compliance?

○ **A.** Allow the athlete to return to rehabilitation when the athlete is ready to make the commitment.

○ **B.** Actively involve the athlete in the goal-setting and rehabilitation planning process.

○ **C.** Call the coach to institute disciplinary measures.

○ **D.** Refuse to work with the athlete until the athlete is dedicated and ready to benefit from your instruction.

○ **E.** Explain to the athlete your rehabilitation philosophy and rationale for selecting specific exercises.

179. How can you best explain to an athlete why, although no longer feeling pain, the athlete is not yet ready to return to competition?

○ **A.** The athlete is in the inflammatory phase of the healing process, and the scar tissue has not yet completely formed, but because of the treatments being received, the athlete is not appreciating the pain.

○ **B.** The athlete is in the fibroblastic repair phase of the healing process, and the scar tissue has created a stable area, but the tissue has not returned to pre-injury type and strength.

○ **C.** The athlete is in the remodeling phase of the healing process, and the scar tissue is just beginning to fill in the matrix, so the tissue will not respond to maximum tensile forces.

○ **D.** The athlete is in the subacute inflammatory phase of the healing process, and the injured area has been walled off and cleaned of all waste and debris, so pain fibers are not being stimulated.

○ **E.** The athlete is in the remodeling phase of the healing process and the A(d) and C fibers are being changed to A(a) and A(b) fibers, so pain is being transmitted despite the presence of injured tissue.

180. What is the most important educational instruction you can provide an athlete regarding the use of over-the-counter medications?

○ **A.** Take the medication as instructed on the label.

○ **B.** Select a medication that addresses multiple symptoms to ensure the most effective treatment.

○ **C.** Understand that dosing is only a recommendation and that doses can be doubled safely.

○ **D.** Take all medications with food and/or a full glass of milk or water to minimize gastrointestinal upset.

○ **E.** Selecting natural medications minimizes adverse reactions and side effects.

181. As an athletic trainer in a hospital-based sports medicine clinic, what is the most important thing you can do when explaining a home exercise program to an 8-year-old patient?

○ **A.** Provide a handout with pictures of the exercises to be completed.

○ **B.** Ask the patient to demonstrate the exercises before leaving the clinic.

○ **C.** Explain the program to the patient and a responsible adult who will assist the child with the program.

○ **D.** Set up a reward system with stickers and prizes to encourage home exercise program compliance.

○ **E.** Explain to the patient that the patient cannot return to sport participation without completing the program.

182. You are concerned that a 12-year-old figure skater, who practices 3 hours each day, may be demonstrating negative psychological consequences of maintaining high-intensity training for an extended period. What potential negative aspect of this training should you explain to the parents of this child?

○ **A.** The child will experience body image issues and may develop an eating disorder.

○ **B.** The child will become self-centered and introverted.

○ **C.** The child may exhibit abnormal sleeping and eating patterns.

○ **D.** The child will likely grow up to be unable to handle failure in life.

○ **E.** The child may experience impaired intellectual development.

183. Which of the following modifications should be made to a rehabilitation program to improve participation of individuals with cognitive impairment?

○ **A.** Repeating skills for enhanced learning and creating nicknames for all exercises to promote familiarity

○ **B.** Minimizing noise and distractions and incorporating familiar, functional activities into the treatment

○ **C.** Providing consistency within the rehabilitation program and adding only one new exercise session

○ **D.** Providing consistency within the rehabilitation environment and setting up a reward system for successful completion of activities

○ **E.** Modifying the pace of activities and scheduling appointments for early in the day

184. You are using electrical stimulation to manage the pain associated with a knee sprain of an athlete with Down's syndrome. You have selected parameters consistent with managing pain via the gate control theory. How will you best explain to the athlete the expected sensation associated with this treatment?

○ **A.** "It will feel like tiny needle pricks, but you can tell me when it hurts."

○ **B.** "It will feel warm and fuzzy, like when you rub your skin."

○ **C.** "It will feel like intermittent electrical shocks, but do not worry because they will not hurt you."

○ **D.** "It will feel tingly and tickly, like when your foot falls asleep."

○ **E.** "It will feel painful at first, but then it will start to feel better."

185. Which of the following factors should be included in a comprehensive substance abuse plan?

○ **A.** Requiring all student athletes to submit to monthly alcohol and drug screens conducted by a local laboratory

○ **B.** Conducting yearly educational programs for student athletes, team managers, coaches, administrators, and team support personnel about substance abuse issues pertaining specifically to student athletes

○ **C.** Establishing a rule preventing student athletes from leaving campus for spring break and other long weekends

○ **D.** Requiring student athletes found guilty of an alcohol- or drug-related offense to write a paper on the health consequences of substance abuse

○ **E.** Requiring student athletes found guilty of using an illegal substance to submit to a 48-hour commitment to a local psychiatric and rehabilitation center

186. Cavanagh and Levitov have developed a six-stage process to be used in the helping interview. What is the first stage in the helping interview process?

○ **A.** Establish an alliance with the person seeking help.

○ **B.** Gather information to find out more about the situation facing the patient.

○ **C.** Determine the patient's symptoms, their causes, their relief, and the patient's readiness for help.

○ **D.** Clarify the roles of each individual, and express the expectations of each person.

○ **E.** Record the progress the patient has been making, and revise the treatment plan accordingly.

187. In which of the following situations should the athletic trainer refer an athlete to an outside health-care provider rather than continue to treat the athlete?

○ **A.** When the relationship with the athlete serves the athletic trainer's needs more than it serves the athlete

○ **B.** When an athlete is frustrated with the progress being made during rehabilitation

○ **C.** When an athlete is pulling away from the team and coaches due to strong feelings of homesickness

○ **D.** When the athletic trainer seems to be thinking about the athlete's needs and ways to address these needs during nonworking hours

○ **E.** When an athlete confesses to taking somebody else's attention deficit–hyperactivity disorder prescription to stay up and study for a mid-term examination

188. In the process of referring an athlete for psychosocial counseling, which of the following poorly demonstrates professional considerations and subsequent actions?

○ **A.** Expressing your concern for the athlete's welfare and optimal well-being

○ **B.** Protecting yourself, others, and the athlete

○ **C.** Continuing to be supportive to the athlete throughout treatment

○ **D.** Assisting as requested in the communication process with the mental health professional

○ **E.** Probing into the current issues about the athlete's therapy

189. You are conducting an educational session for your student athletes on substance abuse. Which of the following signs and symptoms may indicate a substance use disorder?

○ **A.** Increasing mistakes through inattention or poor judgment and unexplained weight loss

○ **B.** Increased appetite and increasing physical complaints of unknown origin or evidence of injury

○ **C.** Arriving late to practice or class and overreacting to real or imagined criticisms

○ **D.** Increasing complaints from teammates and desire to change academic major

○ **E.** Minimizing relationship with parents and bragging about a vibrant social life

190. A four-step screening tool called CAGE is used to inquire about patterns and consequences of alcohol use. For this screening tool, what is the accompanying question for the letter A?

○ **A.** Have you ever attended an Alcoholics Anonymous meeting?

○ **B.** Have your friends or family ever recommended you Abstain from drinking?

○ **C.** Have you ever had your first drink in the A.m. hours?

○ **D.** Have people Annoyed you by criticizing your drinking?

○ **E.** Have you ever Awakened in a strange place and not known where you were after drinking?

191. An athletic trainer is using healing imagery to assist a patient who is progressing slower than anticipated through the repair phase of the healing process. Which of the following images should the athletic trainer teach the athlete to envision?

○ **A.** Visualize the injured ankle successfully responding in a game situation.

○ **B.** Visualize the mast cells releasing histamine to begin to wall off the injured area.

○ **C.** Visualize a happy place to relax and not think about the injury.

○ **D.** Visualize fibroblasts laying down scar tissue to make the injured area stronger and more stable.

○ **E.** Visualize performing rehabilitation exercises without pain and with full strength.

192. Which of the following cognitive-based relaxation strategies is geared at eliminating negative thoughts that are linked to the spiraling effects of anxiety?

○ **A.** Thought stoppage and reframing

○ **B.** Desensitization

○ **C.** Disassociation

○ **D.** Autogenic training

○ **E.** Meditation

193. Which of the following somatic-based relaxation strategies is based on the premise that it is impossible to be nervous or tense if muscles are completely relaxed?

○ **A.** Differential relaxation

○ **B.** Progressive relaxation

○ **C.** Rhythmic breathing

○ **D.** Concentration breathing

○ **E.** 1:2 breathing

194. An athlete, who is a 5th-year senior, has had four shoulder surgeries and is contemplating a fifth surgery. The coach, teammates, and parents are pressuring the athlete to get the surgery as soon as possible. The athlete begins to exhibit physical, psychological, and emotional withdrawal. Which psychosocial conditions is this athlete most likely exhibiting?

○ **A.** Achievement motivation

○ **B.** Anxiety

○ **C.** Adjustment disorder

○ **D.** Burnout

○ **E.** Addiction

Answers for Domain IV: Treatment, Rehabilitation, and Reconditioning

Role A: Administer therapeutic and conditioning exercise(s) using standard techniques and procedures in order to facilitate recovery, function, and/or performance.

1. B

2. A

3. C

4. A

5. E

6. E

7. A

8. B

9. C

10. E

11. B

12. D

13. E

14. A

15. D

16. D

17. E

18. A

19. A

20. B

21. D

22. A

23. C

24. B

25. B

26. E

27. A

28. D

29. B

30. C

31. D

32. A

33. B

34. A

35. B

36. E

37. D

38. C

39. A

40. A

41. E

42. C

43. A

44. B

45. A

46. D

47. B

48. A

49. E

50. C

Role B: Administer therapeutic modalities using standard techniques and procedures in order to facilitate recovery, function, and/or performance.

51. A

52. E

53. C

54. A

55. A

56. C

57. C

58. E

59. B

60. A

61. B

62. C

63. B

64. E

65. E

66. A

67. D

68. A

69. C

70. B

71. D

72. C

73. A

74. A

75. C

76. E

77. D

78. B

79. A

80. C

81. B

82. D

83. E

84. A

85. A

86. B

87. D

88. B

89. E

Role C: Apply braces, splints, or assistive devices in accordance with appropriate standards and practices in order to facilitate recovery, function, and/or performance.

90. D

91. B

92. A

93. D

94. A

95. A

96. D

97. B

98. B

99. A

100. E

101. C

102. D

103. A

104. A

Role D: Administer treatment for general illness and/or conditions using standard techniques and procedures to facilitate recovery, function, and/or performance.

105. E

106. A

107. B

108. D

109. C

110. C

111. E

112. B

113. A

114. B

115. C

116. A

117. A

118. D

119. E

120. B

121. C

122. E

123. A

124. B

125. B

126. D

127. C

128. A

129. E

130. B

131. C

132. B

133. A

134. C

135. A

136. D

137. B

138. C

139. C

140. C

141. E

142. B

143. D

Role E: Reassess the status of injuries, illnesses, and/or conditions using standard techniques and documentation strategies in order to determine appropriate treatment, rehabilitation, and/or reconditioning and to evaluate readiness to return to a desired level of activity.

144. E

145. A

146. C

147. A

148. A

149. D

150. A

151. B

152. E

153. D

154. C

155. B

156. C

157. A

158. C

159. E

160. D

161. D

162. B

163. C

164. A

165. B

166. E

167. C

168. A

169. B

170. A

171. D

172. B

Role F: Educate the appropriate patient(s) in the treatment, rehabilitation, and reconditioning of injuries, illnesses, and/or conditions using applicable methods and materials to facilitate recovery, function, and/or performance.

173. D

174. E

175. A

176. A

177. C

178. B

179. B

180. A

181. C

182. E

183. B

184. D

Role G: Provide guidance and/or counseling for the appropriate patient(s) in the treatment, rehabilitation, and reconditioning of injuries, illnesses, and/or conditions through communication to facilitate recovery, function, and/or performance.

185. B

186. A

187. A

188. E

189. C

190. D

191. D

192. A

193. B

194. D

Domain V: Organization and Administration

1. What risk management areas should be developed with guidelines before the start of a season?

○ **A.** Emergency action plan, exposure control plan, and environmental hazards plan

○ **B.** Treatment procedures, general policies, and emergency medical service protocols

○ **C.** Pregnant athlete policy, employee infectious disease plan, and physician referral protocol

○ **D.** Surgical observation guidelines, phone contact list, and method of recording medication administration

○ **E.** Forms to communicate strength and conditioning, personnel scheduling policies, and dress code

2. An established emergency care plan is an essential element in an institution's policy and procedure manual. Which of the following would be included in your facility's policy and procedure manual but not in your emergency care plan?

○ **A.** Emergency action plan rehearsal schedule

○ **B.** Personnel attire requirements

○ **C.** Roles and responsibilities of essential personnel

○ **D.** Names and contact information for persons with means and authority to unlock various doors and gates

○ **E.** Information that will be communicated during referral processes

3. An athlete is making the complaint of negligence against an athletic trainer you employ. To prove negligence, which of the following conditions must be established?

○ **A.** The conduct of the athletic trainer exceeded duty of care.

○ **B.** The athletic trainer was not working under the direct supervision of a physician.

○ **C.** The Good Samaritan Law was violated.

○ **D.** Damages occurred as a result of the athletic trainer's actions.

○ **E.** An assumption of risk waiver was not signed by the athlete.

4. What does AOASM stand for?

○ **A.** American Orthopedic Academy of Sports Medicine

○ **B.** Association of Organization and Administration in Sports Medicine

○ **C.** American Osteopathic Academy of Sports Medicine

○ **D.** Academy for Orthopedic Assistance in Sports Medicine

○ **E.** Alliance for Outreach and Advancement of Sports Medicine

5. When traveling with your high school football team, which of the following must you bring with you because you cannot assume it will be provided by the host school?

○ **A.** Automated external defibrillator

○ **B.** Spine board

○ **C.** Splints

○ **D.** Blood pressure cuff

○ **E.** Rescue inhaler

6. Which of the following documents would best assist you in justifying a request for additional personnel to provide coverage for your college sports teams?

○ **A.** NCAA Sports Medicine Handbook

○ **B.** State Athletic Training Practice Act

○ **C.** National Center for Catastrophic Sports Injury Research Database

○ **D.** National Safety Council Recommendation for Athlete to Healthcare Provider Ratio

○ **E.** Recommendations and Guidelines for Appropriate Medical Coverage of Intercollegiate Athletics

7. As the director of sports medicine for a small college, you are responsible for assigning your two certified athletic trainers to cover team practices. If there are four practices occurring simultaneously on unconnected fields, on which document should you rely when determining staff placement?

○ **A.** NCAA Injury Surveillance System

○ **B.** National Safety Council Recommendation for Athlete to Healthcare Provider Ratio

○ **C.** National Electronic Injury Surveillance System

○ **D.** Annual Survey of Football Injury Research

○ **E.** American College of Sports Medicine Injury Incidence Report

8. A member of your soccer team carries sickle cell trait. What equipment should be on the sideline while this athlete is practicing to best manage a potential exertional sickling episode?

○ **A.** Isotonic electrolyte beverages

○ **B.** Liquid glucose

○ **C.** Supplemental oxygen

○ **D.** Ice immersion tub

○ **E.** Rescue inhaler

9. A member of your field hockey team has type 1 diabetes. Which of the following should be in your field kit at all times to best provide emergency care for this athlete?

○ **A.** Rescue inhaler

○ **B.** Injectable insulin

○ **C.** Diet soda

○ **D.** Glucose gel

○ **E.** Supplemental oxygen

10. A softball player is referred to an ear, nose, and throat physician after being struck in the nose by a ball. Which is the most important document that should accompany the player to the off-campus health-care facility?

○ **A.** Medical history and injury report

○ **B.** List of contact numbers and medical referral paperwork

○ **C.** Insurance information and list of athlete's allergies

○ **D.** Medical referral paperwork and insurance information

○ **E.** Injury report and parent contact information

11. You are organizing a station-based pre-participation examination prior to the start of the academic year. The first station in the examination will be the review of individuals' medical history. Which health-care provider is best qualified to conduct this review?

○ **A.** Athletic training student

○ **B.** Team manager

○ **C.** Certified athletic trainer

○ **D.** Emergency medical technician

○ **E.** Physical therapist

12. You are organizing a station-based pre-participation examination for your 350 athletes before the start of the academic year. Your team physician, a physician assistant, a nurse from student health services, and the members of your athletic training staff will be conducting the examinations. The athletic training students and team managers have also agreed to assist as needed. Based on limited number of personnel, whom should you assign to conduct the urinalysis station?

○ **A.** Athletic training student

○ **B.** Nurse

○ **C.** Physician assistant

○ **D.** Certified athletic trainer

○ **E.** Physician

13. Your athletic director is investigating options for medical insurance for student athletes and is considering self-insurance. Which of the following is an advantage of self-insurance?

○ **A.** Simplified claims processing

○ **B.** Large claim risk

○ **C.** Ability to predetermine exact insurance costs for the year

○ **D.** Institutional funds are committed prior to request

○ **E.** No catastrophic coverage is needed

14. What measures can you use to help your institution keep insurance premiums to a minimum?

○ **A.** Establish policies that limit the institution's financial obligation, and require physicians to work on a retainer.

○ **B.** Require student athletes to have primary insurance, and conduct an annual risk-assessment audit.

○ **C.** Require athletes to use only physicians approved by their primary insurance plan, and decrease your deductible.

○ **D.** Require each athlete to pay a modest sum for insurance, and require athletes to get three bids for all surgical procedures.

○ **E.** Encourage medical providers to treat athletes on an "insurance-only" basis, and coaches should budget to pay co-pays for all off campus health-care visits.

15. You are working as an athletic trainer in an outpatient physical therapy clinic. Following patient treatment, you must identify which procedures were completed for insurance billing purposes. Which coding system is used to identify these procedures?

○ **A.** ICD-9CM

○ **B.** UB-92

○ **C.** CPT

○ **D.** CMS-1500

○ **E.** EDI

16. What legal term is invoked when an individual fails to act in a reasonable and prudent manner or, as is sometimes stated, "without due care"?

○ **A.** Tort

○ **B.** Negligence

○ **C.** Liability

○ **D.** Felony

○ **E.** Prudence

17. By which clause can employers be held liable for the acts of their employees?

○ **A.** Contributory negligence

○ **B.** Vicarious liability

○ **C.** Charitable immunity

○ **D.** Good Samaritan clause

○ **E.** Assumption of risk

18. An athletic trainer who uses a therapeutic modality in a contraindicated manner could be found guilty of which type of negligence?

○ **A.** Malfeasance

○ **B.** Nonfeasance

○ **C.** Breach of duty

○ **D.** Tort

○ **E.** Misfeasance

19. According the Joint Position Statement of the American Medical Society for Sports Medicine and the American Orthopedic Society for Sports Medicine on HIV and Other Blood-Borne Pathogens in Sports, which of the following variables should be considered when determining whether an HIV-positive athlete should continue competition?

○ **A.** The nature and intensity of training and potential contribution of stress from athletic competition

○ **B.** Potential risk of HIV transmission to others and risk of direct tissue trauma

○ **C.** Nature and intensity of training and the injury exposure rate of the sport

○ **D.** The athlete's current state of health and the athlete's family history of autoimmune disease

○ **E.** Status of HIV infection and ability of the facility to manage blood exposure

20. According the Joint Position Statement of the American Medical Society for Sports Medicine and the American Orthopedic Society for Sports Medicine on HIV and Other Blood-Borne Pathogens in Sports, what is the position of these professional organizations on mandatory HIV testing as a condition for athletic participation or competition?

○ **A.** Mandatory testing would effectively prevent the spread of infection.

○ **B.** Mandatory testing is easily done in athletic populations.

○ **C.** Mandatory testing should be required only for contact sports.

○ **D.** Mandatory testing is not justified.

○ **E.** Mandatory testing is a cost-effective way of promoting health and safety.

21. During a routine blood test, one of your athletes tests positive for hepatitis A virus. What actions must be taken by the physician who ordered the blood test?

○ **A.** The physician must report the athlete's condition to state agencies.

○ **B.** The physician must require the athlete to notify all recent sexual partners.

○ **C.** The physician must notify anyone providing health care to the athlete about potential exposure.

○ **D.** The physician must keep this information confidential.

○ **E.** The physician must notify the athlete's parent or guardian of the recent diagnosis.

22. You have been subpoenaed to provide testimony regarding a previous student athlete's medical condition. Which of the following guidelines should you observe to safeguard your credibility?

○ **A.** Avoid memorizing the testimony, and never refer to medical records while on the stand.

○ **B.** Avoid testifying beyond the boundaries of your experience and, if unsure, making an educated guess.

○ **C.** Discuss your testimony with an attorney prior to giving it in the courtroom, and never guess.

○ **D.** Testify only on issues about which you are an expert, and speak on behalf of the athlete's best interests.

○ **E.** Be truthful when testifying about the athlete's feelings, and avoid overpreparing for your testimony because it will appear rehearsed.

23. Which of the following forms should be signed to minimize potential legal ramifications of the pre-participation physical examination?

○ **A.** A waiver of liability

○ **B.** An HIPAA disclosure form

○ **C.** A permission to bill insurance form

○ **D.** Drug testing consent form

○ **E.** A consent form

24. Which of the following is one of the two overarching goals of the NCAA drug testing program?

○ **A.** To prevent athletes from becoming addicted to drugs

○ **B.** To remove pressure on athletes to take drugs to have a chance to win

○ **C.** To provide a means for promoting order and discipline on a team

○ **D.** To prevent or discourage potentially illegal activity

○ **E.** To prevent athletes from testing positive when they reach the professional sports arena

25. What is the consequence of a student athlete not signing the NCAA drug testing consent form?

○ **A.** The athlete will be disqualified from any NCAA tournaments.

○ **B.** The athlete can participate but will not be eligible for a scholarship.

○ **C.** The athlete will be found guilty of a first positive drug test.

○ **D.** The athlete will be declared ineligible for competition.

○ **E.** The athlete must attend weekly drug education sessions for 1 year.

26. Which of the following statements demonstrates appropriate drug testing specimen handling and chain of custody?

○ **A.** The athlete should produce the specimen in a single toilet stall with the door closed to protect privacy.

○ **B.** The athlete should be allowed to observe the handling of the specimen until it is transferred to a sealed bottle and packaged for shipment.

○ **C.** The athlete must wash hands before and immediately after providing the specimen.

○ **D.** The athlete must sign the bottle, indicating no one has tampered with the specimen.

○ **E.** The athlete may not leave the testing area until an adequate specimen has been provided.

27. To ensure safe operation and minimize the risk of patient injury, to what must whirlpool motors be connected?

○ **A.** Circuit breaker

○ **B.** Ground fault interrupter

○ **C.** Hospital-grade plug

○ **D.** Fast-blow fuse

○ **E.** Dedicated circuit

28. How often should hydrotherapeutic modalities be cleaned?

○ **A.** After each patient use

○ **B.** Twice per day

○ **C.** Once per day

○ **D.** Once per week

○ **E.** Twice per week

29. Regarding athletic facilities, which of the following is outside the intended scope of practice of the athletic trainer?

○ **A.** Informing the coaching staff that the grass is too high

○ **B.** Ensuring that the blocking sled is properly padded

○ **C.** Reporting and/or correcting uneven playing surfaces

○ **D.** Ensuring that goal posts are properly padded

○ **E.** Informing the coaching staff that the practice field was just fertilized

30. What is the most important consideration when determining necessary square footage for a new athletic training room?

○ **A.** Scope of the athletic training program and number of athletes

○ **B.** Number of staff athletic trainers and existence of accredited undergraduate program

○ **C.** Number of teams to be served and expected number of injuries for those sports

○ **D.** Location and size of the current facility

○ **E.** Construction budget and extent of administrative support

31. According to the AHA/ACSM Joint Position Statement: Recommendations for Cardiovascular Screening, Staffing, and Emergency Policies at Health/Fitness Facilities, what is the responsibility of any facility offering exercise equipment or services?

○ **A.** The facility must provide a stress test for all new members or prospective users.

○ **B.** The facility must require all new members to provide proof of a recent comprehensive physical examination.

○ **C.** The facility must require all new members to provide proof of active health insurance.

○ **D.** The facility's personnel should conduct cardiovascular screening of all new members or prospective users.

○ **E.** The facility should deny membership to anyone identified as being at risk for cardiovascular incident.

32. Which branch of the federal government approves and regulates the use of many therapeutic modalities?

○ **A.** Underwriters Laboratories

○ **B.** National Operating Committee on Standards for Athletic Equipment

○ **C.** Federal Trade Commission

○ **D.** Food and Drug Administration

○ **E.** American Physical Therapy Association

33. You are working at a hospital-based sports medicine clinic. Which of the following organizations would be most likely to visit your clinic during an on-site accreditation visit?

○ **A.** The Joint Commission

○ **B.** American Medical Association

○ **C.** Commission on Accreditation of Rehabilitative Facilities

○ **D.** Occupational Safety and Health Administration

○ **E.** Commission on Accreditation and Healthcare Safety

34. What actions should you take if the waste in your biohazardous waste container is putrescible?

○ **A.** Move it to a more convenient location.

○ **B.** Schedule a pickup by a biohazardous material company.

○ **C.** Place a sharps container more proximal to your biohazardous waste container.

○ **D.** Put a sign above it that says "May contain blood or other OPIM."

○ **E.** Move it to an area with less foot traffic.

35. Your athletic training students would like to have a pizza party in the athletic training room during the lunch hour. Which of the following statements best explains your rationale for not allowing the party?

○ **A.** "Food and Drug Administration standards require that food and drink be in work areas only after designated work hours."

○ **B.** "The state health department guidelines for food cleanliness in a public place cannot be met with the cleaning products used in an athletic training programs."

○ **C.** "The athletic training room cannot be closed during working hours because the athletes need ongoing, uninterrupted access."

○ **D.** "Department of Health and Environmental Control guidelines for health-care facilities prohibit ingesting food within 30 minutes of providing health care."

○ **E.** "Occupational Safety and Health Administration regulations prohibit eating and drinking in work areas where there is a reasonable likelihood of occupational exposure."

36. Which of the following components should be included in your facility exposure control plan?

○ **A.** Action steps to take if exposure occurs and method of documenting HIV status of employees

○ **B.** Method for recording every occupational exposure and cost list for personal protection equipment

○ **C.** Annual employee training plan and criteria for identifying individuals most likely to carry blood-borne pathogens

○ **D.** Bloodborne pathogens education and plans for exposure prevention

○ **E.** List of signs and symptoms of bloodborne pathogens and criteria for determining an exposure incident

37. Which of the following statements correctly reflects current recommendations for the placement of electrical outlets in the treatment area of an athletic training room?

○ **A.** Electrical outlets should be placed at least 1 ft from the ground and spaced close to tables and therapeutic modalities.

○ **B.** Electrical outlets should be placed in an area 4 to 6 ft from the ground and every 2 ft throughout the facility.

○ **C.** Electrical outlets should be wired to a master ground fault interrupter to minimize risk of burns and electrocution.

○ **D.** Electrical outlets should be placed at least 3 ft from the ground and spaced every 4 ft throughout the facility.

○ **E.** Electrical outlets should be located next to phone and cable connections to minimize construction costs.

38. In which budgetary category would you place a piece of equipment costing $4000 and having a life span of 3 or more years?

○ **A.** Expendable supplies

○ **B.** Nonexpendable supplies

○ **C.** Capital supplies

○ **D.** Big-ticket supplies

○ **E.** Overhead supplies

39. Although securing goods and services through competitive bidding is generally considered desirable for an athletic department, under what circumstances would direct purchase be preferable?

○ **A.** The buyer has had satisfactory dealings with a specific supplier.

○ **B.** There are a great many suppliers of the item requested.

○ **C.** Some of the previous suppliers have been unsatisfactory.

○ **D.** Only one supplier is available in the immediate area.

○ **E.** The goods or services are known to be available from only one source.

40. Which of the following is essential to maintaining a useful inventory in an athletic training department?

○ **A.** Biannual check of all nonexpendable equipment

○ **B.** Annual check and estimate of expendable and nonexpendable equipment

○ **C.** Listing of nonexpendable equipment lost or misplaced during the year

○ **D.** Listing of all expendable equipment lost or misplaced during the year

○ **E.** Evaluation of the expendable equipment most frequently used during the year

41. What type of insurance should athletic trainers maintain while practicing in the field?

○ **A.** Professional liability

○ **B.** Catastrophic event

○ **C.** Accident

○ **D.** Life

○ **E.** Indemnity

42. What type of analysis is considered a useful tool in the strategic planning of an existing athletic training program?

○ **A.** HCFA analysis

○ **B.** Strengths/weaknesses analysis

○ **C.** WOTS-UP analysis

○ **D.** Samson analysis

○ **E.** Forecast analysis

43. You are creating an advertisement for an open staff athletic trainer position at your facility. Which of the following statements would be most appropriate to include?

○ **A.** Seeking male applicants; minorities are encouraged to apply.

○ **B.** Salary is commensurate with experience.

○ **C.** Our facility provides on-site day care at a fair market rate.

○ **D.** Benefits include state health plan, optional vision coverage, and choice of standard or flexible retirement plan.

○ **E.** Work schedule is 8:30 a.m. to 4:30 p.m. daily with additional evening and weekend hours as assigned.

44. What is the purpose of a job description?

○ **A.** To list specific tasks that must be performed daily by the employee

○ **B.** To protect the institution from a potential lawsuit

○ **C.** To define the expected, allowed, and disallowed duties of employees

○ **D.** To detail benefits provided for the employee

○ **E.** To justify a division's or institution's budget allocation

45. How might you justify hiring a minority candidate who meets the qualifications in a job description but is not the most qualified candidate in the application pool?

○ **A.** Title IX provisions for equal employment encourage this practice.

○ **B.** Equal Opportunity and Affirmative Action guidelines permit direct hiring of minority candidates.

○ **C.** Americans With Disabilities Act guidelines prohibit discrimination of persons on the basis of race and gender.

○ **D.** Federal employment guidelines provide private institutions with autonomy in hiring minorities.

○ **E.** Institutions receive additional state appropriations when minority candidates fill historically nonminority positions.

46. What is the most commonly employed organizational chart in sports medicine settings?

○ **A.** Service-oriented

○ **B.** Matrix

○ **C.** Staff-centered

○ **D.** Function-oriented

○ **E.** Formalistic

47. Which of the following questions is illegal to ask a potential employee during an interview?

○ **A.** Are you older than age 18?

○ **B.** Do you anticipate any absences from work on a regular basis?

○ **C.** Do you have any restrictions on your ability to travel?

○ **D.** Are you available to work on weekends?

○ **E.** How many children are you planning to have?

48. During an interview, the interviewer may use various question types. Which of the following is an example of a close-ended question?

○ **A.** Did you like your last job?

○ **B.** Working on your own does not bother you, does it?

○ **C.** If I call your references, what will they say about you?

○ **D.** How would you organize your team to begin work?

○ **E.** What does it take to challenge you?

49. An employee is complaining of having to work back-to-back weekends and several long days and becomes angry upon being scheduled to work an upcoming holiday. Which component of role strain is this employee demonstrating?

○ **A.** Role conflict

○ **B.** Role incongruity

○ **C.** Role ambiguity

○ **D.** Role overload

○ **E.** Role incompetence

50. In which stage of employee burnout would the first symptoms begin to appear?

○ **A.** First stage: Job contentment

○ **B.** Second stage: Job disappointment

○ **C.** Third stage: Job disillusionment

○ **D.** Fourth stage: Job despair

○ **E.** Fifth stage: Work redefined

51. Which type of budget allocates money for the daily functions of a program?

○ **A.** Capital

○ **B.** Flex

○ **C.** Line-item

○ **D.** Zero-based

○ **E.** Operating

52. Which supervisory model emphasizes the use of formal authority to improve employee efficacy and efficiency?

○ **A.** Clinical supervision

○ **B.** Developmental supervision

○ **C.** Performance evaluation supervision

○ **D.** Inspection-production supervision

○ **E.** Centralized leadership supervision

53. What document can assist a head athletic trainer at a college or university in justifying the hiring of additional staff?

○ **A.** NCAA's Sports Medicine Handbook chapter on Recommended Event Coverage

○ **B.** State Practice Act ratios of health-care providers to participants

○ **C.** NATA's Recommendations and Guidelines for Appropriate Medical Coverage in Intercollegiate Athletics

○ **D.** National Association of Collegiate Directors of Athletics' Recommendations for Risk Management and Hiring Practices

○ **E.** The Intercollegiate Athletics Advisory Panel Recommendations on Necessary Medical Care

54. Which of the following characteristics exemplifies a manager in contrast to a leader?

○ **A.** Creates excitement and develops fresh approaches to problems

○ **B.** Concerned with what events and decisions mean to people

○ **C.** Has impersonal goals that arise from organizational necessity

○ **D.** Develops visions for the future and strategies to produce change

○ **E.** Energizes people to overcome political, bureaucratic, and resource barriers

55. Which of the following characteristics exemplifies a leader in contrast to a manager?

○ **A.** Possesses tough-mindedness, intelligence, and analytical ability

○ **B.** Produces change, often to a dramatic extent

○ **C.** Formulates strategies, makes decisions, manages conflict

○ **D.** Is role-oriented and concerned with how to get things done

○ **E.** Uses planning and organization to solve problems

56. Propriety standards are used during an employee's performance evaluation to ensure that the process is legal and fair. Which of the following is a propriety standard?

○ **A.** Conflict of interest

○ **B.** Constructive orientation

○ **C.** Evaluator credibility

○ **D.** Functional reporting

○ **E.** Follow-up

57. Utility standards are used during an employee's performance evaluation to ensure that the evaluation is useful to workers, employers, and others who need to use the information. Which of the following is a utility standard?

○ **A.** Interaction with those being evaluated

○ **B.** Access to personnel evaluation reports

○ **C.** Formal evaluation guidelines

○ **D.** Defined uses

○ **E.** Service orientation

58. You have just implemented your budget for the upcoming year. What is the next step in the budgeting process?

○ **A.** Evaluate the effectiveness of the budget by determining what is and is not working in the budget process.

○ **B.** Plan the budget based on the goals and objectives of your program.

○ **C.** Gather data, and analyze feedback from staff and other participants.

○ **D.** Present the budget in a clear and concise manner to appropriate administrators.

○ **E.** Build consensus on the proposed budget, and provide possible alternatives to budget decisions.

59. Which of the following records would be protected by the HIPAA but not the FERPA?

○ **A.** Records of counseling sessions with the high school guidance counselor

○ **B.** Official transcript and test scores housed in the vice principal's office

○ **C.** Records of counseling sessions with the high school psychologist

○ **D.** Attendance records indicating absences due to illness housed in the main office

○ **E.** Results of school-wide random drug testing for street drugs housed in the principal's office

60. What is the penalty for a person who violates HIPAA in a noncriminal manner?

○ **A.** May be fined up to $25,000

○ **B.** May face jail time

○ **C.** May be fined up to $250,000

○ **D.** Will be placed on probation by the Department of Justice

○ **E.** Will be required to attend HIPAA educational sessions for 1 year

61. To whom do HIPAA regulations apply?

○ **A.** To anyone providing health care

○ **B.** To covered entities

○ **C.** To licensed health-care providers only

○ **D.** To federally funded health-care facilities only

○ **E.** To facilities that file insurance only

62. According to the National Center for Medical Rehabilitation Research's terminology for disability classification, which of the following is defined as a limitation or inability to perform activities and roles to the levels expected within physical and social contexts?

○ **A.** Disability

○ **B.** Impairment

○ **C.** Functional limitation

○ **D.** Societal limitation

○ **E.** Pathophysiological limitation

63. According to the National Center for Medical Rehabilitation Research's common specific terminology for disability classification, which of the following classifications is illustrated by a patient's inability to reach overhead, squat down to pick something up, or throw a ball?

○ **A.** Disability

○ **B.** Impairment

○ **C.** Societal limitation

○ **D.** Pathophysiological limitation

○ **E.** Functional limitation

64. According to the National Center for Medical Rehabilitation Research's common specific terminology for disability classification, which of the following illustrations would be classified as an impairment?

○ **A.** Patient is unable to reach up for items on the top shelf of kitchen cabinets

○ **B.** Patient is unable to sit for the entire class period

○ **C.** Patient lacks 20° of active shoulder flexion

○ **D.** Patient cannot enter a building due to lack of ramps

○ **E.** Patient has been diagnosed with a rotator cuff tear

65. As an athletic trainer serving as a physician extender for a physician whose practice focuses on joint replacements, you are often required to follow up with in-hospital patients after surgery. You note in a patient's chart that the Functional Independence Measure Scale has progressed from 5 to 6. What does this change indicate?

○ **A.** The patient is now demonstrating complete independence.

○ **B.** The patient can now ambulate with an assistive device.

○ **C.** The patient needs supervision to maintain safety during ambulation.

○ **D.** The patient needs total physical assistance from a health-care provider.

○ **E.** The patient requires 50% physical assistance from a health-care provider.

66. Which of the following pieces of information gathered during an initial patient evaluation is most appropriately recorded in the subjective section of your medical documentation?

○ **A.** Patient's score on Functional Independent Measure Scale

○ **B.** Patient's answer to the following question: "What would you like to be able to do after you complete your rehabilitation sessions?"

○ **C.** Patient's answer to the following question: "On average, how many hours of sleep are you losing each night due to pain?"

○ **D.** Patient's ability to ascend and descend stairs

○ **E.** Patient's score on the Klein-Bell Activities of Daily Living Scale

67. What question does the assessment portion of an initial evaluation medical record answer?

○ **A.** Why does this patient require rehabilitation skills and services?

○ **B.** Does this patient need to be seen by another health-care provider?

○ **C.** When will the patient be ready to return to full activity or sport participation?

○ **D.** How did the patient's injury occur?

○ **E.** What treatments will best benefit the patient?

68. For a patient with workman's compensation reimbursement, what should be included in at least one of the final goals of treatment?

○ **A.** A list of job responsibilities for which 50% must be met

○ **B.** Full pain-free range of motion for all activities completed involving the affected joint

○ **C.** Ability to complete all activities of daily living

○ **D.** Specific workplace task that will allow the patient to return to work with minimal or no work restrictions

○ **E.** Ability to be medication-free for a minimum of 90 days prior to discharge

69. Which of the following is an example of an objective assessment of ambulation that would be included in your medical record?

○ **A.** Adjectives the patient uses to describe pain during ambulation

○ **B.** List of surgical procedures performed on the patient's lower extremity

○ **C.** Location of the activity during which the injury occurred

○ **D.** Day of onset of current alteration from normal ambulatory patterns

○ **E.** Type of surface on which the patient is able to ambulate

70. Which of the following should be included in the plan of care portion of the initial assessment record?

○ **A.** Total number of treatments required and goals by which progress will be measured

○ **B.** Number of visits per week and treatment parameters for each therapeutic modality

○ **C.** Exercises likely to be performed during rehabilitation and methods for encouraging compliance

○ **D.** Date of expected follow-up visit to physician and modalities to be incorporated into the treatment plan

○ **E.** Anticipated time required for each visit and ICD-9 code for patient's exact diagnosis

71. Minimally, how often should a patient's treatment and rehabilitation goals be reassessed to determine progress?

○ **A.** Daily

○ **B.** Once per week

○ **C.** Every 2 weeks

○ **D.** Monthly

○ **E.** Prior to discharge

72. An athletic trainer documents the following in a daily treatment note: 10/9/10 Treatment lasted approximately 35 minutes. Patient reports decreased pain and swelling since the last visit. Knee AROM: 0-135, MMT: Quad ⅗, Hamstrings 4+/5; US 100% 3.0MHz 1.5 w/cm²×8 mins f/b CKC TKE 3×15×BW, 4 way SLR 3×15×2#, Mini-squats 2×20. Patient has reached full AROM goal. Patient iced following treatment and left in a happy mood. *Anna, ATC.* Which of the common errors in documenting daily treatment notes is evident in this documentation?

○ **A.** Failure to list the treatment time in minutes

○ **B.** Failure to document all treatment modalities and procedures used

○ **C.** Failure to include the visit number

○ **D.** Failure to reassess objective data and goals

○ **E.** Failure to sign and date all injuries

73. Which of the following components of documentation of treatment is likely to result in a Medicare audit?

○ **A.** Treatment schedule of three times/week for the first 6 weeks and two times/week for the next 3 weeks

○ **B.** Claims submitted for eight visits on one claim form

○ **C.** Daily treatments for the first 5 days and then treatments three times/week for the next 4 weeks

○ **D.** Modalities integrated into the exercise and functional activity program

○ **E.** Performing the same modality throughout the course of treatment

74. Your athletic training facility has expanded to include an off-campus athletic training room at your outdoor sport fields. How might you best share medical records with staff at both facilities to avoid duplicating records?

○ **A.** Utilize a computer-driven fax system

○ **B.** Utilize a commonly networked printer housed at your main facility to receive hard copies of all medical documentation

○ **C.** Utilize e-mail to transfer medical records between facilities

○ **D.** Utilize a local courier service twice a day to transport hard copies of medical records

○ **E.** Utilize a network or Web-based computerized medical record system

75. An athlete who recently graduated from your university has gone on to a professional athletics career. According to the statute of limitations, what is the recommended length of time this athlete's medical records should be kept?

○ **A.** For the duration of the athlete's professional athletics career if it exceeds your standard retention time frame

○ **B.** 10 years from the date of last activity in the chart

○ **C.** 20 years after the athlete graduates

○ **D.** 15 years after the athlete turns 21

○ **E.** Until the patient dies

76. Before buying computer software, which of the following should an athletic trainer consider?

○ **A.** Features of the software, days between order and receipt of software, and cost of software

○ **B.** User-friendliness, compatibility of software to current hardware, and institutional technical support

○ **C.** Quality of written instructions, availability on a trial basis, and reputation of the software design company

○ **D.** Ability to negotiate a price, views of other users, and ability to network the software program

○ **E.** Quantity of memory on current hard drives, antiviral capability of the software, and amount of training required

77. You have a regularly scheduled preseason meeting with your team physician. What should be the primary purpose of this meeting?

○ **A.** To catch up on personal and professional issues occurring over the summer months

○ **B.** To indicate the physician's roles and responsibilities as a member of the sports medicine team

○ **C.** To revisit your current plan for providing health care to athletes and refine as necessary

○ **D.** To formulate a letter to be distributed to coaches to remind them of your roles

○ **E.** To discuss specific health concerns of the athletes from the previous school year

78. Which of the following would be the most effective method of developing a professional rapport with your team physician?

○ **A.** Present a professional image on days you will be working around the physician.

○ **B.** Develop a professional work atmosphere in which the physician is an important and integral part of the program.

○ **C.** Set up a list of do's and don'ts for the physician, and share it with all program staff.

○ **D.** Have a meeting with the team physician, and indicate the physician's primary roles and responsibilities.

○ **E.** Routinely inquire about the physician's family and personal hobbies.

79. What is the most professionally productive relationship between a coach and the team physician?

○ **A.** There should be mutual confidence and trust between the two.

○ **B.** There should be mutual respect and awe between the two.

○ **C.** There should be mutual admiration along with a healthy degree of suspicion between the two.

○ **D.** There should be mutual approval and affection between the two.

○ **E.** There should be mutual professional courtesy along with some skepticism between the two.

80. The women's cross-country coach has expressed to you her concern for the amount of time one of her athletes is taking to recover from a recently diagnosed injury. The athlete has seen the team physician twice in the past 2 weeks. What should you instruct the coach to do regarding this athlete's injury?

○ **A.** Tell the coach to seek a physician who agrees with her line of thinking and will recommend what she thinks is necessary.

○ **B.** Give the coach the physician's phone number and instruct the coach to schedule a meeting.

○ **C.** Ask the coach to encourage the athlete to express her concerns to her athletic trainer and the team physician.

○ **D.** Tell the coach that you should meet with her and the team physician to discuss the athlete's injury.

○ **E.** Let the coach know that your role is to provide health care for her athletes and that she should focus her attention on coaching.

Answers for Domain V: Organization and Administration

Role A: Establish action plans for response to injury and illness using available resources to provide the required range of health-care services for patients, athletic activities, and events.

1. A

2. B

3. D

4. C

5. E

6. E

7. A

8. C

9. D

10. D

11. C

12. A

13. A

14. B

15. C

Role B: Establish policies and procedures for the delivery of health-care services following accepted guidelines to promote safe participation, timely care, and legal compliance.

16. B

17. B

18. E

19. A

20. D

21. A

22. C

23. E

24. B

25. D

26. B

Role C: Establish policies and procedures for the management of health-care facilities and activity areas by referring to accepted guidelines, standards, and regulations to promote safety and legal compliance.

27. B

28. A

29. A

30. C

31. D

32. D

33. A

34. B

35. E

36. D

37. D

Role D: Manage human and fiscal resources by utilizing appropriate leadership, organization, and management techniques to provide efficient and effective health-care services.

38. C

39. E

40. B

41. A

42. C

43. B

44. C

45. B

46. D

47. E

48. A

49. B

50. B

51. E

52. D

53. C

54. C

55. B

56. A

57. D

58. A

Role E: Maintain records using an appropriate system to document services rendered, provide for continuity of care, facilitate communication, and meet legal standards.

59. C

60. A

61. B

62. A

63. E

64. C

65. B

66. B

67. A

68. D

69. E

70. A

71. B

72. C

73. E

74. E

75. A

76. B

Role F: Develop professional relationships with appropriate patients and entities by applying effective communication techniques to enhance the delivery of health care.

77. C

78. B

79. A

80. C

Domain VI: Professional Responsibility

1. Which individual is ultimately responsible for determining the athlete's medical ability to return to competition?

○ **A.** Physician

○ **B.** Athletic trainer

○ **C.** Parent

○ **D.** Coach

○ **E.** Athletic director

2. Which of the following continuing education credit activities would most likely be denied if submitted by a certified athletic trainer for credit?

○ **A.** Attending a district athletic training symposium in the district in which the certified athletic trainer is a member

○ **B.** Attending a district athletic training symposium in a district in which the certified athletic trainer is not a member

○ **C.** Attending the NATA national symposium

○ **D.** Reading articles and completing continuing education unit quizzes in approved journals

○ **E.** Serving as an athletic trainer for a district all-star game

3. Which of the following continuing education credit activities would most likely be denied if submitted by a certified athletic trainer for credit?

○ **A.** Serving as a panelist at a clinical symposium where the primary audience is allied health-care professionals

○ **B.** Completing college coursework in administration

○ **C.** Completing home study courses offered by a facility listed in the NATA Board of Certification's approved provider directory

○ **D.** Obtaining cardiopulmonary resuscitation recertification

○ **E.** Providing an interview on athletic training for the local newspaper

4. Which of the following documents identifies the primary tasks of an entry-level athletic trainer?

○ **A.** The NATA Education Council's Competencies in Athlete Training

○ **B.** The Board of Certification Standards of Practice

○ **C.** The NATA Code of Ethics

○ **D.** The Board of Certification Role Delineation Study

○ **E.** Commission on Accreditation of Athletic Training Education Guidelines for Entry-Level Athletic Training

5. Which of the following actions falls outside the standard of care of the certified athletic trainer?

○ **A.** Maintaining documentation

○ **B.** Implementing rehabilitation programs

○ **C.** Preventing injuries

○ **D.** Dispensing medications

○ **E.** Educating coaches, athletes, and parents

6. As an athletic trainer, you are responsible for accumulating and maintaining an accurate record of all completed continuing education activities. Which of the following statements might lead you to overestimate the number of accumulated continuing education units (CEUs)?

○ **A.** Each time you become recertified in cardiopulmonary resuscitation, continuing CEUs are awarded.

○ **B.** You can only count CEUs accumulated during a 3-year period.

○ **C.** CEUs may be obtained by attending workshops and seminars hosted by approved providers.

○ **D.** CEUs may be obtained by attending a non–approved provider workshop and seminar

○ **E.** First aid is not a continuing education requirement/

7. You find out that a certified athletic trainer at another school in your town has been consuming alcohol during working hours. Which of the following codes is this individual violating?

○ **A.** Board of Certification Code of Honor

○ **B.** NATA Code of Ethics

○ **C.** Commission on Accreditation of Athletic Training Education Code of Professionalism

○ **D.** NCAA Code of Sports Medicine Practice

○ **E.** American Medical Association Code of Health Care

8. Your basketball team has reached the Sweet 16 round of the NCAA basketball tournament. In yesterday's practice session, your starting All-American point guard sprained an ankle and will not be ready for the game this coming weekend. You share this information at lunch with several close friends. After you share this information, your friends convince you to place a bet against your team because you are sure to make a profit. Which NATA Code of Ethics principle have you violated?

○ **A.** Principle 1: Members shall respect the rights, welfare, and dignity of all.

○ **B.** Principle 2: Members shall comply with the laws and regulations governing the practice of athletic training.

○ **C.** Principle 3: Members shall maintain and promote high standards in their provision of service.

○ **D.** Principle 4: Members shall not engage in conduct that could be construed as a conflict of interest or that reflects negatively on the profession.

○ **E.** Principle 5: Members shall report illegal or unethical practices related to athletic training to the appropriate person or authority.

9. For which of the following actions would a certified athletic trainer found to be noncompliant with the Board of Certification (BOC) Standards of Practice?

○ **A.** Endorsing a student's application to sit for the BOC certification examination in an examination window before the student's last semester of coursework

○ **B.** Completing an institutional review board protocol application before conducting research

○ **C.** Attending an educational conference sponsored by the American Physical Therapy Association

○ **D.** Following standing orders provided by your supervising physician when providing care

○ **E.** Refusing a coach who insists on returning an athlete with a head injury to practice before the athlete meets return-to-play criteria

10. Which of the following NATA position statements should a high school athletic trainer review before the start of preseason football to minimize the risk of heat-related illnesses?

○ **A.** Exertional Heat Illness

○ **B.** Emergency Planning in Athletics

○ **C.** Inter-Association Task Force on Exertional Heat Illness

○ **D.** Youth Football and Heat-Related Illness

○ **E.** Appropriate Medical Care for Secondary School Age Athletes

11. Athletic trainers should be professional. Which of the following behaviors best reflect professionalism?

○ **A.** Conduct research, treat all people with respect, and be consistent.

○ **B.** Avoid being self-serving, take an interest in the personal life of colleagues, and do the best you can.

○ **C.** Admit your mistakes; invite ideas, opinions, and feedback from others; and seek external funding to support your program.

○ **D.** Avoid wearing jewelry, be collaborative, and keep knowledge and skills up to date.

○ **E.** Give people a fair chance; be truthful and forthright; and be active at local, state and national levels.

12. Professional ethos evolves over time as a result of internal and external influences affecting a profession's maturation. Which of the following is considered an internal influence that shaped the profession of athletic training?

○ **A.** Increase in the number of female certified athletic trainers

○ **B.** Athletic trainers serving the needs of recreational athletes

○ **C.** Increased litigation involving athletic trainers

○ **D.** State licensure and certifications requirements

○ **E.** Third-party reimbursement for services

13. Professional ethos evolves over time as a result of internal and external influences affecting a profession's maturation. Which of the following is considered an external influence that shaped the profession of athletic training?

○ **A.** Increase in the number of ethnically diverse athletic trainers

○ **B.** Accreditation of undergraduate athletic training education programs

○ **C.** Increase in the number of post-professional educational programs

○ **D.** Increased reliance on technology

○ **E.** Diversification in the various job settings employing athletic trainers

14. Which of the following is an example of professional enculturation?

○ **A.** When an athletic training student completes a full evaluation and reaches a correct conclusion

○ **B.** When an athletic training student attends the state athletic trainer's association annual meeting

○ **C.** When an athletic training student can name the leadership of the professional organization

○ **D.** When an athletic training student successfully passes the Board of Certification examination

○ **E.** When an athletic training student displays sound reasoning and judgment and applies critical thinking

15. A coach approaches you with concerns that the female athletic trainer assigned to his team may be crossing professional lines with one of the male athletes. Which of the following factors should you consider in evaluating the patient-therapist relationship?

○ **A.** The athlete is undergoing a psychological adjustment to a significant illness or injury, and the athletic trainer is observed laughing and joking with the athlete during treatments.

○ **B.** The athletic trainer is providing multiple treatments per day, and the athlete is still reeling from the recent divorce of his parents.

○ **C.** The athlete is particularly lonely and shy, and the athletic trainer is preoccupied with the athlete.

D. The athlete is suffering from economic difficulty, and the athletic trainer and the athlete spend a lot of time talking about their love for dogs.

E. The athletic trainer accompanies the athlete to all physician's appointments, and the athlete is suffering from the death of his grandmother.

16. Why is it necessary for professions to have a code of ethics?

A. They set boundaries for proper and acceptable behavior.

B. They define punishable actions in the workplace.

C. They assist workers in deciding between right and wrong.

D. They assist in defining roles and responsibilities.

E. They protect workers from legal action.

17. As an experienced athletic trainer, you would like to model good professional behavior. Which of the following actions would you avoid in this effort?

A. Host a monthly journal club for staff members and graduate students.

B. Meet with graduate students at the beginning of their contract to discuss personal and professional expectations.

C. Seek constructive criticism from the staff regarding your decision making.

D. Explain to your colleagues factors that were considered in reaching an ethical decision.

E. Discuss specifics of an athlete's treatment plan at an after-hours staff social function.

18. You are the head athletic trainer at a small university. Your spouse is a sales representative for a national apparel chain. In your position, you encourage the athletics department and coaches to select your spouse's company as its sole uniform and accessories provider. How would this behavior be categorized?

A. Legal and ethical

B. Legal but unethical

C. Illegal and unethical

D. Illegal but ethical

E. Falling short of the criteria for illegal activity

19. Which of the following is an example of a NATA membership sanction that might be levied for unethical conduct?

A. Fine by the NATA

B. Revocation of certification

C. Public censure

D. Revocation of state license

E. Ban from attending annual meetings

20. The foundational behaviors in athletic training permeate every aspect of professional practice and relate to the principle of right conduct or the common values of the professions. Which of the following is an example of a foundational behavior as identified in the NATA Educational Competencies?

A. Purchasing modalities from a reputable dealer

B. Treating all patients the same regardless of their cultural backgrounds by strictly adhering to protocols

C. Using evidence-based practice as a foundation for the delivery of health care

D. Realizing that the patient and family members are not equipped for decision making regarding treatment and rehabilitation

E. Taking a stand against referral of athletes to competing health-care professionals

21. Which of the following best completes the analogy: Technical standards:ethical standards

A. Knowing and doing:being

B. Skill:mastery

C. Professionalism:ethics

D. Math and science:psychology

E. Computers:written documentation

22. An athletic trainer routinely exhibits compassion and empathy when caring for athletes. Under which of the following foundational behaviors of professional practice does this behavior fall?

A. Cultural competence

B. Ethical practice

C. Teamed approach to practice

D. Legal practice

E. Professionalism

23. You are busy completing the staff schedule, and one of your staff members comes to your door requesting 20 minutes to discuss a concern. You stop what you are doing to meet with the staff member. What important interpersonal skill are you demonstrating?

○ **A.** Providing support and encouragement

○ **B.** Being accessible

○ **C.** Demonstrating respect for culturally diverse staff members

○ **D.** Demonstrating confidence

○ **E.** Advocating for patients

24. An athlete on your swim team has been sick and is seeking a referral to a local herbalist, which is typical of the athlete's cultural upbringing. You respond by indicating that there is no evidence in the literature to support such a referral but that you will gladly provide a referral to the general medical clinic to see one of your physicians later that afternoon. What behavior are you demonstrating?

○ **A.** Evidence-based practice

○ **B.** Critical decision making

○ **C.** Ethnocentrism

○ **D.** Cultural awareness

○ **E.** Factualism

25. You are working at an elite soccer camp where some of the participants are international athletes. Which of the following typically accepted communication methods may be interpreted negatively by this population of athletes?

○ **A.** Asking if the athlete is fluent in English or if an interpreter is needed

○ **B.** Avoiding slang or technical terms

○ **C.** Using open-ended questions to provide an opportunity to gather as much information as possible

○ **D.** Maintaining direct eye contact when speaking with the athlete

○ **E.** Asking how the athlete would prefer to be addressed

26. Which branch of the federal government approves and regulates the use of many therapeutic modalities?

○ **A.** Underwriter's Laboratory

○ **B.** National Operating Committee on Standards for Athletic Equipment

○ **C.** Federal Trade Commission

○ **D.** Food and Drug Administration

○ **E.** Federal Health and Therapy Commission

27. Which of the following organizations accredits entry-level athletic training education programs?

○ **A.** Commission on Accreditation of Athletic Training Education

○ **B.** American Academy of Sports Medicine

○ **C.** Commission on Accreditation of Allied Health Education Programs

○ **D.** NATA Research and Education Foundation

○ **E.** Board of Certification

28. According to Title VII of the Civil Rights Act of 1964, when is an unwelcome sexual advance considered sexual harassment?

○ **A.** If submission to the advance is implicitly or explicitly a term or condition of employment

○ **B.** If rejection of the advance results in a display of anger by the advancing party

○ **C.** If submission to the advance results in promotion of the advancing party

○ **D.** If rejection of the advance creates a more professional work environment

○ **E.** If submission to the advance results in guilt and mental anguish for the submitting party

29. Which of the following is an example of inappropriate sexual innuendos in the athletic training workplace?

○ **A.** An athlete thanks you and gives you a hug on the day of discharge from treatment

○ **B.** A long-standing patient brings you homemade cookies

○ **C.** An athletic trainer receives a sincere "thank you" note from a patient for the care provided

○ **D.** Making repeated dormitory room visits to assist an athlete in performing rehabilitation exercises

○ **E.** An athletic trainer makes a copy of a CD a patient has told you is very motivational

30. A female coworker confides in you that she feels she is being sexually harassed by a male colleague. Which of the following is an appropriate action the employee can take?

○ **A.** Call a toll-free national hotline sponsored by a union.

○ **B.** Call Human Resources, and request a meeting to discuss her concerns.

○ **C.** Schedule an appointment with the president of your facility.

○ **D.** Send an e-mail to all female employees warning them about the colleague.

○ **E.** Confront the colleague about his behavior when there are many witnesses.

31. What steps can an employer take to minimize sexual harassment lawsuits?

○ **A.** Be aware that females tend to be more emotional and therefore report harassment at a higher rate.

○ **B.** Conduct required sexual harassment training every 5 years.

○ **C.** Have all employees complete a screening form to determine who is most likely to file a complaint.

○ **D.** Assign same-gender supervisors to complete employee evaluations.

○ **E.** Treat same-sex harassment and a male reporting harassment in the same way you would treat a woman lodging a complaint against a male.

32. After you pass the Board of Certification (BOC) examination, you move to a new state. What governs your athletic training practice in this state?

○ **A.** Certification regulations

○ **B.** Occupational Safety and Health Administration Guidelines

○ **C.** State licensure

○ **D.** State Medical practice act

○ **E.** BOC Standard of Practice

33. Which of the following is an example of NCAA legislation involving health and safety issues as outlined in the NCAA Sports Medicine Handbook?

○ **A.** The pre-participation physical examination should include a relevant musculoskeletal examination.

○ **B.** All participants should be removed from the playing field when the flash-to-bang count reaches 30 seconds.

○ **C.** An institution may cover expenses of counseling related to the treatment of eating disorders.

○ **D.** All athletes should be immunized for the following: MMR, hepatitis B, diphtheria, tetanus, and meningitis.

○ **E.** A team physician has the final responsibility to determine when a student athlete should be removed or withheld from participation.

34. One of your rowers has missed several weeks of classes while being treated for mononucleosis. The mother contacts you and asks you to facilitate obtaining current grades and assignments in each of the athlete's classes. How should you best respond to this request?

○ **A.** Inform her that HIPAA prohibits you from releasing any confidential information without the athlete's permission.

○ **B.** Inform her that the Buckley Amendment prohibits you from obtaining and sharing student grades.

○ **C.** Inform her that you will be glad to access these records for her because FERPA rules do not apply in this situation.

○ **D.** Inform her that you would be happy to help if you had a little more time in your schedule.

○ **E.** Inform her that you will have to check to see if the athlete signed a medical records release; if so, you will get the information to her as soon as possible.

35. When developing an administrative manual, which of the following key areas would include information explaining the need for the policy?

○ **A.** Purpose

○ **B.** Procedures

○ **C.** Documentation

○ **D.** Policies

○ **E.** Practices

36. The team is leaving in 1 hour for a road trip. One of your athlete's patellar tendonitis has flared up. You contact the team physician, who instructs you to provide the athlete with a 7-day course of a prescription COX-2 inhibitor, which is kept in a locked cabinet in your athletic training room. Should you comply with the physician's instructions?

○ **A.** No; physicians cannot delegate to athletic trainers the authority for dispensing prescription medications.

○ **B.** Yes; the drugs are the property of the physician to be dispensed at the physician's discretion.

○ **C.** No; the drugs are a controlled substance that cannot be carried over state lines.

○ **D.** Yes; athletic trainers work under the direct supervision of and are legally covered by physician orders.

○ **E.** No; drugs can be dispensed legally only by a pharmacist.

37. A HIPAA disclosure authorization is included as part of your pre-participation medical paperwork. An athlete with junior standing questions having to re-sign this form because it was completed at a previous pre-participation physical. How should you best respond to this athlete?

○ **A.** The HIPAA disclosure authorization must be completed every other year per NCAA requirements.

○ **B.** The HIPAA disclosure authorization must have been accidentally placed in the athlete's packet, and it can be ignored.

○ **C.** The HIPAA disclosure authorization must be signed, or the athlete will be deemed ineligible by the NCAA.

○ **D.** The HIPAA disclosure authorization must be re-signed now that she is 21 years of age.

○ **E.** The HIPAA disclosure authorization must be completed annually due to its expiration date.

38. A student completing observation hours in anticipation of applying the athletic training education program in the subsequent semester has begun to dress and act like students who are currently enrolled in the program. Which stage of organizational integrity is this student demonstrating?

○ **A.** Stage 1: Social Darwinism

○ **B.** Stage 2: Machiavellianism

○ **C.** Stage 3: Cultural conformity

○ **D.** Stage 4: Allegiance to authority

○ **E.** Stage 5: Democratic participation

39. How does sexual harassment differ from workplace bullying?

○ **A.** Women are more frequently victims of harassment, whereas men are more frequently victims of bullying.

○ **B.** Harassment can have a criminal element, but this tends not to be the case with bullying.

○ **C.** Bullying is primarily physical in nature, whereas harassment is primarily psychological.

○ **D.** Technology is used more in bullying than in sexual harassment.

○ **E.** Harassment can result in a civil lawsuit, whereas bullying is most often handled by administrators.

40. As an athletic trainer working in an outpatient sports medicine clinic, you must ensure that treatments are documented appropriately in order to seek third-party reimbursement. Which of the following documentations would be acceptable for third-party billing purposes?

○ **A.** Patient performed SLR 3×12×1# independently

○ **B.** Patient performed retro-walking in the therapy pool while monitored by an aide

○ **C.** Patient performed D2 UE flexion pattern rhythmic initiation 3×10 with moderate resistance

○ **D.** Patient cycled ×15 min for warm-up and mild cardio-vascular workout

○ **E.** Patient performed flexibility exercises after completing a supervised rehabilitation session

41. As an athletic trainer working in an outpatient sports medicine clinic, you must ensure that modality treatments are documented appropriately in order to seek third-party reimbursement. Which of the following must be included when documenting modality treatments when seeking reimbursement?

○ **A.** Evidence that the patient has been screened for all known contraindications to each modality utilized

○ **B.** Evidence of prior treatment effectiveness for every visit in which the modality is used

○ **C.** Evidence that low-cost modalities have been attempted prior to initiating more expensive modalities

○ **D.** Modality utilization summarization form at discharge

○ **E.** Clinical rationale for using the modality for the particular patient problem for every visit in which the modality is used

42. What is the role of the primary care physician in an HMO insurance program?

○ **A.** To provide referrals for nonemergency services

○ **B.** To provide health care for patients who cannot afford to see a specialist

○ **C.** To order all diagnostic tests prior to referral to specialists

○ **D.** To ensure that only generic prescription medications are utilized

○ **E.** To select the health-care providers that will be included in a patient's network

43. How does a PPO differ from an HMO?

○ **A.** A patient with a PPO must secure a referral from the primary care physician before being seen by a specialist.

○ **B.** A patient with an HMO will overall pay more in premiums but will have more coverage and more convenience.

○ **C.** A patient with a PPO typically has no out-of-network benefits.

○ **D.** A patient with a PPO will have coverage for wellness and preventive care.

○ **E.** A patient with a PPO has the right to choose which services they elect to receive and who is providing the services.

44. When does a person become eligible for Medicare benefits?

○ **A.** Upon showing proof of financial need

○ **B.** Upon turning 65 years of age and being eligible for Social Security benefits

○ **C.** Upon being dropped from the employer's health plan

○ **D.** Upon being unemployed and receiving state unemployment benefits

○ **E.** Upon choosing to pay the premium associated with the program

45. You are reviewing an athlete's chart, and you see that the athlete has Medicaid as primary insurance coverage. What does this mean?

○ **A.** The athlete's parents are older than 65 years and are eligible for Social Security benefits.

○ **B.** The athlete has a documented disability.

○ **C.** The athlete has met the criteria for federal and state regulated insurance coverage.

○ **D.** The athlete's parents have selected an insurance plan with high premiums and low out-of-pocket costs.

○ **E.** The athlete is in a state-limited network with a small number of choices for health-care providers.

46. You are in the process of bidding out your institution's secondary insurance program. Which of the following is the least likely inclusion to be added as a rider to the secondary insurance policy?

○ **A.** Heart and circulatory benefit

○ **B.** Preexisting conditions benefit

○ **C.** HMO denial clause

○ **D.** PPO denial clause

○ **E.** Cancerous condition benefit

47. You have just interviewed a potential hire who will not begin your contract until the fall semester (in approximately 3 months). The candidate is concerned about being without health coverage during the summer months. What recommendation can you make to this candidate?

○ **A.** Investigate the possibility of a COBRA plan provided by the candidate's current employer.

○ **B.** Purchase a short-term major medical policy for coverage.

○ **C.** Investigate the Family Medical Leave Act through the human resources office at the candidate's current employer.

○ **D.** Request a pre-employment insurance retainer provided through your institution.

○ **E.** Go without any coverage because the candidate appears healthy and leads a low-risk lifestyle.

48. One of your coworkers, who has been on the job for only 3 months, has a parent who has just been diagnosed with pancreatic cancer. The coworker's sick leave is exhausted, but the individual wants to have additional time to help the parent without having to quit the job. What may the coworker do according to the Family and Medical Leave Act of 1993?

○ **A.** Apply for funds through Human Resources to hire a temporary athletic trainer to fulfill the job responsibilities

○ **B.** Take up to 12 weeks of unpaid leave within a 12-month period

○ **C.** Bank the hours owed as long as they are made up within 12 months

○ **D.** Receive 50% of days currently available from the sick leave pool

○ **E.** Use own funds to hire a temporary athletic trainer to fulfill the job responsibilities

49. Civil rights legislation has led to the identification of protected classes or characteristics. These are traits that the law prohibits employers from considering when making employment decisions. Which of the following traits are recognized as protected classes or characteristics?

○ **A.** Disability, age, and IQ score

○ **B.** Military status, gender identity, and marital status

○ **C.** Race, number of children, and sexual orientation

○ **D.** Health status, color, and pregnancy

○ **E.** National origin, weight, and religion

50. A bona fide occupational qualification (BFOQ) is a trait that is integral or essential to a job. A BFOQ can be used to legally disqualify individuals who may have applied for a specific position. In which of the following examples is a BFOQ applied correctly?

○ **A.** Only female candidates will be considered for an athletic training position with a women's lacrosse team.

○ **B.** Only African-American males will be considered for an athletic training position at a training center that caters to National Basketball Association prospects.

○ **C.** Only candidates fluent in Spanish and English will be considered for an athletic training position with the Spanish national soccer team training in the United States.

○ **D.** Only devout Christians will be considered for an athletic training position at a conservative southern public institution.

○ **E.** Only heterosexual candidates will be considered for a Division I multisport, gender-diverse athletic program.

51. You are speaking to the Parent-Teacher Association at a local high school on why members should lobby for a full-time athletic trainer to care for their athletes. Which of the following is the best argument for why certified athletic trainers are essential in sport?

○ **A.** They can prevent athletic injuries.

○ **B.** They decrease the odds against negative outcomes from an injury, thus decreasing potential liability issues.

○ **C.** They can decrease the time required to return injured athletes to competition by accelerating the healing process.

○ **D.** They can force coaches to make better decisions that affect the health and safety of their athletes.

○ **E.** They lead to more conference championships and athletes being awarded college scholarships.

52. The marketing company contracted by your sports medicine clinic is designing a section for the clinic's Web sites that will highlight the unique services provided by athletic trainers. Which of the following is the best statement for this section of the Web site?

○ **A.** When it comes to working with injured athletes, certified athletic trainers are more knowledgeable and more highly skilled than physical therapists.

○ **B.** Quality health care is vital for individuals engaged in physical activity, and athletic trainers are the only health-care providers specially trained to provide this level of care.

○ **C.** The profession of athletic training was recognized by the American Medical Association in 1990 as an allied health-care profession.

○ **D.** All certified athletic trainers have at least a bachelor of science degree in athletic training, making them the most qualified health-care professionals to care for athletes.

○ **E.** Given the knowledge and skills acquired through nationally regulated educational programs, athletic trainers can provide quality health care to athletes and others engaged in physical activity.

53. Which of the following qualities are exemplified by athletic trainers functioning as effective educators?

○ **A.** Technology awareness

○ **B.** Sound oral communication skills

○ **C.** Effective pedagogical skills

○ **D.** Fair grading skills

○ **E.** Authoritative and demanding

54. You are explaining the difference between a physical therapist and an athletic trainer to an undergraduate student who is weighing career options. Which of the following statements best describes this difference in terms of scope of practice?

○ **A.** Physical therapists are qualified to treat a broader patient population.

○ **B.** Athletic trainers are limited to the care of the athletic population.

○ **C.** Physical therapists are more highly skilled in rehabilitation programs.

○ **D.** Athletic trainers can treat any athletic patient without needing a prescription.

○ **E.** Physical therapists can see patients for an unlimited number of visits pre-surgery under a physician's standing orders.

55. When communicating with an athlete whose English-speaking skills are poor, which of the following actions would likely result in a miscommunication?

○ **A.** Walking away while finishing your thought

○ **B.** Assuming the athlete is unfamiliar with commonly used terms

○ **C.** Speaking slowly and loudly

○ **D.** Using slang or technical terms

○ **E.** Writing out specific instructions

56. You are explaining the difference between a physical therapist and an athletic trainer to an undergraduate student who is weighing career options. Which of the following statements best describes the difference between the two career fields?

○ **A.** Physical therapists provide comprehensive health care for spine and musculoskeletal injuries.

○ **B.** Athletic trainers are responsible for every aspect of an athlete's health care.

○ **C.** Athletic trainers treat all injured athletes except postsurgical patients.

○ **D.** Physical therapists can bill for services, whereas athletic trainers cannot.

○ **E.** Athletic trainers are not as highly trained as physical therapists.

57. You have noticed that an athletic training colleague has begun to exhibit the behaviors listed below. Which behavior is least associated with professional burnout?

○ **A.** Self preoccupation

○ **B.** Insomnia

○ **C.** Anger

○ **D.** Lack of motivation

○ **E.** Manic episodes

58. Which of the following job characteristics is least likely to result in an athletic trainer experiencing burnout?

○ **A.** Long work hours

○ **B.** Role ambiguity

○ **C.** High expectations from superiors

○ **D.** High number of athletes to care for

○ **E.** Time away from family

59. Which of the following should be included when explaining the term "sports medicine" to the general public?

○ **A.** Umbrella term

○ **B.** Medical specialty

○ **C.** Athlete exclusive

○ **D.** Orthopedic

○ **E.** Surgical

60. Which of the following correctly defines the application of the term "direct supervision"?

○ **A.** As the responsible athletic trainer, I can communicate in person or by phone with the student at any time.

○ **B.** As the responsible athletic trainer, I can intervene on behalf of the athlete and the student at any time.

○ **C.** As the responsible athletic trainer, I can see and touch the athletic training student at all times.

○ **D.** As the responsible athletic trainer, I should provide the student autonomy to make non–life-threatening mistakes.

○ **E.** As the responsible athletic trainer, I am able to decrease the number of athletes I see per hour.

61. What landmark event for the athletic training profession occurred in 1990?

○ **A.** NATA became a 501c corporation.

○ **B.** NATA-REF was established.

○ **C.** The American Medical Association recognized athletic training as an allied health-care profession.

○ **D.** Two educational paths to certification were eliminated.

○ **E.** The Board of Certification split from the NATA.

62. Which of the following types of listening should a health-care professional employ when communicating with a patient?

○ **A.** Passive

○ **B.** Moderate

○ **C.** Critical

○ **D.** Active

○ **E.** Cynical

63. What was the impetus behind the fair practice anti-trust lawsuit of 2008 between the NATA and the American Physical Therapy Association (APTA)?

○ **A.** The APTA's actions to restrict athletic trainers' use of therapeutic modalities in a clinical setting

○ **B.** The APTA's actions to prevent athletic trainers from billing insurance for services

○ **C.** The APTA's actions to limit the type of patient athletic trainers can treat to the physically active.

○ **D.** The APTA's actions to prohibit athletic trainers from working in sports medicine clinics

○ **E.** The APTA's actions to restrict athletic trainers' education in and practice of manual therapy techniques

64. Through which of the following means do physical therapists gain professional qualifications?

○ **A.** Graduate from a master's or doctoral-level program accredited by the Commission on Accreditation in Physical Therapy Education and pass a licensure examination

○ **B.** Graduate from an entry-level program accredited by the Commission on Accreditation in Physical Therapy Education and pass a licensure examination

○ **C.** Graduate from an entry-level program recognized by the American Physical Therapy Association and pass a state licensure examination

○ **D.** Graduate from an entry-level master's program recognized by the American Physical Therapy Association and pass a certification examination

○ **E.** Graduate in the top 50% of the class from an accredited physical therapy program and pass a national-level examination

65. What is the role of the National Federation of State High School Associations as it relates to the pre-participation physical examination?

○ **A.** Establish rules and procedures

○ **B.** Mandate frequency of required examinations

○ **C.** Establish disqualifying conditions

○ **D.** Determine qualifications of authorizing professionals

○ **E.** Make recommendations only

66. You are hosting a lecture series for students in your athletic training education program. The speakers are all credentialed medical and allied health professionals. You have invited all the approved clinical instructors in your program to attend as well. Based on Board of Certification (BOC) guidelines, can these clinical instructors count these lectures toward continuing education unit credits?

○ **A.** Yes, as nonapproved provider credit as long as the presentation is made by a credentialed medical professional

○ **B.** No, because the primary audience is students

○ **C.** Yes; as long as you submit a list of their names and certification numbers to the BOC

○ **D.** No, because it is not being conducted at a conference center

○ **E.** Yes; as long as the content of the lecture falls within the Role Delineation Study

67. A student graduating with an undergraduate major in the Department of Athletic Training and Sport Studies asks about eligibility to sit for the Board of Certification (BOC) examination. What is the correct response?

○ **A.** Yes, if the student is graduating from a Commission on Accreditation of Athletic Training Education–accredited program

○ **B.** Yes, if the student's degree is in sports medicine and the student has all the prerequisite courses required by the BOC

○ **C.** Yes, if the student has taken all the athletic training classes listed on the Commission on Accreditation of Athletic Training Education's Web site and has spent at least 800 hours working under the supervision of a certified athletic trainer

○ **D.** No, because a master's degree is required to sit for the BOC certification examination

○ **E.** No, because the student is not graduating from a degree program in a department of sports medicine or rehabilitation sciences

68. Your team physician is a strong supporter of athletic trainers and would like to become a member of the NATA. Is this possible?

○ **A.** Yes; the physician can be a member in the category of Career Starter

○ **B.** Yes; the physician can be a member in the category of Medical Professionals

○ **C.** No; the physician must be a certified athletic trainer or student to be a member

○ **D.** Yes; the physician can be a member in the category of Associate

○ **E.** No; physicians must be invited by the NATA to become members

69. What benefits are provided by the NATA to a newly certified member employed for the first time in an athletic training position?

○ **A.** 50% reduction in the registration fee for the annual meeting

○ **B.** 4 years instead of 3 to complete requirements for first continuing education unit cycle

○ **C.** Reduction in dues for the first full billing cycle

○ **D.** Special considerations when applying for NATA-sponsored grants

○ **E.** Reception at the NATA annual meeting

70. What does the designation FNATA indicate?

○ **A.** Foundation status in the NATA

○ **B.** Fellow status in the NATA

○ **C.** Founding member of the NATA

○ **D.** Future member of the NATA

○ **E.** Former member of the NATA

71. In conjunction with the medical director at your school's student health services, you are planning an informational session for student athletes on the topic of sickle cell trait. Athletes of what descent should be targeted for this information?

○ **A.** European, Indian, and African-American

○ **B.** Mediterranean, African-American, and Caribbean

○ **C.** African-American, Asian, and Central American

○ **D.** Middle Eastern, African-American, and eastern European

○ **E.** South American, African-American, and North American

72. If you desire to work as an athletic trainer in the industrial setting, which of the following knowledge and skill sets would be most helpful?

○ **A.** Workplace ergonomics

○ **B.** Pedagogical techniques

○ **C.** Mechanical systems

○ **D.** Insurance programs

○ **E.** Stress management

73. When communicating with a patient, what type of question may result in the patient rationalizing or becoming defensive?

○ **A.** Questions that begin with "What"

○ **B.** Questions that begin with "How"

○ **C.** Questions that begin with "Why"

○ **D.** Questions that begin with "Who"

○ **E.** Questions that begin with "Where"

74. Which of the following is characteristic of an empathetic listener?

○ **A.** Focusing on the speaker's emotions and body language

○ **B.** Expressing interest in specific thoughts and appreciating logical presentation of information

○ **C.** Concentrating on the speaker's information and identifying with the speaker

○ **D.** Listening analytically and formulating questions while listening

○ **E.** Listening for pleasure and becoming disenchanted with a lack of humor

75. Which of the following is the best example of the application of active listening?

○ **A.** Establish your authority by sitting behind your desk while meeting an athlete.

○ **B.** Acknowledge that you hear the athlete speaking while you continue caring for other athletes.

○ **C.** When you feel you have enough information, interrupt the athlete to provide suggestions or solutions.

○ **D.** Sugarcoat your responses to avoid crushing the athlete's self-esteem.

○ **E.** Reflect back what the athlete has said using phrasing such as "What I'm hearing you say is . . . ."

Answers for Domain VI: Professional Responsibility

Role A: Demonstrate appropriate professional conduct by complying with applicable standards and maintaining continuing competence to provide quality athletic training services.

1. A

2. E

3. E

4. D

5. D

6. A

7. B

8. D

9. A

10. A

11. E

12. A

13. D

14. B

15. C

16. A

17. E

18. B

19. C

20. C

21. A

22. E

23. B

24. C

25. D

Role B: Adhere to statutory and regulatory provisions and other legal responsibilities relating to the practice of athletic training by maintaining an understanding of these provisions and responsibilities in order to contribute to the safety and welfare of the public.

26. D

27. A

28. A

29. D

30. B

31. E

32. D

33. C

34. B

35. A

36. A

37. E

38. C

39. B

40. C

41. E

42. A

43. E

44. B

45. C

46. E

47. A

48. B

49. B

50. C

Role C: Educate appropriate individuals and entities about the role and standards of practice of the Athletic Trainer through informal and formal means to improve the ability of those individuals and entities to make informed decisions.

51. B

52. E

53. C

54. A

55. D

56. B

57. E

58. C

59. A

60. B

61. C

62. D

63. E

64. A

65. E

66. B

67. A

68. D

69. C

70. B

71. B

72. A

73. C

74. A

75. E

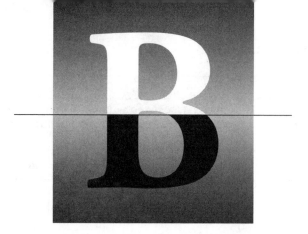

Athletic Training Practice Domains

I. Prevention			
A. Educate the appropriate patient(s) about risk associated with participation and specific activities using effective communication techniques to minimize the risk of injury and illness.			
Knowledge of:	**I Got That**	**Sort of Comfortable**	**No Clue**
Appropriate Patients (e.g., administrators, management, parents, guardians, family members, coaches, participants, and members of the healthcare team)	❑	❑	❑
Common risks (e.g., musculoskeletal, integumentary, neurological, respiratory, and medical)	❑	❑	❑
Catastrophic risk (e.g., cardiorespiratory, neurological, thermoregulatory, endocrinological, and immunological)	❑	❑	❑
Behavioral risk (e.g., nutritional, sexual, substance abuse, blood-borne pathogens, sedentary lifestyle, and overtraining)	❑	❑	❑
Mechanisms of common and catastrophic injury	❑	❑	❑
Preventative measures (e.g., safety rules, accepted biomechanical techniques, ergonomics, and nutritional guidelines)	❑	❑	❑
Epidemiology data related to participation	❑	❑	❑
Effective Communication techniques (e.g. multimedia videos, pamphlets, posters models, handouts, and oral communication	❑	❑	❑

Reprinted with permission from the *Role Delineation Study, Fifth Edition*. Copyright © Board of Certification, Inc. All Rights Reserved.

(table continues on page 156)

I. Prevention (continued)

A. Educate the appropriate patient(s) about risk associated with participation and specific activities using effective communication techniques to minimize the risk of injury and illness.

Skill in:	I Got That	Sort of Comfortable	No Clue
Identifying risks	❑	❑	❑
Communicating effectively	❑	❑	❑
Educating effectively	❑	❑	❑
Identifying appropriate resources	❑	❑	❑

B. Interpret pre-participation and other relevant screening information in accordance with accepted guidelines to minimize the risk of injury and illness.

Knowledge of:	I Got That	Sort of Comfortable	No Clue
Pre-participation evaluation process and procedures	❑	❑	❑
Established Laws, regulations and policies (e.g. institutional, state, and national	❑	❑	❑
Established Guidelines for recommended participation	❑	❑	❑
Privacy laws	❑	❑	❑

Skill in:	I Got That	Sort of Comfortable	No Clue
Identifying conditions that may limit or compromise participation	❑	❑	❑
Collecting and appropriately applying pre-participation screening information	❑	❑	❑
Identifying and applying established guidelines and regulations	❑	❑	❑

C. Instruct the appropriate patient(s) about standard protective equipment using effective communication techniques to minimize the risk of injury and illness.

Knowledge of:	I Got That	Sort of Comfortable	No Clue
Legal risks and ramifications of making equipment modifications	❑	❑	❑
Rules pertaining to the use of protective equipment	❑	❑	❑
Manufacturer's guidelines regarding selection, fit, inspection, and maintenance of equipment	❑	❑	❑
Established Standards pertaining to protective equipment (e.g., NOCSAE and ASTM)	❑	❑	❑
Intended purpose, limitations, and capabilities of protective equipment	❑	❑	❑

I. Prevention (continued)

C. Instruct the appropriate patient(s) about standard protective equipment using effective communication techniques to minimize the risk of injury and illness.

Effective Communication techniques	❏	❏	❏
Effective Instructional techniques	❏	❏	❏
Skill in:	**I Got That**	**Sort of Comfortable**	**No Clue**
Educating patients on the selection of standard protective equipment	❏	❏	❏
Communicating effectively	❏	❏	❏
Fitting standard protective equipment	❏	❏	❏
Interpreting rules regarding protective equipment	❏	❏	❏

D. Apply appropriate prophylactic/protective measures using commercial products or custom-made devices to minimize the risk of injury and illness.

Knowledge of:	**I Got That**	**Sort of Comfortable**	**No Clue**
Commercially available protective products	❏	❏	❏
Materials and methods for fabricating custom-made protective devices	❏	❏	❏
Effective Use of prophylactic/protective measures	❏	❏	❏
Physical properties of the protective equipment materials(e.g., absorption, dissipation, and transmission of energy)	❏	❏	❏
Mechanisms of injury	❏	❏	❏
Legal and safety risks involved in the construction and use of custom protective devices	❏	❏	❏
Legal and safety risks involved in the use and modification of commercial devices	❏	❏	❏
Skill in:	**I Got That**	**Sort of Comfortable**	**No Clue**
Identifying injuries, illnesses and conditions that warrant the application of custom-made or commercially available devices	❏	❏	❏
Fabricating and fitting custom-made devices	❏	❏	❏
Selecting and applying commercial devices	❏	❏	❏

E. Identify safety hazards associated with activities, activity areas, and equipment by following accepted procedures and guidelines in order to make appropriate recommendations and to minimize the risk of injury and illness.

Knowledge of:	**I Got That**	**Sort of Comfortable**	**No Clue**
Hazards common to activities	❏	❏	❏

(table continues on page 158)

I. Prevention (continued)

E. Identify safety hazards associated with activities, activity areas, and equipment by following accepted procedures and guidelines in order to make appropriate recommendations and to minimize the risk of injury and illness.

Hazards common in activity areas (e.g., surface irregularities, obstructions, inadequate offsets, moisture and other foreign objectives, inadequate lighting, inadequate ingress and egress)	❏	❏	❏
Hazards common to equipment (e.g., shoulder pads, goal posts, computer keyboards)	❏	❏	❏
Emergency communication systems	❏	❏	❏
Rules governing play and established standards and practices	❏	❏	❏
Policies and procedures for addressing facility hazards	❏	❏	❏
Corrective measures for facility hazards	❏	❏	❏
Ergonomics	❏	❏	❏
Policy statements and guidelines pertaining to safety hazards (e.g., NATA and NCAA)	❏	❏	❏
Skill in:	**I Got That**	**Sort of Comfortable**	**No Clue**
Conducting inspections for hazards	❏	❏	❏
Recognizing hazards	❏	❏	❏
Recommending and implementing appropriate methods for addressing hazards	❏	❏	❏

F. Maintain clinical and treatment areas by complying with safety and sanitation standards to minimize the risk of injury and illness.

Knowledge of:	**I Got That**	**Sort of Comfortable**	**No Clue**
Situations and conditions that pose risk	❏	❏	❏
Laws, regulations, and policies (e.g., institutional, state and national) regarding safety and sanitation	❏	❏	❏
Manufacturer's guidelines for maintaining equipment and devices	❏	❏	❏
Skill in:	**I Got That**	**Sort of Comfortable**	**No Clue**
Operating or applying therapeutic modalities and rehabilitation equipment	❏	❏	❏
Recognizing noncompliance with safety and sanitation standards	❏	❏	❏
Recognizing malfunction or disrepair of therapeutic modalities, rehabilitation equipment, or furnishings in clinical and treatment areas	❏	❏	❏

I. Prevention (continued)			
F. Maintain clinical and treatment areas by complying with safety and sanitation standards to minimize the risk of injury and illness.			
Complying with manufacturer's recommendations for maintenance of equipment	❑	❑	❑
Maintaining a safe and sanitary environment in compliance with established standards (e.g., OSHA, universal precautions, local health department, and institutional policy)	❑	❑	❑
G. Monitor participants and environmental conditions by following accepted guidelines to promote safe participation.			
Knowledge in:	**I Got That**	**Sort of Comfortable**	**No Clue**
Conditions of participants that predispose them to environmentally caused illness (e.g., prior heat illness, sickle cell trait, asthma, recent viral infection, use of medication, ergogenic aids, obesity, and dehydration)	❑	❑	❑
Environmental conditions that create risk (e.g., heat, humidity, cold, altitude, pollution, weather extremes, insect swarms, infectious pathogens, and ergonomic conditions)	❑	❑	❑
Policies and procedures for removing participants from environmental risk situations (e.g., heat index, lightning, and activity scheduling)	❑	❑	❑
Monitoring techniques (e.g., weight charts, fluid intake, and body composition)	❑	❑	❑
Established Standards regarding environmental risks (e.g., governing body rules/regulations, NATA, NCAA, ACSM, etc.)	❑	❑	❑
Methods for reducing risk from environmental conditions (e.g., activity scheduling, clothing selection, and fluid replacement)	❑	❑	❑
Ergonomic and epidemiological factors as they relate to participation	❑	❑	❑
Skill in:	**I Got That**	**Sort of Comfortable**	**No Clue**
Recognizing characteristics in participants that would predispose them to environmental and ergonomic risk	❑	❑	❑
Using available resources to gather/interpret information regarding environmental data	❑	❑	❑
Recognizing environmental and ergonomic risks	❑	❑	❑
Facilitating appropriate action in response to environmental and ergonomic risk	❑	❑	❑

(table continues on page 160)

I. Prevention (continued)

H. Facilitate physical conditioning by designing and implementing appropriate programs to minimize the risk of injury and illness.

Knowledge of:	I Got That	Sort of Comfortable	No Clue
Physiological adaptation to exercises (e.g., space and attitude)	❑	❑	❑
Components of a physical conditioning program	❑	❑	❑
Various conditioning stages and program intervals	❑	❑	❑
Current strength and conditioning techniques	❑	❑	❑
Ergonomics	❑	❑	❑
Skill in:	**I Got That**	**Sort of Comfortable**	**No Clue**
Addressing the components of a comprehensive conditioning program	❑	❑	❑
Educating appropriate patients in the effective application of conditioning programs (e.g., guardian and administration)	❑	❑	❑
Assessing appropriateness of participation in conditioning programs	❑	❑	❑
Instructing in the use of appropriate conditioning equipment (e.g., bikes, weight machines, and treadmills)	❑	❑	❑
Correcting or modifying inappropriate, unsafe, or dangerous activities undertaken in conjunction with physical conditioning programs	❑	❑	❑

I. Facilitate healthy lifestyle behaviors using effective education, communication, and interventions to reduce the risk of injury and illness and promote wellness.

Knowledge of:	I Got That	Sort of Comfortable	No Clue
Accepted Guidelines for exercise prescription and sound nutritional practices	❑	❑	❑
Professional Resources for stress management and behavior modification	❑	❑	❑
Nutritional disorders, inactivity-related diseases, overtraining, and stress-related disorders	❑	❑	❑
Predisposing factors for nutritional and stress-related disorders	❑	❑	❑
Appropriate Use of exercise in stress management	❑	❑	❑
Skill in:	**I Got That**	**Sort of Comfortable**	**No Clue**
Recognizing signs and symptoms of nutritional and stress-related disorders	❑	❑	❑

I. Prevention (continued)

I. Facilitate healthy lifestyle behaviors using effective education, communication, and interventions to reduce the risk of injury and illness and promote wellness.

Educating appropriate patients on nutritional disorders, maladaptation, substance abuse, and overtraining	❏	❏	❏
Accessing information concerning accepted guidelines for nutritional practices	❏	❏	❏
Communicating with appropriate professionals regarding referral and treatment for patients with nutritional and stress-related disorders	❏	❏	❏
Addressing the issue of special nutritional needs in regard to competition or activity (e.g., pre- and post-game meals, and nutritional supplements	❏	❏	❏

II. Clinical Evaluation and Diagnosis

A. Obtain a history through observation, interview, and/or review of relevant records to assess current or potential injury, illness, or condition.

Knowledge of:	I Got That	Sort of Comfortable	No Clue
Pathomechanics of injury	❏	❏	❏
Relationship between predisposing factors and injuries, illnesses, and health-related conditions	❏	❏	❏
The body's immediate and delayed physiological response to injuries, illnesses, and conditions	❏	❏	❏
Signs and symptoms of injuries, illness, and conditions	❏	❏	❏
Relationship between nutrition and injuries, illnesses, and conditions	❏	❏	❏
Relationship between ergogenic aids and injuries, illnesses, and conditions	❏	❏	❏
Relationship between medications and injuries, illnesses, and conditions	❏	❏	❏
Communication techniques in order to elicit information	❏	❏	❏
Infectious agents	❏	❏	❏
Standard medical nomenclature and terminology	❏	❏	❏
Medical records as a source of information	❏	❏	❏
Injuries, illnesses, and conditions associated with specific activities	❏	❏	❏
Biomechanical factors associated with specific activities	❏	❏	❏
Pathophysiology of illnesses and conditions	❏	❏	❏

(table continues on page 162)

II. Clinical Evaluation and Diagnosis (continued)

A. Obtain a history through observation, interview, and/or review of relevant records to assess current or potential injury, illness, or condition.

Skill in:	I Got That	Sort of Comfortable	No Clue
Identifying the extent and severity of injuries, illnesses, and conditions	❏	❏	❏
Relating signs and symptoms to specific injuries, illnesses, and conditions	❏	❏	❏
Obtaining and recording information related to injuries, illnesses, and conditions	❏	❏	❏
Recognizing predisposing factors to specific injuries, illnesses, and conditions	❏	❏	❏
Identifying anatomical structures involved in injuries, illnesses, and conditions	❏	❏	❏
Interpreting medical records and related reports	❏	❏	❏
Identifying psychosocial factors associated with injuries, illnesses, and conditions	❏	❏	❏
Identifying nutritional factors related to injuries, illnesses, and conditions	❏	❏	❏
Identifying the impact of supplements and prescription and nonprescription medications associated with injuries, illnesses, and conditions	❏	❏	❏
Interviewing and communication for the purpose of gathering information related to the condition	❏	❏	❏

B. Inspect the involved area(s) visually to assess the injury, illness, or health-related condition.

Knowledge of:	I Got That	Sort of Comfortable	No Clue
Bony landmarks and soft tissues	❏	❏	❏
Signs of injuries, illnesses, and health-related conditions	❏	❏	❏
Response to injuries, illnesses, and health-related conditions	❏	❏	❏
Principles of visual inspection	❏	❏	❏
Normal and abnormal structural relationships to the pathomechanics of injuries and conditions	❏	❏	❏
Skill in:	**I Got That**	**Sort of Comfortable**	**No Clue**
Properly Exposing the area in order to evaluate the involved area	❏	❏	❏
Assessing immediate and delayed physiological responses to injuries, illnesses, and health-related conditions	❏	❏	❏

II. Clinical Evaluation and Diagnosis (continued)

B. Inspect the involved area(s) visually to assess the injury, illness, or health-related condition.

Identifying bony surface landmarks and soft tissue abnormalities of specific/special injuries, illnesses, and health-related conditions	❑	❑	❑
Identifying the relationship and severity of pathological signs of injuries, illnesses, and health-related conditions	❑	❑	❑
Assessing the pre-existing structural abnormalities and relating them to pathomechanics of injuries, illnesses, and health-related conditions	❑	❑	❑

C. Palpate the involved area(s) using standard techniques to assess the injury, illness, or health-related condition.

Knowledge of:	I Got That	Sort of Comfortable	No Clue
Human anatomy with emphasis on bony landmarks and soft tissue structures	❑	❑	❑
Immediate and delayed physiological response to injuries, illnesses, and health-related conditions	❑	❑	❑
Principles of palpation techniques	❑	❑	❑

Skill in:	I Got That	Sort of Comfortable	No Clue
Locating and palpating bony landmarks, articulations, ligamentous structures, musculotendinous units and other soft tissues	❑	❑	❑
Recognizing severity of pathological signs and symptoms of injuries, illnesses, and health-related conditions	❑	❑	❑
Assessing immediate and delayed physiological response to injuries, illnesses, and health-related conditions	❑	❑	❑
Palpating appropriate structures in order to assess the integrity of human anatomical/physiological systems	❑	❑	❑

D. Perform specific tests in accordance with accepted procedures to assess the injury, illness, or health-related condition.

Knowledge of:	I Got That	Sort of Comfortable	No Clue
Mechanics, principles, and techniques of specific/special tests (ligamentous, neurological, manual, fracture, and functional tests)	❑	❑	❑
Standard/patient special tests for range of motion, muscular strength, structural integrity, and functional capacity	❑	❑	❑

(table continues on page 164)

II. Clinical Evaluation and Diagnosis (continued)

D. Perform specific tests in accordance with accepted procedures to assess the injury, illness, or health-related condition.

	I Got That	Sort of Comfortable	No Clue
Signs and symptoms of systemic requirements and failure during exercise	❏	❏	❏
Signs, symptoms, and interpretations of specific, special tests	❏	❏	❏

Skill in:	I Got That	Sort of Comfortable	No Clue
Assessing muscular strength through the use of manual or nonmanual muscle tests	❏	❏	❏
Assessing joint range of motion using test and measurement techniques	❏	❏	❏
Identifying structural and functional integrity of anatomical structures	❏	❏	❏
Identifying appropriate specific/special tests for particular injuries	❏	❏	❏
Assessing neurological function	❏	❏	❏
Identifying the signs and symptoms related to specific/special tests	❏	❏	❏
Identifying location, type, function and action of each joint	❏	❏	❏
Using equipment associated with specific/special tests	❏	❏	❏
Performing specific/special tests	❏	❏	❏
Interpreting the information gained from specific/special tests	❏	❏	❏

E. Formulate a clinical impression by interpreting the signs, symptoms, and predisposing factors of the injury, illness, or condition to determine the appropriate course of action.

Knowledge of:	I Got That	Sort of Comfortable	No Clue
Signs, symptoms, and predisposing factors related to injuries, illnesses, and health-related conditions	❏	❏	❏
Basic pharmacological considerations	❏	❏	❏
Pathomechanics of injuries and/or health-related conditions	❏	❏	❏
Psychosocial dysfunction and implications associated with injuries, illnesses, and health-related conditions	❏	❏	❏
Medical terminology and nomenclature	❏	❏	❏

II. Clinical Evaluation and Diagnosis (continued)

E. Formulate a clinical impression by interpreting the signs, symptoms, and predisposing factors of the injury, illness, or condition to determine the appropriate course of action.

	I Got That	Sort of Comfortable	No Clue
Indications for referral	❑	❑	❑
Guidelines for return to participation	❑	❑	❑
Skill in:	**I Got That**	**Sort of Comfortable**	**No Clue**
Interpreting the pertinent information from the evaluation	❑	❑	❑
Synthesizing applicable information from an evaluation	❑	❑	❑
Identifying appropriate courses of action	❑	❑	❑

F. Educate the appropriate patient(s) regarding the assessment by communicating information about the current or potential injury, illness, or health related condition to encourage compliance with recommended care.

Knowledge of:	I Got That	Sort of Comfortable	No Clue
Communication skills and techniques	❑	❑	❑
Patient confidentiality rules and regulations	❑	❑	❑
Medical terminology and nomenclature	❑	❑	❑
Commonly accepted practices regarding the care and treatment of injuries, illnesses, and conditions	❑	❑	❑
Potential complications and expected outcomes	❑	❑	❑
Appropriate Treatment options	❑	❑	❑
Skill in:	**I Got That**	**Sort of Comfortable**	**No Clue**
Using both verbal and written forms of communication	❑	❑	❑
Interpreting medical terminology and describing the nature of injuries, illnesses, and health-related conditions in basic terms	❑	❑	❑
Utilizing appropriate counseling techniques	❑	❑	❑

G. Share assessment findings with other healthcare professionals using effective means of communication to coordinate appropriate care

Knowledge of:	I Got That	Sort of Comfortable	No Clue
Patient confidentiality rules and regulations	❑	❑	❑
Medical terminology and nomenclature	❑	❑	❑
Communication skills and techniques	❑	❑	❑

(table continues on page 166)

II. Clinical Evaluation and Diagnosis (continued)

G. Share assessment findings with other healthcare professionals using effective means of communication to coordinate appropriate care

Role and scope of practice of various healthcare professionals	❑	❑	❑
Commonly accepted Practices regarding the care and treatment of injuries, illnesses, and health-related conditions	❑	❑	❑

Skill in:	I Got That	Sort of Comfortable	No Clue
Communicating with healthcare professionals	❑	❑	❑
Collaborating with healthcare professionals	❑	❑	❑
Using medical terminology and nomenclature	❑	❑	❑
Directing a referral to other medical personnel	❑	❑	❑

III. Immediate Care

A. Employ life-saving techniques through the use of standard emergency procedures in order to reduce morbidity and the incidence of mortality.

Knowledge of:	I Got That	Sort of Comfortable	No Clue
Human anatomy: normal and compromised structures	❑	❑	❑
Human physiology: normal and compromised structures	❑	❑	❑
Biomechanics/kinesiology: mechanisms of catastrophic conditions	❑	❑	❑
Common life-threatening medical situations (e.g., respiratory, central nervous, and cardiovascular	❑	❑	❑
Appropriate Management techniques for life-threatening conditions (e.g., respiratory and central nervous systems)	❑	❑	❑
Emergency action plan(s)	❑	❑	❑
Federal and state occupational, safety, and health guidelines	❑	❑	❑
Standard Protective equipment and removal devices and procedures	❑	❑	❑
Appropriate use of Emergency equipment and techniques(e.g., AED, CPR masks and BP cuff)	❑	❑	❑

Skill in:	I Got That	Sort of Comfortable	No Clue
Performing cardiopulmonary resuscitation techniques and procedures	❑	❑	❑
Implementing federal and state occupational, safety and health guidelines	❑	❑	❑

III. Immediate Care (continued)

A. Employ life-saving techniques through the use of standard emergency procedures in order to reduce morbidity and the incidence of mortality.

Removing protective equipment and using removal devices	❑	❑	❑
Using emergency equipment	❑	❑	❑
Implementing immobilization and transfer techniques	❑	❑	❑
Implementing emergency action plan(s)	❑	❑	❑
Managing common life-threatening emergency situations/conditions (e.g., evaluation, monitoring, and provision of care)	❑	❑	❑
Transferring care to appropriate medical and/or allied health professionals and/or facilities	❑	❑	❑
Measure and monitor vital signs	❑	❑	❑

B. Prevent exacerbation of non–life-threatening condition(s) through the use of standard procedures in order to reduce morbidity.

Knowledge of:	I Got That	Sort of Comfortable	No Clue
Human anatomy: normal and compromised structures	❑	❑	❑
Human physiology: normal and compromised functions	❑	❑	❑
Biomechanics/kinesiology: mechanism of common, non–life-threatening conditions	❑	❑	❑
Common non–life-threatening conditions (e.g., respiratory, general medical, central nervous, musculoskeletal, and cardiovascular)	❑	❑	❑
Appropriate Management techniques for non-life–threatening conditions (e.g., respiratory, general medical, central nervous, musculoskeletal, and cardiovascular)	❑	❑	❑
Indications and contraindications for participation	❑	❑	❑
Emergency action plan(s)	❑	❑	❑
Federal and state occupational, safety and health guidelines	❑	❑	❑
Standard Protective equipment and removal devices and procedures	❑	❑	❑
Appropriate Use of standard medical equipment and techniques (e.g., BP cuff, spine board, cervical collar, splints, and stethoscope)	❑	❑	❑
Pharmacological and therapeutic modality usage for acute conditions	❑	❑	❑

(table continues on page 168)

III. Immediate Care (continued)

B. Prevent exacerbation of non–life-threatening condition(s) through the use of standard procedures in order to reduce morbidity.

Skill in:	I Got That	Sort of Comfortable	No Clue
Implementing federal and state occupational, safety and health guidelines standards and guidelines	❑	❑	❑
Using standard medical equipment	❑	❑	❑
Removing protective equipment and the use of removal devices	❑	❑	❑
Implementing immobilization and transfer techniques	❑	❑	❑
Obtaining vital signs	❑	❑	❑
Managing non–life-threatening conditions (e.g., evaluation, monitoring, provision of care)	❑	❑	❑
Using standard medical equipment	❑	❑	❑
Implementing emergency action plan(s)	❑	❑	❑
Transferring care to appropriate medical and/or allied health professionals and/or facilities	❑	❑	❑
Determining appropriateness for return to activity	❑	❑	❑
Applying pharmacological and therapeutic modalities			

C. Facilitate the timely transfer of care for conditions beyond the scope of practice of the athletic trainer by implementing appropriate referral strategies to stabilize and/or prevent exacerbation of the condition(s).

Knowledge of:	I Got That	Sort of Comfortable	No Clue
Emergency action plan(s)	❑	❑	❑
Conditions beyond the scope of the athletic trainer	❑	❑	❑
Roles of medical and allied healthcare providers	❑	❑	❑
Common management strategies for life- and non–life-threatening conditions	❑	❑	❑

Skill in:	I Got That	Sort of Comfortable	No Clue
Implementing emergency action plan(s)	❑	❑	❑
Recognizing acute conditions beyond the scope of the athletic trainer	❑	❑	❑
Communicating with other medical and allied health-care providers	❑	❑	❑
Managing life- and non–life-threatening conditions until transfer to appropriate medical providers and facilities	❑	❑	❑

III. Immediate Care (continued)

D. Direct the appropriate patient(s) in standard immediate care procedures using formal and informal methods to facilitate immediate care.

Knowledge of:	I Got That	Sort of Comfortable	No Clue
Roles of patient members of the medical management team	❑	❑	❑
Components of the emergency action plan(s)	❑	❑	❑
Effective Communication techniques	❑	❑	❑

Skill in:	I Got That	Sort of Comfortable	No Clue
Communicating effectively with appropriate patients	❑	❑	❑
Implementing the emergency action plan(s)	❑	❑	❑
Educating patients regarding standard emergency care procedures	❑	❑	❑

E. Execute the established emergency action plan using effective communication and administrative practices to facilitate efficient immediate care.

Knowledge of:	I Got That	Sort of Comfortable	No Clue
Emergency action plan(s)	❑	❑	❑
Communication techniques	❑	❑	❑
Pertinent administrative practices	❑	❑	❑

Skill in:	I Got That	Sort of Comfortable	No Clue
Communicating effectively	❑	❑	❑
Identifying the need to implement the emergency action plan(s)	❑	❑	❑
Implementing relevant administrative practices	❑	❑	❑

IV. Treatment, Rehabilitation, and Reconditioning

A. Administer therapeutic and conditioning exercise(s) using standard techniques and procedures in order to facilitate recovery, function, and/or performance

Knowledge of:	I Got That	Sort of Comfortable	No Clue
The Structure, growth, development, and regeneration of tissue	❑	❑	❑
Principles of adaptation and overload of tissues	❑	❑	❑
Principles of adaptation systems	❑	❑	❑
Principle of therapeutic exercise (e.g., isometric, isotonic, isokinetic, work, power, and endurance)	❑	❑	❑
Principles of strength and conditioning exercises (e.g., plyometrics, core stabilization, speed, agility, and power)	❑	❑	❑

(table continues on page 170)

IV. Treatment, Rehabilitation, and Reconditioning (continued)

A. Administer therapeutic and conditioning exercise(s) using standard techniques and procedures in order to facilitate recovery, function, and/or performance

	I Got That	Sort of Comfortable	No Clue
Neurology related to treatment, rehabilitation, and reconditioning	❏	❏	❏
The Inflammatory process related to treatment, rehabilitation, and reconditioning	❏	❏	❏
Proprioception and kinesthesis related to treatment, rehabilitation, and reconditioning	❏	❏	❏
Available Equipment and tools related to treatment, rehabilitation, and reconditioning	❏	❏	❏
Adaptation of the cardiovascular and muscular systems related to treatment, rehabilitation, and reconditioning	❏	❏	❏
Indications and contraindications related to treatment, rehabilitation, and reconditioning	❏	❏	❏
Pharmacology related to treatment, rehabilitation, and reconditioning	❏	❏	❏
Surgical procedures and implications for treatment, rehabilitation, and reconditioning	❏	❏	❏
Age-specific considerations related to treatment, rehabilitation, and reconditioning	❏	❏	❏
Psychology related to treatment, rehabilitation, and reconditioning	❏	❏	❏

Skill in:	I Got That	Sort of Comfortable	No Clue
Applying exercise prescription in the development and implementation of treatment, rehabilitation, and reconditioning (e.g., aquatics, isokinetics, and closed-chain)	❏	❏	❏
Evaluating criteria for return to activity	❏	❏	❏

B. Administer therapeutic modalities using standard techniques and procedures in order to facilitate recovery, function, and/or performance.

Knowledge of:	I Got That	Sort of Comfortable	No Clue
Indications and contraindications for therapeutic modalities	❏	❏	❏
Principles of mechanical, electromagnetic, and acoustical energy	❏	❏	❏
Structure, growth, development, and regeneration of tissue	❏	❏	❏
Inflammatory process related to therapeutic modalities	❏	❏	❏
Available therapeutic modalities related to treatment, rehabilitation, and reconditioning	❏	❏	❏

IV. Treatment, Rehabilitation, and Reconditioning (continued)

B. Administer therapeutic modalities using standard techniques and procedures in order to facilitate recovery, function, and/or performance.

Physiological response to therapeutic modalities	❏	❏	❏
Pharmacology related to therapeutic modalities	❏	❏	❏
Theories of pain	❏	❏	❏
Skill in:	**I Got That**	**Sort of Comfortable**	**No Clue**
Applying thermal, electrical, mechanical, and acoustical modalities	❏	❏	❏
Applying manual therapy techniques			

C. Apply braces, splints, or assistive devices in accordance with appropriate standards and practices in order to facilitate recovery, function, and/or performance.

Knowledge of:	**I Got That**	**Sort of Comfortable**	**No Clue**
Commercially available soft goods	❏	❏	❏
Materials and methods for fabricating custom-made devices	❏	❏	❏
Pathomechanics of the injury or condition	❏	❏	❏
Legal standards for bracing	❏	❏	❏
Functions of bracing	❏	❏	❏
Skill in:	**I Got That**	**Sort of Comfortable**	**No Clue**
Applying braces, splints, or assistive devices	❏	❏	❏
Fabricating braces, splints, or assistive devices	❏	❏	❏

D. Administer treatment for general illness and/or conditions using standard techniques and procedures to facilitate recovery, function, and/or performance.

Knowledge of:	**I Got That**	**Sort of Comfortable**	**No Clue**
Pathophysiology associated with systemic illness, communicable disease; bacterial, viral, fungal, and parasitic infections	❏	❏	❏
Structure, growth, development, and regeneration of tissue	❏	❏	❏
Pharmacology related to treatment of injuries, illnesses, and conditions	❏	❏	❏
Medical and allied healthcare professionals involved in the treatment of injuries, illnesses, and conditions	❏	❏	❏
Available Reference sources related to injuries, illnesses, and conditions	❏	❏	❏

(table continues on page 172)

IV. Treatment, Rehabilitation, and Reconditioning (continued)

D. Administer treatment for general illness and/or conditions using standard techniques and procedures to facilitate recovery, function, and/or performance.

	I Got That	Sort of Comfortable	No Clue
Psychological reaction to injuries, illnesses, and conditions	❏	❏	❏

Skill in:	I Got That	Sort of Comfortable	No Clue
Applying topical wound or skin-care products	❏	❏	❏
Applying universal precautions	❏	❏	❏
Referring to appropriate healthcare providers	❏	❏	❏
Recognizing the status of systemic illnesses	❏	❏	❏
Recognizing the status of bacterial, viral, fungal, and parasitic infections	❏	❏	❏
Recognizing atypical psychosocial conditions	❏	❏	❏

E. Reassess the status of injuries, illnesses, and/or conditions using standard techniques and documentation strategies in order to determine appropriate treatment, rehabilitation, and/or reconditioning and to evaluate readiness to return to a desired level of activity.

Knowledge of:	I Got That	Sort of Comfortable	No Clue
Standard Assessment procedures and techniques	❏	❏	❏
Techniques and procedures to modify, continue, or discontinue treatment plans	❏	❏	❏
Functional criteria for return to activity	❏	❏	❏
Posture, biomechanics, and ergonomics	❏	❏	❏
Appropriate Documentation procedures	❏	❏	❏

Skill in:	I Got That	Sort of Comfortable	No Clue
Interpreting assessment information necessary to modify, continue, or discontinue treatment plans	❏	❏	❏
Applying functional criteria for return to activity	❏	❏	❏

F. Educate the appropriate patient(s) in the treatment, rehabilitation, and reconditioning of injuries, illnesses, and/or conditions using applicable methods and materials to facilitate recovery, function, and/or performance.

Knowledge of:	I Got That	Sort of Comfortable	No Clue
Available Psychosocial, community, family, and healthcare support systems related to treatment, rehabilitation, and reconditioning	❏	❏	❏
Applicable Methods and materials for education	❏	❏	❏
Learning process across the lifespan	❏	❏	❏
Ethnicity and culture	❏	❏	❏

IV. Treatment, Rehabilitation, and Reconditioning (continued)

F. Educate the appropriate patient(s) in the treatment, rehabilitation, and reconditioning of injuries, illnesses, and/or conditions using applicable methods and materials to facilitate recovery, function, and/or performance.

Skill in:	I Got That	Sort of Comfortable	No Clue
Identifying appropriate patients to educate	❑	❑	❑
Communicating appropriate information	❑	❑	❑
Disseminating information to patients at an appropriate level	❑	❑	❑

G. Provide guidance and/or counseling for the appropriate patient(s) in the treatment, rehabilitation, and reconditioning of injuries, illnesses, and/or conditions through communication to facilitate recovery, function, and/or performance.

Knowledge of:	I Got That	Sort of Comfortable	No Clue
Psychological effects related to rehabilitation, recovery, and performance	❑	❑	❑
Referral resources	❑	❑	❑
Psychosocial dysfunction	❑	❑	❑

Skill in:	I Got That	Sort of Comfortable	No Clue
Identifying appropriate patients for guidance and counseling	❑	❑	❑
Using appropriate psychosocial techniques (e.g., goal setting and stress management) in rehabilitation	❑	❑	❑
Referring to appropriate healthcare professionals	❑	❑	❑
Using effective communication skills	❑	❑	❑
Providing guidance/counseling for the patient during the treatment, rehabilitation, and reconditioning process	❑	❑	❑

V. Organization and Administration

A. Establish action plans for response to injury and illness using available resources to provide the required range of healthcare services for patients, athletic activities, and events.

Knowledge of:	I Got That	Sort of Comfortable	No Clue
Organizational preparticipation screening policies and procedures	❑	❑	❑
Institutional guidelines for referring patients to healthcare services	❑	❑	❑
Local and out-of-area medical services	❑	❑	❑
Institutional and local hierarchy for delivery of healthcare services	❑	❑	❑

(table continues on page 174)

V. Organization and Administration (continued)

A. Establish action plans for response to injury and illness using available resources to provide the required range of healthcare services for patients, athletic activities, and events.

	I Got That	Sort of Comfortable	No Clue
Staff preparedness	❏	❏	❏
Environmental hazards	❏	❏	❏
Reimbursement issues	❏	❏	❏
Institutional policies regarding substance abuse	❏	❏	❏
Legal standards and scope of practice	❏	❏	❏
Relevant position statements (e.g., NATA, ACSM, AOASM, AOSSM, AMSSM, NCAA, NFHS, and NAIA)	❏	❏	❏
Appropriate Medical equipment and supplies	❏	❏	❏
Relevant Epidemiology studies	❏	❏	❏
Site-specific access issues	❏	❏	❏
Pre-existing conditions of patient participants	❏	❏	❏

Skill in:	I Got That	Sort of Comfortable	No Clue
Organizing resources and personnel	❏	❏	❏
Interacting with appropriate administration leadership	❏	❏	❏
Obtaining appropriate policies, guidelines, and regulations	❏	❏	❏
Interpreting regulatory policies	❏	❏	❏

B. Establish policies and procedures for the delivery of healthcare services following accepted guidelines to promote safe participation, timely care, and legal compliance.

Knowledge of:	I Got That	Sort of Comfortable	No Clue
Institutional review boards, policies, and procedures regarding informed consent guidelines	❏	❏	❏
Guidelines and regulations for decreasing exposure to environmental hazards	❏	❏	❏
Institutional, governmental, and appropriate organizational guidelines for safety, healthcare delivery, and legal compliance	❏	❏	❏
Guidelines for development of risk management policies and procedures	❏	❏	❏
Institutional risk management policies and procedures	❏	❏	❏
Institutional and governmental regulations regarding drug use, substance abuse, and mental illness	❏	❏	❏

V. Organization and Administration (continued)

B. Establish policies and procedures for the delivery of healthcare services following accepted guidelines to promote safe participation, timely care, and legal compliance.

	I Got That	Sort of Comfortable	No Clue
Prescreening participation guidelines	❏	❏	❏
Institutional drug testing and substance abuse policies	❏	❏	❏
Relevant evidence-based and epidemiology studies	❏	❏	❏
Statutory, regulatory, and other legal provisions pertaining to delivery of healthcare services	❏	❏	❏
Relevant position statements (e.g., NATA, ACSM, AOSSM, AMSSM, NCAA, NFHS, and NAIA)	❏	❏	❏
Skill in:	**I Got That**	**Sort of Comfortable**	**No Clue**
Applying existing guidelines	❏	❏	❏
Interacting with appropriate patients			
Completing the documentation process	❏	❏	❏
Organizing policies and procedures in a logical fashion	❏	❏	❏
Ascertaining appropriate policies, guidelines, and regulations	❏	❏	❏
Applying evidence-based and epidemiology studies	❏	❏	❏
Applying statutory, regulatory, and other legal provision	❏	❏	❏

C. Establish policies and procedures for the management of healthcare facilities and activity areas by referring to accepted guidelines, standards, and regulations to promote safety and legal compliance

Knowledge of:	**I Got That**	**Sort of Comfortable**	**No Clue**
Institutional, professional, and governmental guidelines for maintenance of facilities and equipment	❏	❏	❏
Manufacturer's operational guidelines	❏	❏	❏
Appropriate Inspection procedures and documentation	❏	❏	❏
Safe playing and treatment environments	❏	❏	❏
OSHA guidelines	❏	❏	❏
Skill in:	**I Got That**	**Sort of Comfortable**	**No Clue**
Complying with equipment manufacturer's operational regulations/guidelines	❏	❏	❏

(table continues on page 176)

V. Organization and Administration (continued)

C. Establish policies and procedures for the management of healthcare facilities and activity areas by referring to accepted guidelines, standards, and regulations to promote safety and legal compliance

Complying with institutional and governmental policies and procedures for maintenance of facilities and equipment	❑	❑	❑
Applying OSHA standards	❑	❑	❑
Recognizing potential safety and environmental hazards	❑	❑	❑
Assuring compliance of involved staff	❑	❑	❑

D. Manage human and fiscal resources by utilizing appropriate leadership, organization, and management techniques to provide efficient and effective healthcare services.

Knowledge of:	I Got That	Sort of Comfortable	No Clue
Human resource management	❑	❑	❑
Institutional budgeting and procurement process	❑	❑	❑
Institutional and federal employment regulations (e.g. EEOC, ADA, Title IX)	❑	❑	❑
Staff scheduling, patient flow, and allocation of resources	❑	❑	❑
Credentialing systems and general requirements for pertinent professions	❑	❑	❑
Appropriate Computer software applications	❑	❑	❑
Leadership styles	❑	❑	❑
Management techniques	❑	❑	❑
Strategic planning and goal setting	❑	❑	❑
Storage and inventory procedures	❑	❑	❑
Facility design and operation	❑	❑	❑
Revenue generation strategies	❑	❑	❑
Skill in:	I Got That	Sort of Comfortable	No Clue
Managing human resources (e.g., delegating, planning, staffing, hiring, firing, and conducting performance evaluations)	❑	❑	❑
Managing financial resources (e.g., planning, budgeting, resource allocation, revenue generation	❑	❑	❑
Facility design, operation, and management (e.g., planning, organizing, designing, schedule, coordinating budgeting	❑	❑	❑

V. Organization and Administration (continued)

D. Manage human and fiscal resources by utilizing appropriate leadership, organization, and management techniques to provide efficient and effective healthcare services.

	I Got That	Sort of Comfortable	No Clue
Using computer software applications (e.g., word processing, database spreadsheet, and Internet applications)	❏	❏	❏

E. Maintain records using an appropriate system to document services rendered, provide for continuity of care, facilitate communication, and meet legal standards.

Knowledge of:	**I Got That**	**Sort of Comfortable**	**No Clue**
Institutional informed consent policies and procedures	❏	❏	❏
Documentation protocol			
Accepted medical terminology and abbreviations	❏	❏	❏
Computer technology as it relates to record keeping and documentation	❏	❏	❏
Institutional, local, state, federal regulations/ other legal provisions pertaining to medical records	❏	❏	❏
Evidence-based practice and clinical outcomes assessment	❏	❏	❏
Skill in:	**I Got That**	**Sort of Comfortable**	**No Clue**
Creating and completing the documentation process	❏	❏	❏
Dictating medical records	❏	❏	❏
Using computer applications for record keeping	❏	❏	❏
Applying knowledge of medical terminology and abbreviations	❏	❏	❏
Interpreting medical records	❏	❏	❏
Adhering to legal requirements/procedures pertaining to medical records	❏	❏	❏

F. Develop professional relationships with appropriate patients and entities by applying effective communication techniques to enhance the delivery of healthcare.

Knowledge of:	**I Got That**	**Sort of Comfortable**	**No Clue**
Various effective communication styles and techniques	❏	❏	❏
Institutional chain of command	❏	❏	❏
Confidentiality policies	❏	❏	❏

(table continues on page 178)

V. Organization and Administration (continued)

F. Develop professional relationships with appropriate patients and entities by applying effective communication techniques to enhance the delivery of healthcare.

Effective Meeting planning	❏	❏	❏
Appropriate Personal behaviors	❏	❏	❏
Credentialing systems and general requirements for pertinent professions	❏	❏	❏
Community resources	❏	❏	❏
Skill in:	**I Got That**	**Sort of Comfortable**	**No Clue**
Mitigating conflict	❏	❏	❏
Planning meetings	❏	❏	❏
Respecting diversity of opinions and positions	❏	❏	❏
Interpreting medical terminology for appropriate patients	❏	❏	❏
Nurturing professional relationships	❏	❏	❏
Using effective communication styles and techniques			
Networking and recruiting qualified medical team members	❏	❏	❏

VI. Professional Responsibility

A. Demonstrate appropriate professional conduct by complying with applicable standards and maintaining continuing competence to provide quality athletic training services.

Knowledge of:	**I Got That**	**Sort of Comfortable**	**No Clue**
The BOC Standards of Practice	❏	❏	❏
NATA Code of Ethics	❏	❏	❏
Relevant Policy and position statements of the NATA and other appropriate organizations (e.g., ACSM, AOASM, AOSSM, AMSSM, NCAA, NFHSA, NAIA, USOC)	❏	❏	❏
Resources for continuing education (e.g., current and pertinent research, journals, courses, conferences)	❏	❏	❏
Skill in:	**I Got That**	**Sort of Comfortable**	**No Clue**
Obtaining, interpreting, evaluating, and applying relevant research data, literature, and/or other forms of information	❏	❏	❏

VI. Professional Responsibility (continued)			
A. Demonstrate appropriate professional conduct by complying with applicable standards and maintaining continuing competence to provide quality athletic training services.			
Obtaining, interpreting, evaluating, and applying relevant policy and position statements	❑	❑	❑
Obtaining, interpreting, and applying the BOC Standards of Practice	❑	❑	❑
Obtaining, interpreting, and applying NATA Code of Ethics	❑	❑	❑
Applying evidence-based medicine (EBM)	❑	❑	❑
B. Adhere to statutory and regulatory provisions and other legal responsibilities relating to the practice of athletic training by maintaining an understanding of these provisions and responsibilities in order to contribute to the safety and welfare of the public.			

Knowledge of:	I Got That	Sort of Comfortable	No Clue
State statutes, regulations, and adjudication that directly govern the practice of athletic training (e.g., state practice and title acts, state professional conduct and misconduct acts, liability, and negligence)	❑	❑	❑
Federal and state statutes, regulations, and adjudication that apply to the practice and/or organization and administration of athletic training (e.g., OSHA, DEA, Title IX, Civil Rights Act, HIPAA, Buckley Amendment, labor practices, patient confidentiality, insurance, record keeping)	❑	❑	❑
State statutes, regulations, and adjudication governing *other* professions which impact the practice of athletic training (e.g., medicine, physical therapy, nursing, pharmacology)	❑	❑	❑
Criteria for determining the legal standard of care in athletic training (e.g., state statutes and regulations, professional standards and guidelines, publications, customs, practices, and societal expectations)	❑	❑	❑

Skill in:	I Got That	Sort of Comfortable	No Clue
Researching and applying state and federal statutes, regulations, and adjudications	❑	❑	❑
Researching professional standards and guidelines (e.g., BOC, NATA, state organizations)	❑	❑	❑
Researching practice methods and procedures	❑	❑	❑

(table continues on page 180)

VI. Professional Responsibility (continued)

C. Educate appropriate patients and entities about the role and standards of practice of the athletic trainer through informal and formal means to improve the ability of those patients and entities to make informed decisions.

Knowledge of:	I Got That	Sort of Comfortable	No Clue
Appropriate Patients and entities (e.g., employers, supervisor, administrators, governing boards, parents, participants/patients, coaches, other allied healthcare professionals, and other interested parties)	❑	❑	❑
Communication techniques	❑	❑	❑
The credentialing process and laws for athletic training	❑	❑	❑
Scope of practice of the athletic training profession	❑	❑	❑
Current healthcare issues relevant to athletic training	❑	❑	❑
Accepted Guidelines for different practice settings (e.g., medical care for secondary school–aged athletes, medical coverage in intercollegiate athletics)	❑	❑	❑
Federal and state statutes, regulations, and adjudication which apply to the practice and/or organization and administration of athletic training (e.g., OSHA, DEA, Title IX, Civil Rights Act, HIPAA, Buckley Amendment, Fair Labor Standards Act)	❑	❑	❑

Skill in:	I Got That	Sort of Comfortable	No Clue
Communicating information through various methods	❑	❑	❑
Identifying the appropriate patients and/or entities	❑	❑	❑
Applying relevant information to specific employment and/or practice settings	❑	❑	❑

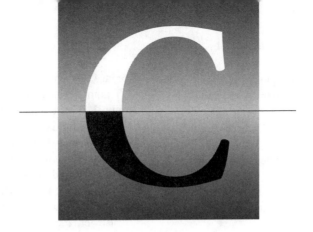

Study Sources and Reference List

The following is a reference list that includes sources compiled by the Board of Certification (BOC) and used in the examination development process as well as sources provided by the authors that were used in the development of this text. The list is divided by domain for use in preparing for the certification examination and to serve as documentation for correct answers to questions in the text. The sources are listed under the relevant primary domains. Note that there may be information in each source that applies to other domains. See the BOC Web site for the most current examination reference list.

Domain I: Prevention

American College of Sports Medicine: ACSM's Guidelines for Exercise Testing & Prescription, ed. 8. Lippincott Williams & Wilkins, 2009.

Anderson, M, Hall, S, and Parr, G: Foundations of Athletic Training, ed. 4. Lippincott Williams & Wilkins, 2008.

Antonio, J, and Stout, J: Sports Supplements. Lippincott Williams & Wilkins, 2001.

Baechle, T, and Earle, R: NSCA's Essentials of Strength Training and Conditioning, ed. 4. Human Kinetics, 2008.

Beam, J: Orthopedic Taping, Wrapping, Bracing & Padding, FA Davis, 2006.

Benardot D: Advanced Sports Nutrition. Human Kinetics, 2006.

Burke, L: Practical Sports Nutrition. Human Kinetics, 2007.

Cummings, N, Stanley-Green, S, and Higgs, P: Perspectives in Athletic Training. Mosby Elsevier, 2009.

Durstine, JL, Moore, G, Painter, P, et al: ACSM's Exercise Management for Persons With Chronic Diseases and Disabilities, ed. 3. Human Kinetics, 2009.

Ehrlich, A, and Schroeder, C: Medical Terminology for Health Professions, ed. 6. Thomson Delmar Learning, 2009.

Garrett, W, Kirkendall, D, and Squire, D: Principles and Practice of Primary Care Sports Medicine. Lippincott Williams & Wilkins, 2001.

Guyton, A, and Hall, J: Textbook of Medical Physiology, ed. 11, Elsevier Science, 2005.

Hall, S: Basic Biomechanics, ed. 5. Mosby, 2006.

Hillman, S: Introduction to Athletic Training, ed. 2. Human Kinetics, 2005.

Howley, E, and Franks, B: Health Fitness Instructor's Handbook, ed. 4. Human Kinetics, 2003.

Jenkins, DB: Hollinshead's Functional Anatomy of the Limbs & Back, ed. 9. WB Saunders, 2008.

Klossner, D: NCAA Sports Medicine Handbook. NCAA, 2009.

Landry, G, and Bernhardt, D: Essentials of Primary Care Sports Medicine. Human Kinetics, 2003.

McArdle, W, Katch, F, and Katch, V: Exercise Physiology: Energy, Nutrition and Human Performance, ed. 6. Lippincott Williams & Wilkins, 2006.

McArdle, W, Katch, F, and Katch, V: Sports and Exercise Nutrition. Lippincott Williams & Wilkins, 2008.

Mellion, M, Walsh, W, Madden, C, et al: Team Physician's Handbook, ed. 3. Hanley and Belfus, 2001.

Moore, K, and Agur, A: Essential Clinical Anatomy, ed. 3. Lippincott Williams & Wilkins, 2006.

Moore, K, Dalley, A, and Agur, A: Clinically Oriented Anatomy, ed. 6. Lippincott Williams & Wilkins, 2009.

NATA Position, Consensus, Official and Support Statements. NATA, 2008.

Perrin, D: Athletic Taping and Bracing, ed. 2. Human Kinetics, 2005.

Pfeiffer, R, and Mangus, B: Concepts of Athletic Training, ed. 5. Jones and Bartlett, 2007.

Prentice, W, and Arnheim, D: Arnheim's Principles of Athletic Training, ed. 13. McGraw-Hill, 2009.

Stanfield, P, Hui, Y, and Cross, N: Essential Medical Terminology, ed. 3. Jones and Bartlett, 2008.

Starkey, C: Athletic Training and Sports Medicine, ed. 4. Jones and Bartlett, 2005.

Street, S, and Runkle, D: Athletic Protective Equipment: Care, Selection and Fitting. McGraw-Hill, 2000.

Tortora, G, and Derrickson, B: Principles of Human Anatomy and Physiology, ed.12. John Wiley and Sons, 2009.

Venes, D: Taber's Cyclopedic Medical Dictionary, ed. 21. FA Davis, 2010.

Williams, M: Nutrition for Health, Fitness, and Sport, ed. 9. McGraw-Hill, 2009.

Wilmore, J, Costill, D, and Kenney, WL: Physiology of Sport and Exercise, ed. 4. Human Kinetics, 2008.

Domain II: Clinical Evaluation and Diagnosis

Anderson, M, Hall, S, and Parr, G: Foundations of Athletic Training, ed. 4. Lippincott Williams & Wilkins, 2008.

Baranoski, S, and Ayello, E: Wound Care Essentials: Practice Principles, ed. 2. Lippincott Williams & Wilkins, 2007.

Booher, J, and Thibodeau, G: Athletic Injury Assessment, ed. 4. McGraw-Hill, 2000.

Brunet, M: Unique Considerations of the Female Athlete. Delmar Cengage Learning, 2010.

Ciccone, C: Pharmacology in Rehabilitation, ed. 4. FA Davis, 2007.

Clarkson H: Musculoskeletal Assessment: Joint Range of Motion and Manual Muscle Strength, ed. 2. Lippincott Williams & Wilkins, 1999.

Cummings, N, Stanley-Green, S, and Higgs, P: Perspectives in Athletic Training. Mosby Elsevier, 2009.

Cuppett, M, and Walsh, K: General Medical Conditions in the Athlete. Mosby Elsevier, 2005.

Ehrlich, A, and Schroeder, C: Medical Terminology for Health Professionals, ed. 5. Thomson Delmar Learning, 2005.

Gallaspy, J, and May, JD: Signs & Symptoms of Athletic Injuries. Mosby, 1995.

Garrett, W, Kirkendall, D, and Squire,D: Principles and Practice of Primary Care Sports Medicine. Lippincott Williams & Wilkins, 2001.

Guyton, A, and Hall, J: Textbook of Medical Physiology, ed. 11, Elsevier Science, 2005.

Hislop, H, and Montgomery J: Daniels and Worthington's Muscle Testing: Techniques of Manual Examination, ed.8. Saunders Elsevier, 2007.

Hoppenfeld, S, Hutton, T, and Thomas, H: Physical Examination of the Spine & Extremities, Prentice Hall, 1976.

Houglum, J, Harrelson, G, and Leaver-Dunn, D: Principles of Pharmacology for Athletic Trainers. Slack, 2005.

Jenkins, DB: Hollinshead's Functional Anatomy of the Limbs & Back, ed. 9. Saunders Elsevier, 2008.

Kendall, F, McCreary, E, Provance, P, et al: Muscles: Testing and Function, With Posture and Pain, ed. 5. Lippincott Williams & Wilkins, 2005.

Kettenbach, G: Writing SOAP Notes With Patient/Client Management Formats, ed. 3. FA Davis, 2003.

Klossner, D: NCAA Sports Medicine Handbook. NCAA, 2009.

Konin, J, and Frederick, M: Documentation for Athletic Training. Slack, 2005.

Konin, J, Wikstein, D, Isear, J, et al: Special Tests for Orthopedic Examination, ed. 3. Slack, 2006.

Landry, G, and Bernhardt, D: Essentials of Primary Care Sports Medicine. Human Kinetics, 2003.

Levangie, P, and Norkin, C: Joint Structure and Function: A Comprehensive Analysis, ed. 4. FA Davis, 2005.

Magee, D: Orthopedic Physical Assessment, ed.5. Saunders Elsevier, 2007.

McArdle, W, Katch, F, and Katch, V: Exercise Physiology: Energy, Nutrition and Human Performance, ed. 6. Lippincott Williams & Wilkins, 2006.

Mellion, M, Walsh, W, Madden, C, et al: Team Physician's Handbook, ed. 3. Hanley and Belfus, 2001.

Moore, K, Dalley, A, and Agur, A: Clinically Oriented Anatomy, ed. 6. Lippincott Williams & Wilkins, 2009.

NATA Position, Consensus, Official and Support Statements. NATA, 2008.

Norkin, C: Measurement of Joint Motion, ed. 4. FA Davis, 2009.

Pfeiffer, R, and Mangus, B: Concepts of Athletic Training, ed. 5. Jones and Bartlett, 2007.

Prentice, W, and Arnheim, D. Arnheim's Principles of Athletic Training, ed. 13. McGraw-Hill, 2009.

Seidel, H, Ball, J, Dains, J, et al: Mosby's Guide to Physical Examination, ed. 6. Elsevier, 2006.

Shultz, S, Houglum, P, and Perrin, D: Examination of Musculoskeletal Injuries, ed. 3. Human Kinetics, 2010.

Stanfiel, P, Hui, Y, and Cross, N: Essential Medical Terminology, ed. 3. Jones and Bartlett, 2008.

Starkey, C: Athletic Training and Sports Medicine, ed. 4. Jones and Bartlett, 2005.

Starkey, C, Brown S, and Ryan, J: Examination of Orthopaedic & Athletic Injuries, ed. 3. FA Davis, 2009.

Starkey, C, Brown S, and Ryan, J: Orthopedic and Athletic Injury Examination Handbook, ed. 2. FA Davis, 2010.

Tortora, G, and Derrickson, B: Principles of Human Anatomy and Physiology, ed. 12. John Wiley and Sons, 2009.

Venes, D: Taber's Cyclopedic Medical Dictionary, ed. 21. FA Davis, 2010.

Wolff, K, and Johnson, RA: Fitzpatrick's Color Atlas and Synopsis of Clinical Dermatology, ed. 6. McGraw-Hill Inc, 2009.

Ziegler, T: Management of Bloodborne Infections in Sport: A Practical Guide for Sports Healthcare Providers and Coaches. Human Kinetics, 1996.

Domain III: Immediate Care

American Red Cross: CPR for the Professional Rescuer, ed. 3. StayWell, 2006.

American Safety and Health Institute: Complete Emergency Care. Human Kinetics, 2007.

Anderson, M, Hall, S, and Parr, G: Foundations of Athletic Training, ed. 4. Lippincott Williams & Wilkins, 2008.

Baranoski, S, and Ayello, E: Wound Care Essentials: Practice Principles, ed. 2. Lippincott Williams & Wilkins, 2007.

Booher, J, and Thibodeau, G: Athletic Injury Assessment, ed. 4. McGraw-Hill, 2000.

Cummings, N, Stanley-Green, S, and Higgs, P: Perspectives in Athletic Training. Mosby Elsevier, 2009.

Cuppett, M, and Walsh, K: General Medical Conditions in the Athlete. Mosby Elsevier, 2005.

Ehrlich, A, and Schroeder, C: Medical Terminology for Health Professionals, ed. 5. Thomson Delmar Learning, 2005.

Gorse, K, Blanc, R, Feld, F, et al: Emergency Care in Athletic Training. FA Davis, 2010.

Gulli, B: AAOS Emergency Care and Transportation of the Sick and Injured, ed. 9. Jones and Bartlett, 2009.

Houglum, J, Harrelson, G, and Leaver-Dunn, D: Principles of Pharmacology for Athletic Trainers. Slack, 2005.

Kettenbach, G: Writing SOAP Notes With Patient/Client Management Formats, ed. 3. FA Davis, 2003.

Klossner, D: NCAA Sports Medicine Handbook. NCAA, 2009.

Konin, J, and Frederick, M: Documentation for Athletic Training. Slack, 2005.

Landry, G, and Bernhardt, D: Essentials of Primary Care Sports Medicine. Human Kinetics, 2003.

Mellion, M, Walsh, W, Madden, C, et al: Team Physician's Handbook, ed. 3. Hanley and Belfus, 2001.

NATA Position, Consensus, Official and Support Statements. NATA, 2008.

National Safety Council: Bloodborne Pathogens—A Scenario-Based Approach. Jones and Bartlett, 1998.

Pfeiffer, R, and Mangus, B: Concepts of Athletic Training, ed. 5. Jones and Bartlett, 2007.

Prentice, W, and Arnheim, D. Arnheim's Principles of Athletic Training, ed. 13. McGraw-Hill, 2009.

Rankin, J, and Ingersoll, C: Athletic Training Management: Concepts & Application, ed. 2. McGraw-Hill, 2001.

Ray, R: Management Strategies in Athletic Training, ed. 3. Human Kinetics, 2005.

Ray, R, and Wiese-Bjornstal, D: Counseling in Sports Medicine. Human Kinetics, 1999.

Rehberg, R: Sports Emergency Care: A Team Approach. Slack, 2007.

Schottke, D: AAOS First Responder: Your First Response in Emergency Care, ed. 4. Jones and Bartlett, 2007.

Stanfield, P, Hui, Y, and Cross, N: Essential Medical Terminology, ed. 3. Jones and Bartlett, 2008.

Starkey, C: Athletic Training and Sports Medicine, ed. 4. Jones and Bartlett, 2005.

Venes, D: Taber's Cyclopedic Medical Dictionary, ed. 21. FA Davis, 2010.

Ziegler, T: Management of Bloodborne Infections in Sport: A Practical Guide for Sports Healthcare Providers and Coaches. Human Kinetics, 1996.

Domain IV: Treatment, Rehabilitation, and Reconditioning

American College of Sports Medicine: ACSM's Guidelines for Exercise Testing & Prescription, ed. 8. Lippincott Williams & Wilkins, 2009.

Anderson, M, Hall, S, and Parr, G: Foundations of Athletic Training, ed. 4. Lippincott Williams & Wilkins, 2008.

Andrews, J, Harrelson, G, and Wilk, K: Physical Rehabilitation of the Injured Athlete, ed. 3. Saunders Elsevier, 2004.

Baechle, T, and Earle, R: Essentials of Strength Training and Conditioning From the National Strength and Conditioning Association, ed. 3. Human Kinetics, 2008.

Bandy, W, and Sanders, B: Therapeutic Exercise: Techniques for Intervention. Lippincott Williams & Wilkins, 2001.

Baranoski, S, and Ayello, E: Wound Care Essentials: Practice Principles, ed. 2. Lippincott Williams & Wilkins, 2007.

Benardot, D: Advanced Sports Nutrition. Human Kinetics, 2006.

Burke, L: Practical Sports Nutrition. Human Kinetics, 2007.

Ciccone, C: Pharmacology in Rehabilitation, ed. 4. FA Davis, 2007.

Clarkson, H: Musculoskeletal Assessment: Joint Range of Motion and Manual Muscle Strength, ed. 2. Lippincott Williams & Wilkins, 1999.

Coppard, B, and Lohman, H: Introduction to Splinting: A Clinical-Reasoning & Problem-Solving Approach, ed. 2. Mosby, 2001.

Crossman, J: Coping With Sports Injuries: Psychological Strategies for Rehabilitation. Oxford University Press, 2001.

Cummings, N, Stanley-Green, S, and Higgs, P: Perspectives in Athletic Training. Mosby Elsevier, 2009.

Cuppett, M, and Walsh, K: General Medical Conditions in the Athlete. Mosby Elsevier, 2005.

Denegar, C, Saliba, E, and Saliba, S: Therapeutic Modalities for Musculoskeletal Injuries, ed. 3. Human Kinetics, 2010.

Durstine, JL, Moore, G, Painter, P, et al: ACSM's Exercise Management for Persons With Chronic Diseases and Disabilities, ed. 3. Human Kinetics, 2009.

Ehrlich A, and Schroeder, C: Medical Terminology for Health Professionals, ed. 5. Thomson Delmar Learning, 2005.

Ellenbecker, T, and Davies, G: Closed Kinetic Chain Exercise—A Comprehensive Guide to Multiple Joint Exercises. Human Kinetics, 2001.

Ellenbecker, T, De Carlo, T, and DeRosa, C: Effective Functional Progressions in Sport Rehabilitation. Human Kinetics, 2009.

Fritz, S: Mosby's Fundamentals of Therapeutic Massage, ed. 3. Mosby, 2004.

Garrett, W, Kirkendall, D, Squire, D: Principles and Practice of Primary Care Sports Medicine. Lippincott Williams & Wilkins, 2001.

Hall, S: Basic Biomechanics, ed. 5. Mosby, 2006.

Heil J: Psychology of Sport Injury, Human Kinetics, 1995.

Houglum, J, Harrelson, G, and Leaver-Dunn, D: Principles of Pharmacology for Athletic Trainers. Slack, 2005.

Houglum, P: Therapeutic Exercise for Musculoskeletal Injuries, ed. 2. Human Kinetics, 2005.

Kendall, F, McCreary, E, Provance, P, et al: Muscles: Testing and Function, With Posture and Pain, ed. 5. Lippincott Williams & Wilkins, 2005.

Kettenbach, G.: Writing SOAP Notes With Patient/Client Management Formats, ed. 3. FA Davis, 2003.

Kisner, C, and Colby, L: Therapeutic Exercise: Foundations & Techniques, ed. 5. FA Davis, 2007.

Klossner, D: NCAA Sports Medicine Handbook. NCAA, 2009.

Koester, M: Therapeutic Medications in Athletic Training, ed. 2. Human Kinetics, 2007.

Konin, J, and Frederick, M: Documentation for Athletic Training. Slack, 2005.

Levangie, P, and Norkin, C: Joint Structure and Function: A Comprehensive Analysis, ed. 4. FA Davis, 2005.

Mangus, B, and Miller, M: Pharmacology Application in Athletic Training. FA Davis, 2005.

McArdle, W, Katch, F, and Katch, V: Exercise Physiology: Energy, Nutrition and Human Performance, ed. 6. Lippincott Williams & Wilkins, 2006.

McArdle, W, Katch, F, and Katch, V: Sports and Exercise Nutrition. Lippincott Williams & Wilkins, 2008.

Mellion, M, Walsh, W, Madden, C, et al: Team Physician's Handbook, ed. 3. Hanley and Belfus, 2001.

Mensch, J, and Miller, G: The Athletic Trainer's Guide to Psychosocial Intervention and Referral. Slack, 2008.

Michlovitz, S, and Nolan, T: Modalities for Therapeutic Intervention, ed. 4. FA Davis, 2005.

Moore, K, Dalley, A, and Agur, A: Clinically Oriented Anatomy, ed. 6. Lippincott Williams & Wilkins, 2009.

Murphy, S: Sport Psychology Interventions. Human Kinetics, 1995.

NATA Position, Consensus, Official and Support Statements. NATA, 2008.

Norkin, C, and White J: Measurement of Joint Motion: A Guide to Goniometry, ed. 4. FA Davis, 2009.

Perrin, D: Athletic Taping and Bracing, ed. 2. Human Kinetics, 2005.

Pfeiffer, R, and Mangus, B: Concepts of Athletic Training, ed. 5. Jones and Bartlett, 2007.

Prentice, W: Rehabilitation Techniques in Sports Medicine, ed. 4. McGraw-Hill, 2005.

Prentice, W: Therapeutic Modalities in Rehabilitation, ed. 3. McGraw-Hill, 2005.

Prentice, W: Therapeutic Modalities in Sports Medicine, ed. 4. McGraw-Hill, 1999.

Prentice, W, and Arnheim, D: Arnheim's Principles of Athletic Training, ed. 13. McGraw-Hill, 2009.

Prenctice, W, and Voight, M: Techniques in Musculoskeletal Rehabilitation. McGraw-Hill, 2001.

Stanfield, P, Hui, Y, and Cross, N: Essential Medical Terminology, ed. 3. Jones and Bartlett, 2008.

Starkey, C: Athletic Training and Sports Medicine, ed. 4. Jones and Bartlett, 2005.

Starkey, C: Therapeutic Modalities, ed. 2. FA Davis, 1999.

Street, S, and Runkle, D: Athletic Protective Equipment: Care, Selection and Fitting. McGraw-Hill, 2000.

Tortora, G, and Derrickson, B: Principles of Human Anatomy and Physiology, ed. 12. John Wiley and Sons, 2009.

Venes, D: Taber's Cyclopedic Medical Dictionary, ed. 21. FA Davis, 2010.

Williams, M: Nutrition for Health, Fitness, and Sport. McGraw-Hill, 2009.

Wilmore, J, Costill, D, and Kenney, W: Physiology of Sport and Exercise, ed. 4. Human Kinetics, 2008.

Ziegler, T: Management of Bloodborne Infections in Sport: A Practical Guide for Sports Healthcare Providers and Coaches. Human Kinetics, 1996.

Domain V: Organization and Administration

Anderson, M, Hall, S, and Parr, G: Foundations of Athletic Training, ed. 4. Lippincott Williams & Wilkins, 2008.

Arnold, B, Gansneder, B, and Perrin, D: Research Methods in Athletic Training. FA Davis, 2005.

Cummings, N, Stanley-Green, S, and Higgs, P: Perspectives in Athletic Training. Mosby Elsevier, 2009.

Harrelson, G, Gardner, G, and Winterstein, A: Administrative Topics in Athletic Training: Concepts to Practice. Slack, 2009.

Herbert, DL: Legal Aspects of Sports Medicine. PRC Publishing, Inc., 1994.

Klossner, D: NCAA Sports Medicine Handbook. NCAA, 2009.

Mellion, M, Walsh, W, Madden, C, et al: Team Physician's Handbook, ed. 3. Hanley and Belfus, 2001.

Mensch, J, and Miller, G: The Athletic Trainer's Guide to Psychosocial Intervention and Referral. Slack, 2008.

NATA Position, Consensus, Official and Support Statements. NATA, 2008.

Pfeiffer, R, and Mangus, B: Concepts of Athletic Training, ed. 5. Jones and Bartlett, 2007.

Prentice, W, and Arnheim, D. Arnheim's Principles of Athletic Training, ed. 13. McGraw-Hill, 2009.

Rankin, J, and Ingersoll, C: Athletic Training Management: Concepts & Application, ed. 3. McGraw-Hill, 2005.

Ray, R: Management Strategies in Athletic Training, ed. 3. Human Kinetics, 2005.

Ray, R, and Wiese-Bjornstal, D: Counseling in Sports Medicine. Human Kinetics, 1999.

Schlabach, G, and Peer, K: Professional Ethics in Athletic Training. Mosby Elsevier, 2008.

Starkey, C: Athletic Training and Sports Medicine, ed. 4. Jones and Bartlett, 2005.

Venes, D: Taber's Cyclopedic Medical Dictionary, ed. 21. FA Davis, 2010.

Domain VI: Professional Responsibility

Anderson, M, Hall, S, and Parr, G: Foundations of Athletic Training, ed. 4. Lippincott Williams & Wilkins, 2008.

Arnold, B, Gansneder, B, and Perrin, D: Research Methods in Athletic Training. FA Davis, 2005.

Baumgartner, T, and Hensley L: Conducting & Reading Research in Health & Human Performance, ed. 4. McGraw-Hill, 2006.

Board of Certification: Role Delineation Study for the Entry-Level Certified Athletic Trainer, ed. 5. Board of Certification, 2004.

Harrelson, G, Gardner, G, and Winterstein, A: Administrative Topics in Athletic Training: Concepts to Practice. Slack, 2009.

Ingersoll, C: Research in Athletic Training. Slack, 2001.

Klossner, D: NCAA Sports Medicine Handbook. NCAA, 2009.

Mellion, M, Walsh, W, Madden, C, et al: Team Physician's Handbook, ed. 3. Hanley and Belfus, 2001.

NATA Code of Ethics.

NATA Position, Consensus, Official and Support Statements. NATA, 2008.

Pfeiffer, R, and Mangus, B: Concepts of Athletic Training, ed. 5. Jones and Bartlett, 2007.

Prentice, W, and Arnheim, D. Arnheim's Principles of Athletic Training, ed. 13. McGraw-Hill, 2009.

Rankin, J, and Ingersoll, C: Athletic Training Management: Concepts & Application, ed. 3. McGraw-Hill, 2005.

Ray, R: Management Strategies in Athletic Training, ed. 3. Human Kinetics, 2005.

Ray, R, and Wiese-Bjornstal, D: Counseling in Sports Medicine. Human Kinetics, 1999.

Starkey, C: Athletic Training and Sports Medicine, ed. 4. Jones and Bartlett, 2005.

Venes, D: Taber's Cyclopedic Medical Dictionary, ed. 21. FA Davis, 2010.

Weidner, T: The Athletic Trainer's Pocket Guide to Clinical Teaching. Slack, 2009.

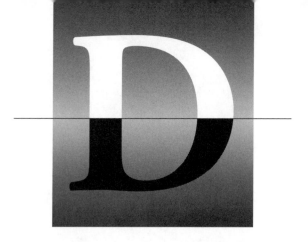

Personal Study
Plan Worksheets

See the Rozzi Web page at http://davisplus.fadavis.com for
printable Personal Study Plan Worksheets.